Neurology and Ophthalmology

For UKMLA and Medical Exams

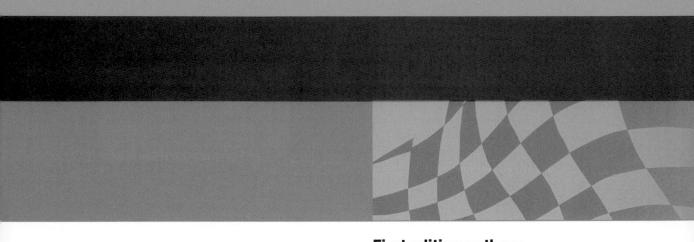

First edition authors

Anish Bahra

Katia Cikurel

Second and third edition author

Christopher Turner

Fourth edition author

Mahinda Yogarajah

Fifth edition author

Umesh Vivekananda

6th Edition

CRASH COURSE

SERIES EDITOR

Philip Xiu

MA (Cantab), MB BChir, MRCP, MRCGP, MScClinEd, FHEA, MAcadMEd, RCPathME
Honorary Senior Lecturer
Leeds University School of Medicine
PCN Educational Lead
Medical Examiner
Leeds Teaching Hospital Trust
Leeds, UK

FACULTY ADVISORS

Umesh Vivekananda

MA, MRCP, PhD
Consultant neurologist
National Hospital for Neurology and Neurosurgery, Queen Square
London UK

Jon Yu

MA (Cantab), MB BChir, FRCOphth
Consultant Ophthalmologist.
Manchester Royal Eye Hospital
Manchester, UK

Neurology and Ophthalmology

For UKMLA and Medical Exams

Rubika Balendra

MA (Cantab), MRCP, PhD
Academic Clinical Lecturer University College
London
Specialist Registrar in Neurology National
Hospital for Neurology and Neurosurgery
Queen Square London, UK

Lakhan S. V. A. Ajmeria

BMBS
Foundation Year 2 Doctor
University Hospital of Wales
Cardiff, UK

ELSEVIER

First edition 1999

Second edition 2006

Third edition 2009

Fourth edition 2013

Fifth edition 2019

Sixth edition 2025

Notices

Practitioners and researchers must always rely on their own experience and knowledge in evaluating and using any information, methods, compounds or experiments described herein. Because of rapid advances in the medical sciences, in particular, independent verification of diagnoses and drug dosages should be made. To the fullest extent of the law, no responsibility is assumed by Elsevier, authors, editors or contributors for any injury and/or damage to persons or property as a matter of products liability, negligence or otherwise, or from any use or operation of any methods, products, instructions, or ideas contained in the material herein.

ISBN: 978-0-443-11556-1

Content Strategist: Trinity Hutton
Content Project Manager: Taranpreet Kaur
Design: Miles Hitchen
Marketing Manager: Deborah Watkins

Printed in India

Last digit is the print number: 9 8 7 6 5 4 3 2 1

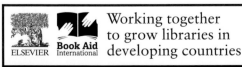

Working together to grow libraries in developing countries

www.elsevier.com • www.bookaid.org

Series editor's foreword

With great honour and pride, we present the latest edition of the *Crash Course* series. This series has traversed a journey of nearly a quarter-century, stemming from the vision of Dr. Dan Horton-Szar, and his legacy continues to walk with us on this pathway of knowledge.

The series has been popular with students worldwide, selling over **1 million copies** and being translated into more than **8 languages**, reinforcing our commitment to global learning.

We remain extremely grateful for your unwavering trust. The series has once again been refreshed and fully upgraded in accordance with the rapidly changing medical guidelines, ensuring the content is comprehensive, accurate and fully up-to-date.

This latest series continues our tradition of integrating clinical practice with basic medical sciences, tailored meticulously for today's medical undergraduate curriculum. A central highlight of this instalment is our emphasis on high-yield exam content designed specifically for the UKMLA curriculum.

The addition of the **Rapid UKMLA Index** at the beginning of the book enhances this offering, serving as a valuable aid to students to track their exam preparation efficiently. We have also revised all self-assessment questions to align with the single best answer format in line with the latest UKMLA examination style. We have also added ***High-Yield Association Tables***. These are essential tools designed to aid students in recognizing clinical patterns and acing vignette-style exam questions. By condensing complex medical scenarios into digestible, manageable insights, these tables ensure efficient learning. They connect symptoms, diagnosis and treatment, bolstering understanding and confidence in tackling the rigorous UKMLA exams. This comprehensive approach makes these tables an indispensable asset in your exam preparations.

Utilizing student feedback, we have strived to maintain the core principles of this series: delivering precise and readable text that brings together depth and clarity. The authors are experienced junior doctors who successfully navigated these exams recently, ensuring practical and tested guidance. A team of expert faculty advisors from across the United Kingdom ensures the content's accuracy, making it resilient and reliable.

As we turn a new chapter with the latest edition, we honour the past, cherish the present, and embrace the promise of the future. We wish you every success in your journey of learning and growth and hope that this series adds value to your life, both as students and as future medical professionals.

Philip Xiu

Prefaces

It is increasingly apparent that a significant proportion of clinical presentations both in primary care (10%) and the acute medical take (20%) has a neurological basis. In addition, neurological complications post-surgery and in intensive care are commonplace. It is our experience that neurology is treated with trepidation and is frequently overcomplicated amongst medical students and junior doctors. This book aims to consolidate the core skills required in neurology of systematic history taking and neurological examination and provide a logical and simple approach to understanding the fundamental concepts that underlie most common neurological diseases.

Neurology is an ever-evolving field; technological advances such as in neurogenetics and imaging have enabled new conditions to be identified and other established conditions to be much better characterized. This sixth edition aims to reflect the recent significant advancement in neurology. It intimately combines both neurology and neuroscience, to provide a strong basis for understanding the pathogenesis of common neurological pathologies. The first part of the book focuses on the history taking, examination and investigations relevant to neurology. The second part of the book provides a framework for analyzing and formulating a differential diagnosis of common presenting symptoms such as headache, dizziness, speech disturbance and limb weakness. In the final part of the book, the clinical features, investigation and management of specific neurological disorders are discussed in more detail.

This edition includes new sections on neurological emergencies, functional neurological disorders and autoimmune neurological diseases. A number of new single best answer questions have also been written in the self-assessment section at the end of the book. We are confident that this sixth edition of Crash Course: Neurology and Ophthalmology will provide not only a solid foundation for medical students preparing for exams and postgraduates working towards MRCP, but also an excellent reference book for those working in hospital medicine and general practice.

Rubika Balendra and Umesh Vivekananda

The importance of Ophthalmology extends beyond the confines of specialized medical practice, making it a vital field for medical students and practitioners alike. Proficiency in ophthalmic knowledge and skills is crucial for every medical professional, as eye-related issues often manifest as symptoms in various medical conditions. Ophthalmology plays a pivotal role in preventive healthcare, early disease detection, and overall patient well-being. The sixth edition of Crash Course: Neurology and Ophthalmology is a comprehensive and dynamic guide designed not only to fortify your understanding of the intricacies of Ophthalmology for final exams but also to specifically address the nuanced requirements of the Medical Licensing Assessment (UKMLA).

In this edition, we have incorporated substantial enhancements, including single best answer questions (SBAQs) and Objective Structured Clinical Examination (OSCE) content, to enrich your preparation for contemporary medical assessments.

Furthermore, the new inclusion of numerous visuals, including over 80 pictures, illustrations, and diagrams within this edition, aims to facilitate a more comprehensive understanding of ophthalmic concepts. As you engage with the material in this book, we encourage you to embrace the visual elements as dynamic aids in your learning journey.

We extend our sincere wishes for success in your studies and future endeavours. May this edition be your trusted companion as you navigate the challenges of the UKMLA and embark on a fulfilling career in the fascinating and ever-evolving field of Ophthalmology.

Lakhan S.V.A Ajmeria and Jon Yu

Acknowledgements

Thank you to Umesh Vivekananda for his invaluable guidance and assistance with this Edition.

For everything, thank you to Vasanthini Balendra, Thanabalasingam Balendra and Shiama Balendra, and to Judi Watkin and Jeff Watkin, and to Harry Watkin and Ravi Jude Watkin.

Rubika Balendra

I would like to express my profound gratitude to Dr Philip Xiu, the editor-in-chief, for providing me with the extraordinary opportunity to contribute to this medical textbook at the early stage of my medical career. This enriching journey has underscored the importance of medical education in shaping our understanding of healthcare. Thank you to Dr Sohaib Rufai, whose unwavering passion for medical education served as a beacon, inspiring me to surpass conventional expectations and delve deeper into the subject matter. The credit for embarking on this academic voyage goes to Dr Jade Scott-Blagrove, founder of the Widening Participation Medics Network (WPMN). Her tireless efforts in advocating for underrepresented groups and dismantling barriers within medicine have not only bolstered my confidence but also empowered me to actively seek and embrace such invaluable opportunities.

A special acknowledgment is reserved for Mr. Jonathan Yu, whose patience and unwavering support have been instrumental in guiding me through the intricacies of ophthalmology and shaping the content of the Ophthalmology section.

I extend my heartfelt appreciation and apologies to my family, friends, and colleagues for being so understanding during this project. Your unwavering support, boundless love, and resilience have been the pillars that supported me to move forward and allowed me to bring the Ophthalmology section within the sixth edition to fruition.

Lakhan S.V.A Ajmeria

For Elizabeth, Noah and Phoebe. Thank you for your utmost patience and encouragement.

Umesh Vivekananda

Series editor's acknowledgement

We would like to express our sincere gratitude to those who have provided their support and expertise in preparing this sixth edition of the *Crash Course* series. Our junior doctor contributors' participation in crafting the manuscript has been indispensable. Their first-hand experience and current medical knowledge have infused realism and practicality into our content.

Our faculty editors deserve a special note of thanks. They have extensively validated the correctness of the information, ensuring that the content is not just accurate but also contemporaneous, credible, and aligns with the latest medical standards.

We extend our heartfelt thanks to our publisher, Elsevier. Their staff have demonstrated an unwavering commitment to quality, maintaining the high standards set since the first edition. Their insights have routinely enriched the content and process alike.

Our Commissioning Editor, Jeremy Bowes, deserves a special mention for his consistent support and guiding hand throughout the development process. His directions and advice have bettered this edition and spurred us on our quest for excellence.

We are greatly indebted to Alex Mortimer for her wisdom, practical insights and valuable guidance. A big thank you to our Content Strategists, Trinity Hutton and Cloe Holland-Borosh, who need special acknowledgement for meticulously outlining the direction and scope of the content. They've managed to mix details with a strategic plan, keeping our readers in mind.

Lastly, much gratitude is owed to our Content Product Managers, Taranpreet Kaur, Ayan Dhar, Shivani Pal and Tapajyoti Chaudhuri, who have juggled the numerous day-to-day tasks with utmost dedication and perseverance. Despite the ever-approaching deadlines, they have shown remarkable patience and steadfast determination, ensuring that each step of the book's development was accomplished seamlessly.

In conclusion, we sincerely thank each of these wonderful people for their outstanding contributions and support, without which this work wouldn't have been achieved. Their passion, commitment and collaborative effort have helped us bring this edition together.

Philip Xiu

Rapid UKMLA Index

The UKMLA Curriculum Conditions Priority levels have been based on the below:

Level 1: Conditions that a newly qualified doctor should have a good knowledge of and be able to recognise and manage.
Level 2: Conditions requiring knowledge for recognising and confirming diagnosis and planning first-line management in straightforward cases.
Level 3: Conditions where recognition of clinical presentation and describing principles of management are important.

NEUROLOGY

Table 1 UKMLA Conditions and Where to Find Them

Priority List	UKMLA Conditions	Chapter	Page
2	Acoustic neuroma	Chapter 9: Facial sensory loss and weakness Chapter 10: Deafness, tinnitus, dizziness and vertigo Chapter 31: Neuro-oncology	70 75 216
1	Bell's palsy	Chapter 9: Facial sensory loss and weakness	72, 73
3	Brain abscess	Chapter 32: Infections of the nervous system	226, 229
2	Brain metastases	Chapter 31: Neuro-oncology	217, 218
3	Cerebral palsy and hypoxic-ischaemic encephalopathy	Chapter 16: Disorders of gait Chapter 22: Epilepsy	112, 113 148
1	Dementias	Chapter 6: Disorders of higher cerebral function Chapter 21: Dementia Chapter 23: Parkinson's disease and other extrapyramidal disorders Chapter 25: Motor neurone disease Chapter 34: The effects of vitamin deficiencies and toxins on the nervous system Chapter 36: Hereditary conditions affecting the nervous system	51 141-146 156 171 242 249
2	Diabetic neuropathy	Chapter 14: Limb weakness Chapter 15: Limb sensory symptoms Chapter 27: Disorders of the peripheral nerves	103 106 184
2	Encephalitis	Chapter 21: Dementia Chapter 32: Infections of the nervous system Chapter 35: Autoimmune conditions affecting the nervous system	141, 142 224, 225 245, 246
1	Epilepsy	Chapter 4: Neurological emergencies Chapter 5: Disturbances of consciousness Chapter 22: Epilepsy Chapter 36: Hereditary conditions affecting the nervous system	37 43 147-153 249
3	Essential tremor	Chapter 13: Movement disorders	90
1	Extradural haemorrhage	Chapter 30: Vascular diseases of the nervous system	210, 211
3	Febrile convulsion	Chapter 22: Epilepsy	148
1	Malaria	Chapter 32: Infections of the nervous system	232
1	Ménière's disease	Chapter 10: Deafness, tinnitus, dizziness and vertigo	78
1	Meningitis	Chapter 4: Neurological emergencies Chapter 32: Infections of the nervous system	37 221-224

continued

continued

OPHTHALMOLOGY

Table 3 UKMLA Conditions and Where to Find Them

Priority List	UKMLA Conditions	Chapter	Page
1	Acute glaucoma	Chapter 17: The red, painful eye Chapter 40: Glaucoma	119 275, 276
2	Benign eyelid disorders	Chapter 20: Eyelid problems and the bulging eye Chapter 38: Adnexal (eyelids, lacrimal system and orbit)	136, 137 259
2	Blepharitis	Chapter 38: Adnexal (eyelids, lacrimal system and orbit) Chapter 39: Anterior segment (cornea and cataract)	258, 259 267
1	Cataracts	Chapter 18: Gradual change in vision Chapter 39: Anterior segment (cornea and cataract)	123 269-272
3	Central retinal arterial occlusion	Chapter 19: Sudden change in vision Chapter 41: Retina	130, 132 284, 285
3	Chronic glaucoma	Chapter 18: Gradual change in vision Chapter 40: Glaucoma	123 273-278
1	Conjunctivitis	Chapter 17: The red, painful eye	117, 118
1	Diabetic eye disease	Chapter 19: Sudden change in vision Chapter 41: Retina	131 279-282
3	Infective keratitis	Chapter 17: The red, painful eye Chapter 39: Anterior segment (cornea and cataract)	115, 118 265, 266, 267
3	Iritis	Chapter 17: The red, painful eye Chapter 42: Medical ophthalmology and uveitis	117, 120 294, 295
3	Macular degeneration	Chapter 18: Gradual change in vision Chapter 41: Retina	123, 126 285, 286, 287
3	Optic neuritis	Chapter 18: Gradual change in vision Chapter 19: Sudden change in vision Chapter 43: Neuro-ophthalmology	126 131 307, 308, 309
3	Periorbital and orbital cellulitis	Chapter 20: Eyelid problems and the bulging eye Chapter 38: Adnexal (eyelids, lacrimal system and orbit)	136, 137 264
3	Retinal detachment	Chapter 19: Sudden change in vision Chapter 41: Retina	129, 130, 131 287, 288
2	Scleritis	Chapter 17: The red, painful eye	117, 118, 119
3	Thyroid eye disease	Chapter 19: Sudden change in vision Chapter 20: Eyelid problems and the bulging eye Chapter 38: Adnexal (eyelids, lacrimal system and orbit)	131 137 263, 264
2	Uveitis	Chapter 17: The red, painful eye Chapter 42: Medical ophthalmology and uveitis	120, 121 294-297
3	Visual field defects	Chapter 18: Gradual change in vision Chapter 19: Sudden change in vision Chapter 40: Glaucoma Chapter 41: Retina Chapter 43: Neuro-ophthalmology	125 130, 131 273, 274 288 301, 302

Contents

Section 3 Diseases and Disorders

Contents

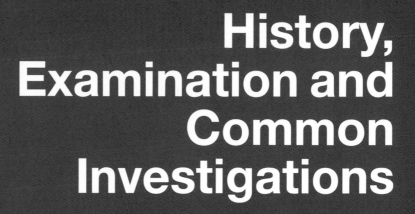

History, Examination and Common Investigations

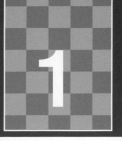
THE NEUROLOGICAL HISTORY

The patient's neurological history is the most crucial aspect in reaching a diagnosis. Many common conditions, such as headache and epilepsy, can be diagnosed solely from the clinical history. To start a neurological history, you would:

- Introduce yourself and explain who you are.
- Ask for permission to talk to and examine the patient.
- Ask the patient's age and occupation.
- Ask whether the patient is right- or left-handed (if you do not ask this at the beginning, you might forget). Handedness is important because the left hemisphere controls language in right-handed patients and in about 75% of left-handed or ambidextrous patients.

Within the first few minutes of the consultation you should be able to make some inferences about the patient's mood and cognitive state:

- Does the patient respond appropriately (indicating probable preservation of important higher mental functioning)?
- Does he or she appear to be depressed (which can either be part of the patient's neurological condition or might indicate a reaction to it) or behaving inappropriately (as in patients who have frontal lobe dysfunction)?
- Is the patient's speech normal?

HINTS AND TIPS

The history is the most important part of the neurological assessment, and the time course of the symptoms will often give an insight into the underlying pathological process. The history should be used to construct diagnostic hypotheses that are then tested using the neurological examination.

STRUCTURE OF THE HISTORY

As with history taking for other systems, the following schema applies.

The presenting complaint

Consider the presenting complaint (PC) from the patient's point of view. Ask:

- What is the main problem/what caused you to seek medical attention?

When presenting the history to others, use the patient's language (e.g., 'This woman complains of seeing double') not the medical terminology (e.g., 'This woman complains of horizontal diplopia').

History of the presenting complaint

Establish the history of the presenting complaint (HPC) by asking:

- When did the patient first notice it?
- Was the onset sudden (over seconds or minutes), subacute (over hours or days) or insidious and gradual (over weeks, months, or years)? The time course of onset of symptoms gives an important insight into the underlying pathological process. For example, a sudden onset unilateral visual loss over seconds might suggest amaurosis fugax or vascular aetiology; onset over 10 to 15 minutes followed by a headache might suggest migraine; onset over 1 to 2 days associated with pain on eye movement and resolution over 6 weeks would suggest optic neuritis and an inflammatory aetiology.
- Is the symptom episodic, constant, and progressive, or constant with fluctuations in intensity?
- Has it worsened, improved, or stayed the same since?
- What is the character of the symptom (e.g., headache may be throbbing, stabbing or pressure-like) and its distribution (unilateral, bilateral, frontal, occipital, etc.)?
- Is there anything that makes it better (e.g., medications, sleep, exercise) or worse (e.g., movement, coughing, posture)?
- Are there associated symptoms that are recognized as part of a particular syndrome? For example, in a patient with parkinsonian gait, there may also be an associated tremor and slowness in performing everyday tasks such as handwriting.
- Has the patient ever had other neurological symptoms in the past? These might be related (e.g., an episode of transient

visual loss 5 years previously in a young woman now complaining of difficulty in walking is indicative of possible multiple sclerosis).

- Are there any relevant risk factors? For example, in a patient presenting with a likely stroke, ask about stroke risk factors such as smoking, diabetes, hypertension and a history of atrial fibrillation.

Once the HPC has been elucidated, it is useful to ask general questions pertaining to neurological dysfunction including:

- a history of dizziness, blackouts or falls;
- difficulties with memory or other cognitive functions;
- problems with vision;
- difficulties in speech, swallowing, chewing;
- weakness or sensory symptoms in the limbs;
- sphincter function (bowels, bladder, sexual function);
- a history of headache;
- symptoms of autonomic nervous system function (dizziness/ fainting, urinary symptoms, sexual dysfunction, early satiety, sweating too much or too little, cool peripheries).

COMMON PITFALLS

Sometimes it is critical to acquire a collateral history in patients. For example, in patients who have had episodes of altered awareness or loss of consciousness, a witness account of events will be critical to differentiate between seizures and syncope. Similarly, in patients with cognitive decline it is important to also get a history from family members to aid diagnosis.

Medical history

Some clinicians prefer to take the medical history (MH) before considering the PC because there might be important background information. The following may be relevant in neurological cases:

- birth history and childhood development (e.g., motor and verbal milestones)
- major illnesses during childhood (e.g., meningitis)
- hypertension, ischaemic heart disease, diabetes
- a systemic disorder (e.g., systemic lupus erythematosus)

Drug history

To determine the drug history (DH), find out from the patient:

- Is he or she taking any medicines now, or any longstanding medication in the past?
- Are there any known drug allergies?

Prior and current exposure to drugs can be important in several conditions. For example, parkinsonism can occur as a side effect of antipsychotic use, or some peripheral neuropathies can be caused by previous chemotherapeutic agent exposure.

Review of systems

Review of systems (ROS) should include questions such as:

- Gastrointestinal: appetite, weight loss or gain, swallowing, change in bowel function.
- Cardiovascular: chest pain, breathlessness, palpitations, claudication.
- Respiratory: cough, breathlessness.
- Genitourinary: bladder function, impotence, sexual function.
- Musculoskeletal: joint pain, stiffness.
- Systemic symptoms: weight loss, fatigue, night sweats.

Family history

Many neurological disorders are familial and have a genetic basis. To determine the family history (FH), find out from patients:

- If there are any 'family illnesses', especially in relatives younger than the age of 60 years.
- If their parents, siblings and children are alive and well and, if not, what they died of and at what age.
- If their parents could possibly be related (i.e., a consanguineous marriage). This is especially important in autosomal recessive conditions when related patients may carry the same defective gene and pass both to their children.

Social history

The social history (SH) can be important, because depending on the neurological problem, the impact will vary according to the social circumstances of the individual. For example, in a patient with difficulty walking, it will be important to have knowledge of home circumstances (e.g., number of stairs). To determine the SH, ask the patient about:

- Home circumstances: house or flat, stairs, help from Social Services.
- Smoking history.

- Alcohol intake (units/week): is there a past history of heavy alcohol consumption/tendency to binge?
- Recreational drug use including nitrous oxide.
- Diet (vegetarian or vegan).
- Sexual history or orientation: this might be relevant in certain cases.
- Occupation.

THE OPHTHALMIC HISTORY

Start an ophthalmic history the same way you would a neurological history as mentioned above. Including introduction and assurance of confidentiality throughout the consultation. Follow the structure as above:

The presenting complaint

Start by asking general questions:

- 'What is the problem with your eyes?'
- 'Is one or both eyes affected?'

Remember to screen for common ophthalmic symptoms including:

- Visual disturbances – 'Has there been any changes in vision recently?'
- Red eye – 'Have you noticed changes in the colour of your eye?'
- Eye discharge/watering – 'Any discharge from your eye (clear/watery/sticky/yellow)?'
- Grittiness/dryness of eyes – 'Do you feel your eyes are dry?'
- Itching – 'Are you rubbing your eye more than usual?'
- Photophobia – 'Do you have to close your curtains during daylight?'
- Swelling or tenderness of eye – 'Have you noticed any swelling or pain around your eye(s)?'

RED FLAG

Key red flag symptoms
- Acute pain
- Photophobia
- Visual disturbances
- Red eye
- Trauma

History of the presenting complaint

Ascertain how long the problem has been there for, as timing is very important to differentiate between acute and chronic ocular problems. Ask:

- 'When did you first notice the problem?' – (is it acute or chronic?)
- 'When was the first or last episode?'
- 'Is it getting worse or better?'
- 'Does anything make it worse/better?'

For exploring pain symptoms, the acronym **SOCRATES** is commonly used.

- **S**ite
- **O**nset
- **C**haracter
- **R**adiation
- **A**ssociated symptoms
- **T**ime course
- **E**xacerbating/relieving factors
- **S**everity

Family history

Ask about any eye conditions that occurred to other family members with similar presentations, or any history of other formal diagnoses. Ask specifically about:

- diabetes mellitus;
- hypertension;
- autoimmune conditions.

Past ocular history

It is important to find out whether the patient has had any issues with their eyes in the past (any formal diagnoses?). Any prior intraocular surgery in the past?

Medical history

Ask about what their past MH is, and how well it is being managed. Relevant medical condition to ask about include:

- diabetes mellitus;
- hypertension;
- autoimmune conditions: hyper/hypothyroidism, SLE, rheumatoid arthritis;
- atopy: asthma, allergic rhinitis, eczema.

Medications

Same as above. However, it is important to note if the patient is currently on any anticoagulant medication, as these are contra-indicated in eye surgery.

Allergies

Ask about any allergies including drugs. Important to note if they have previously been on any topical eye medications, and if they had any issues with them in the past.

Social history

An important risk factor to identify is whether the patient is smoking. Smoking increases the likelihood of many ocular conditions including retinal and optic nerve vascular occlusive diseases.

Formulating a summary

Summarizing a patient history to colleagues is a very important skill and should not take longer than 2 to 3 minutes. It is worth investing time to practice condensing and communicating a history succinctly. It is best to start with a general summary such as: 'Miss Randolph is a 40-year-old administrator who complains of numbness in the feet'. The HPC, MH and ROS should then be described. You do not have to mention all negative points, but it is worth pointing out those that are important (e.g., 'She has no history of diabetes' in a patient who has a peripheral neuropathy).

Describe the DH and FH, if relevant; if it is not, state: 'There is no relevant family history'. Describe important social points: 'She drinks only moderate amounts of alcohol and has never smoked'.

You will then move on to your examination findings.

Chapter Summary

- A comprehensive neurological/ocular history is vital in formulating a list of differential diagnoses.
- If the patient cannot give a history themselves then a collateral history is required.
- Use the acronym SOCRATES to explore pain symptoms.
- In ophthalmic history, asking about diabetes mellitus, hypertension, rheumatological conditions and smoking is key to produce a list of differentials.

UKMLA Presentation
Family history of possible genetic disorder

THE NEUROLOGICAL EXAMINATION

The neurological examination consists of the following elements, which should be carried out in sequence:

1. Assessing mental state and higher cerebral functions
2. Assessing speech
3. Assessing gait
4. Testing the cranial nerves
5. Testing motor function
6. Testing sensory function
7. Examining related structures

MENTAL STATE AND HIGHER CEREBRAL FUNCTIONS

Consciousness

Consciousness is the state of being aware of self and the environment. A number of ill-defined terms are used to describe different levels of consciousness:

- **Alert:** full wakefulness and immediate and appropriate responsiveness. The patient is orientated in person, time and place.
- **Confusion:** the inability to think with the usual speed and clarity. There may be lack of attention, disorientation in time and place and impairment of memory. Delirium is a confusional state characterized by fluctuant hyperactivity.
- **Obtundation:** the patient is drowsy and indifferent to the environment, but responsive to verbal stimuli.
- **Stupor:** the patient is unconscious but rousable when stimulated.
- **Coma:** the patient is unaware of self and the environment and is not rousable.

The terms described above are often used differently by different clinicians. The level of consciousness is therefore more objectively assessed using the Glasgow Coma Scale (see Chapter 5

Appearance and affect

Assessment of the patient's mental state begins as soon as you meet the patient. You should note:

- Physical appearance. Self-neglect is common but may be masked by caring relatives.
- Does the patient seem depressed?
- Signs of delusions or hallucinations (seen in, e.g., delirium, Lewy body dementia)?
- Loss of interest, euphoria or social disinhibition (frontal lobe dysfunction).
- Emotional lability, or uncontrollable laughing or crying (seen in, e.g., motor neurone disease, Parkinson's disease).

Cognitive function

The clarity with which a patient presents their history and cooperates with the examination may convey a sense of their intellectual capacity. This should be compared with one's own estimate of their premorbid ability given their job and educational history. If after taking the history there is no suggestion of a defect of higher cerebral function, then further testing is not required. However, if there is any doubt, more extensive testing with for example, the Mini-Mental State Examination should be carried out. The history should also be corroborated with independent witnesses if possible.

Mini-Mental State Examination

The Mini-Mental State Examination is a screening test for cognitive function (Table 2.1). Any score greater than or equal to 24 points (out of 30) indicates a normal cognition. Below this, scores can indicate severe (≤9 points), moderate (10–18 points) or mild (19–23 points) cognitive impairment.

Formal neuropsychometric testing should be performed for all patients suspected of having impaired cognition.

SPEECH

The content and articulation of speech should be evident when taking the history. If there is any suggestion that it is abnormal, further examination is necessary. Speech production is organized at three levels:

1. Phonation
2. Articulation
3. Language production

The anatomy involved in speech production is illustrated in Fig. 2.1.

Table 2.1 Mini-Mental State Examination

Domain	Test	Score	Further points
Orientation		10	Establishes awareness of self and environment
Registration		3	Immediate memory. Verbal memory (short sentence) or visual memory (objects on table) could also be assessed
Attention and calculation		5	This is dependent on patient's premorbid arithmetic ability
Recall		3	
Language		8	Comprehension of speech and written language
Constructional/spatial		1	

Orientation

1. What is the year, season, date, month, day? (One point for each correct answer)
2. Where are we? Country, county, town, hospital, floor? (One point for each answer)

Registration

3. Name three objects, taking 1 second to say each. Then ask the patient to name all three. One point for each correct answer. Repeat the question until the patient learns all three, e.g., 'bus', 'rose', 'door'

Attention and calculation

4. Serial sevens. One point for each correct answer. Stop after five answers. Alternative: spell 'world' backwards

Recall

5. Ask for names of the three objects asked in question 3. One point for each correct answer

Language

6. Point to a pencil and a watch. Ask the patient to name them for you. One point for each correct answer
7. Ask the patient to repeat 'No ifs, ands or buts'. One point
8. Ask the patient to follow a three-stage command: 'Take the paper in your right hand; fold the paper in half; put the paper on the floor with your left hand'. Three points
9. Ask the patient to read and obey the following: CLOSE YOUR EYES. (Write this in large letters.) One point
10. Ask the patient to write a sentence of his or her own choice. (The sentence must contain a subject and an object and make some sense). Ignore spelling errors when scoring. One point

Constructional/spatial

11. Ask the patient to copy two intersecting pentagons with equal sides. Give one point if all the sides and angles are preserved and if the intersecting sides form a quadrangle
Maximum score = 30 points

Phonation: dysphonia

Phonation is the production of sounds as the air passes through the vocal cords and resonating sound boxes. A disorder of this process is called dysphonia and is caused by:

- local vocal cord pathology (e.g., laryngitis)
- abnormality of the nerve supply via the vagus nerve.

Assessment

- Coughing should be tested in patients with dysphonia as it relies on normal vocal cord function.
- Sustained vowels like 'eeeee' can be tested as fatigability is seen in myasthenia gravis.

Articulation: dysarthria

Voice production requires the coordination of breathing, vocal cords, larynx, palate, tongue and lips. A disorder of this process is called dysarthria.

- Lesions in the basal ganglia or cerebellum affect the speech rhythm.
- Lesions of the cranial nerves critical to voice production produce disturbance in articulation but the rhythm is normal.

Assessment

Articulation is assessed from the patient's spontaneous speech during history taking. Ask the patient to repeat a series of phrases:

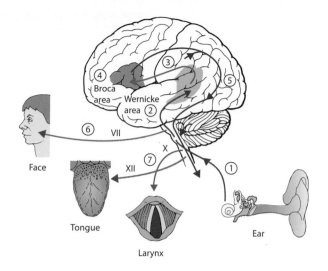

Fig. 2.1 The pathways involved in language formation. 1. Ear and cochlear nerve; 2. Wernicke area; 3. arcuate fasciculus; 4. Broca area; 5. central motor output pathways; and 6. peripheral motor output pathways. (From Fuller G, Manford, M. *Neurology: An Illustrated Colour Text*. 3rd ed. Churchill Livingstone: Elsevier; 2010.)

	Site	Function	Abnormality
①	Ear and auditory nerve	Hearing	Deafness
②	Wernicke area	Understanding	Fluent aphasia
③	Arcuate fasciculus	Repetition	Loss of repetition
④	Broca area	Language production	Nonfluent aphasia
⑤	Motor output pathways, central: cerebellum Corticospinal tracts	Articulation of speech	Dysarthria
⑥	Motor output pathways, peripheral: facial, hypoglossal, vagus nerves, face and tongue	Articulation of speech	Dysarthria
⑦	Larynx	Voice production	Dysphonia

- 'Baby Hippopotamus' or 'British Constitution' tests labial (lip) sounds.
- 'Yellow Lorry' or 'West Register Street' tests lingual (tongue) sounds.
- 'Peter Piper picked a peck of pickled pepper' can be used to test cerebellar function, which is necessary to coordinate the muscles of speech articulation.

Before attributing dysarthria to a neurological cause, non-neurological causes (such as an inflammatory or infective process affecting the mucosal surfaces) should be excluded. Ill-fitting or absent dentures can also cause the patient to sound dysarthric.

Dysarthria may result from a lesion of the:

- **Upper motor neurone** (UMN; pseudobulbar palsy): spasticity of the tongue, palate and mouth produces a slow, high-pitched and forced and often described as 'hot potato speech' because the patient talks as if they have a hot potato in their mouth.
- **Lower motor neurone** (LMN; bulbar palsy): paralysis of the soft palate causes slurred and indistinct speech, with nasal intonation due to the nasal escape of air; labial (lip) and lingual (tongue) sounds are affected.
- **Basal ganglia:** slow, low-pitched and monotonous (akinetic-rigid syndromes); loud, harsh and with

variable intonation (chorea and myoclonus); loud, slow and indistinct consonants (athetoid).

- **Cerebellum:** slow and slurred, scanning (equal emphasis on each syllable) or 'staccato' quality if there is also involvement of the corticobulbar tracts.
- **Muscle and neuromuscular junction:** similar to those of a bulbar palsy. In myasthenia gravis, there might be a deterioration in the quality of speech (fatigability) during prolonged speech or over the course of the day.

Dysarthria is further discussed in Chapter 11.

Language production: dysphasia

Language production is the organization of phonemes into words and sentences. It is controlled by the speech centres in the dominant hemisphere (Broca and Wernicke areas). A disorder of this process is called dysphasia.

Assessment
To assess language production:

- Listen to the patient's spontaneous speech, assessing its fluency and content.
- Assess the patient's comprehension by observing response to simple commands, e.g., 'Open your mouth', 'Look up to the ceiling'. Then try more complicated two- or three-stage commands, e.g., 'with your right index finger touch your nose and then your left ear'.
- Assess the patient's ability to name familiar objects: use your wristwatch (face, hands, strap, buckle). Start with easy objects, before moving onto objects that are used less frequently.
- Assess the patient's ability to repeat sentences, e.g., 'No ifs, ands or buts'.
- Assess the patient's ability to read and write.

The clinical features of the different types of dysphasia are summarized in Table 2.2 and also discussed in Chapter 11.

GAIT

Normal gait requires input from the motor, somatosensory, visual, cerebellar and vestibular systems. Assessing the gait carefully can therefore provide the examiner with a great deal of information about each of these systems, which can be examined in detail later in the examination. The assessment and abnormalities of gait are described in Chapter 16.

CRANIAL NERVES

Olfactory nerve (first, I)

To test the olfactory nerve, first ask the patient about any recent change in the sense of smell or taste. A characteristic-smelling object (e.g., peppermint, clove oil) is held under each nostril in turn while the other is occluded and the patient keeps the eyes closed. An individual who has intact olfaction can not only detect the smell but also discriminate and name it. The recommended special testing bottles are rarely available when needed and most clinicians perform preliminary assessment with accessible objects such as fruit, a coffee jar or cigarette packet. Avoid using irritating odours such as ammonia or camphor because these can nonspecifically activate fifth nerve receptors in the nasal mucosa.

Unilateral loss of smell is usually asymptomatic. Bilateral loss of smell may be associated with an altered sensation of taste (dysgeusia or ageusia).

When examining patients who have anosmia, it is important to look carefully for frontal lobe signs and evidence of optic nerve or chiasmal damage, as these structures are anatomically close to the pathways that subserve smell.

The most common cause of impaired smell is pathology in the nasal passages or sinuses.

Optic nerve (second, II)

Visual acuity
Visual acuity (VA) is tested using a Snellen chart in a well-lit room. Seat or stand the patient 6 m from the chart. Small, hand-held Snellen charts can be read at a distance of 2 m.

Table 2.2 Classification of dysphasia

Type	Lesion	Speech fluency	Speech content	Comprehension	Repetition
Expressive	Broca area	Nonfluent	Impaired	Normal	Variable
Nominal	Angular gyrus	Fluent	Impaired	Normal	Normal
Receptive	Wernicke area	Fluent	Impaired	Impaired	Impaired
Conductive	Arcuate fasciculus	Fluent	Impaired	Normal	Impaired
Global	Frontal, parietal and temporal lobe	Nonfluent	Impaired	Impaired	Impaired

10

Correct the patient's refractive error with glasses or a pinhole. Ask the patient to cover each eye in turn with their palm, and find which line of print the patient can read comfortably. VA is expressed as the distance between the chart and the patient and the number of the smallest visible line on the chart. The numbers associated with each line on the chart correspond to the distance (in metres) at which a normal patient should be able to read that line of letters. So, 6/6 is normal and 6/24 means that from 6 m away the patient can only read letters that a normal individual can read from 24 m. If the patient is unable to read characters of line 60 (VA less than 6/60), assess his or her ability to count your fingers at 1 m (VA:CF), see your hand movements (VA:HM) or perceive a torch light (VA:PL). If unable to perceive light (VA:NPL), then the patient is blind. The VA is a measure of the integrity of central macular vision.

COMMON PITFALLS

When testing visual acuity, patients who already wear glasses should keep them on to correct for refractive error.

Colour vision

Colour vision is tested using Ishihara plates in a day-lit room. Test each eye separately. If at least 15 of 17 plates are read correctly, colour vision can be regarded as normal. This test is designed principally to detect congenital colour vision defects, but is sensitive in detecting mild degrees of optic nerve dysfunction, where the red colours are often lost first.

Attention

Sit about 1 m from the patient with your eyes at the same horizontal level. Start by testing for visual inattention (see Chapter 6). Ask the patient to look into your eyes; hold your hands halfway between you and the patient. Stimulate the patient's visual fields by moving each hand separately and then both hands together, and ask the patient to indicate which of your hands has moved each time.

In patients with a nondominant parietal lobe lesion, a visual stimulus presented in isolation to the contralateral field is perceived, but it may be missed when a comparable stimulus is presented simultaneously to the ipsilateral field.

Visual fields

Visual fields are then examined by confrontation, during which you compare your own visual fields with the patient's on the assumption that yours are normal. The patient's visual field will match yours only if your head positions are exactly comparable and if your hand is exactly halfway between you and the patient.

Visual fields in poorly cooperative patients are assessed by the response to visual threat (sudden, unexpected hand movement into the patient's visual field).

Examine each eye in turn. To test the patient's right visual field, ask the patient to cover the left eye with their left palm and to look into your left eye throughout the examination. Initially ask the patient if any part of your face is missing or distorted. Then cover your right eye with your right hand, and test the patient's peripheral field by bringing the moving fingers of your left hand into the upper and then the lower quadrants of the patient's temporal fields. Ask the patient to inform you as soon as they see your fingers. Now cover your right eye with your left hand and examine the patient's nasal fields with your right hand, using the same method. The peripheral fields can be tested more sensitively by using a white hat pin instead of fingers and asking the patient to say when they first perceive the pin. A red hat pin is more sensitive to defects of central vision and can be used to map the blind spot. Lesions of different parts of the visual pathway produce characteristic field defects (see Chapter 438).

Blind spot

Routine testing is unnecessary, but enlargement of the blind spot may be an important finding in patients with raised intracranial pressure. The blind spot is tested using a red hatpin. Ask the patient to cover their left eye, and move the pin from the central into the temporal field, along the horizontal meridian, having explained to the patient that the pin will disappear briefly and then reappear again, and that the patient indicates when this happens. Once you have found the patient's blind spot, you can map its shape and compare its size with yours.

Central field

The central field is tested by moving a red hatpin along the central visual field (fixation area) in the horizontal meridian. Ask the patient to indicate if the pin disappears (absolute central scotoma) or if the colour appears diminished (relative scotoma). A central scotoma may extend temporally from the fixation area into the blind spot (centrocaecal scotoma).

Fundoscopy

Ask the patient to fixate on a distant target in dimmed light. Using a direct ophthalmoscope, examine the patient's right eye using your right eye and the patient's left eye using your left eye.

Adjust the ophthalmoscope lens until the retinal vessels are in focus, and trace them back to the optic disc. Assess the cupping, colour and contour of the optic disc, and the clarity of its margins. The temporal disc margins are normally slightly paler than the nasal margins. The physiological cup varies in size but does not extend to the disc margins. The retinal vessels should then be assessed. The arteries are narrower than the veins and redder in colour. The vessels should not be obscured as they cross the disc margins. Look for retinal vein pulsation, which is present in about 80% of normal individuals and is an index of normal intracranial pressure. This is seen best at the disc margins where the veins cross over the arteries. Note the width of the blood vessels and look for arteriovenous nipping at the cross-over points. Fig. 2.2 illustrates a normal optic disc on fundoscopy.

Assess the rest of the retina, noting any evidence of discoloration, haemorrhages or white patches of exudate. Ask the patient to look at the light of the ophthalmoscope, which brings the macula into view. Classify fundoscopic abnormalities into those affecting the optic disc, the retinal vessels or the retina (Table 2.3).

Oculomotor (third, III), trochlear (fourth, IV) and abducens (sixth, VI) nerves

Eyelids

Ptosis is drooping of the upper eyelid and the drooping is usually partial. A full ptosis (complete closure of the eyelid) is usually due to a third nerve palsy. Examination of pupil responses and eye movements provide essential information about the cause of the ptosis (Table 2.4).

Pupils

Size and shape

Assess the size and shape of the pupils. They should be circular and symmetrical (see Chapter 43). A discrepancy between the size of the pupils is called anisocoria. The most common cause of an irregular pupil is disease or trauma directly to the anterior chamber of the eye (e.g., anterior uveitis or postsurgical). The Argyll Robertson pupil is associated with tertiary syphilis and consists of irregular pupils that have an accommodation reflex but an absent light reflex. This abnormality occurs more often in examinations than in everyday practice.

Light response

Light responses should be assessed using a bright torchlight. Ask the patient to fixate on a distant target, then shine the light into each eye in turn, bringing the torch beam quickly onto the pupil from the lateral side. Observe the direct (ipsilateral) and the consensual (contralateral) responses.

Assess the presence of an afferent pupillary defect by swinging the light from one eye to the other, pausing 3 s on each (see Chapter 43).

Accommodation

The accommodation reflex consists of two components. The first involves convergence of the eyes, which requires simultaneous adduction of both eyes. The second involves bilateral

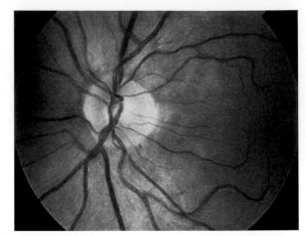

Fig. 2.2 Appearances of a normal fundus. (From Fuller G, Manford, M. *Neurology: An Illustrated Colour Text.* 3rd ed. Churchill Livingstone: Elsevier; 2010.)

simultaneous constriction of the pupils. This reflex is required for actions such as reading a book or walking downstairs. To test this reflex, ask the patient to look into the distance and then bring an object to within 10 cm of the patient's eyes and ask the patient to fixate on the object. Both components of the reflex should be observed on near fixation.

Eye movements

Inspect the eyes and note the position of the eyelids and the presence of any strabismus (misalignment of the visual axes). Strabismus is nonparalytic or paralytic (see Chapter 43). There are two main types of eye movement:

- Pursuit eye movements are used to follow an object smoothly.
- Saccadic ('jump') eye movements are used to look from one object to a distant object without focusing on objects in between.

Conjugate eye movements occur when the visual axes stay correctly aligned during either pursuit or saccadic movements. If the visual axes are misaligned, the patient experiences diplopia. Sometimes, the brain tries to correct a partial failure of gaze with a saccadic movement. The cycle of failure to sustain gaze and correction by saccadic movement is called nystagmus.

Pursuit eye movements

To test pursuit eye movements, ask the patient to focus on an object, such as a finger or pen, held approximately 50 cm in front of the patient's nose. Any strabismus, ptosis, or nystagmus in the 'primary position' should be noted. The patient should be asked to follow the object as it describes the shape of an 'H' in front of

Table 2.3 Common fundoscopic abnormalities

Structure	Abnormality	Pathology
Optic disc	Papilloedema – the optic disc is 'swollen' with blurring of the disc margin and engorgement of the retinal veins; there may be flame-shaped haemorrhages near the disc	Raised intracranial pressure (space-occupying lesions, e.g., tumours, particularly of the posterior fossa, hydrocephalus subsequent to meningitis or subarachnoid haemorrhage), venous obstruction (e.g., cavernous sinus thrombosis), malignant hypertension, idiopathic intracranial hypertension
	Optic atrophy – the disc is paler than usual, particularly on the temporal side, with fewer small vessels crossing its margins	Any cause of chronic optic nerve disease – central retinal artery occlusion, optic neuritis (multiple sclerosis, ischaemia), chronic glaucoma, vitamin B_{12} deficiency, toxins (e.g., methyl alcohol, tobacco), hereditary (e.g., Leber optic atrophy), lesion of the optic chiasm and or tract
Retinal arteries	Silver-wiring, increased tortuosity, arteriovenous nipping	Hypertension
	Gross narrowing with retinal pallor and reddened fovea	Central retinal artery occlusion
	Cholesterol or platelet emboli	Cerebrovascular disease
	New vessel formation (on the surface of the optic disc or retina): new vessels develop subsequent to widespread retinal ischaemia; they do not affect vision, but are fragile and may bleed	Diabetes, central or branch retinal vein occlusion
Retinal veins	Venous engorgement	Papilloedema (see above), central retinal vein occlusion
Retina	Haemorrhages	Superficial flame-shaped and deep dot-shaped (hypertension, diabetes); subhyaloid between the retina and the vitreous (subarachnoid haemorrhage)
	Exudates	'Soft cotton-wool spots' (retinal infarcts) and hard exudates (lipid accumulation within the retina from leaking blood vessels in hypertension and diabetes)
	Pigmentation	Retinitis pigmentosa (e.g., Refsum disease, Kearns–Sayre syndrome), choroidoretinitis (e.g., toxoplasmosis, sarcoidosis, syphilis), following laser treatment (diabetes)

Table 2.4 Assessment of ptosis

Cause	Additional clinical features	Pupil responses	Eye movements
Congenital	Hereditary; unilateral or bilateral	Normal	Normal
Neurogenic			
Third nerve palsy (see Chapter 43)	Complete ptosis	Dilated pupil, absent response to light and accommodation	Eye looks 'down and out' ophthalmoplegia with diplopia in all positions of gaze
Horner syndrome	Partial ptosis, apparent enophthalmos; ipsilateral anhidrosis	Constricted pupil, impaired response to light and accommodation	Normal
Myogenic			
Senile	This is due to degenerative changes in the levator superioris muscle of the upper eyelid	Normal; senile pupil – constricted with impaired dilatation in the dark	Normal
Myasthenia gravis	Fatigable and therefore variable ptosis	Normal	Variable diplopia and ophthalmoplegia
Myopathy	Associated bulbar/limb weakness	Normal	Abnormal if extraocular muscles involved

the patient and to inform the examiner of any double vision. In the presence of diplopia, identify the direction of the maximum separation of images and the two muscles responsible for moving the eyes in this direction (see Chapter 43). Cover each eye in turn and observe when the outer image disappears. The outer image is always produced by the pathological eye, irrespective of where the double vision occurs. The presence of nystagmus should also be noted, whether it is horizontal or vertical, and in which direction it is maximal. The smoothness and speed of pursuit eye movements should also be noted.

Saccadic eye movements

To test saccadic eye movements, hold a finger approximately 50 cm in front of the patient's nose and a fist approximately 50 cm lateral to the finger. Ask the patient to move his or her gaze rapidly back and forth between the fist and finger. This is repeated in all four directions keeping a finger in front of the patient and moving the fist in the appropriate direction. Assess the velocity and the accuracy of these movements. The presence of slow or absent adduction in the horizontal plane is consistent with internuclear ophthalmoplegia (see Chapter 43). There may also be horizontal gaze-evoked nystagmus in the abducting eye.

> ### HINTS AND TIPS
>
> Normal pursuit movements depend on intact posterior cortical areas and cerebellum. Normal saccadic eye movements depend on intact basal ganglia, cerebellum, anterior cortical areas and the superior colliculi of the midbrain.

Oculocephalic reflex (doll's eye movements)

If pursuit or saccadic eye movements are absent, the oculocephalic reflex will differentiate between supranuclear and nuclear gaze palsy. The oculocephalic reflex is tested by asking the patient to fixate on your eyes while you rotate the patient's head in the horizontal and the vertical planes. The reflex in supranuclear lesions is intact, allowing the patient's eyes to remain fixated on the examiner's eyes. This reflex is intact because the afferent (information from neck muscle and vestibular apparatus) and efferent (nerves and muscles controlling eye movements) loop is intact. If there is a nuclear or peripheral lesion (i.e., pathology in the brainstem, nerves or muscles) then the reflex loop is broken and doll's eye movements are absent.

Ocular nerve palsies

Clinical signs and causes of ocular nerve palsies are discussed in Chapter 43.

Nystagmus

Nystagmus is an involuntary, rhythmic oscillation of the eyes caused by lesions affecting the vestibular apparatus, the vestibulocochlear (eighth) nerve, brainstem centres involved in controlling gaze or the cerebellum. Nystagmus is usually asymptomatic, but patients sometimes describe an unpleasant experience of alternating movements of their visual fields, which is called oscillopsia.

In normal individuals a few beats of nystagmus can often be observed at the extremes of gaze. This is not pathological or sustained. It may also occur during voluntary rapid oscillation of the eyes. These physiological movements are called nystagmoid jerks.

Nystagmus should be looked for in the primary position of gaze (i.e., when the patient is looking straight ahead) and also during the testing of eye movements. Nystagmus can be jerky (the oscillation has a fast and a slow phase) or pendular (the oscillation occurs with equal velocity in all directions). The nystagmus may be horizontal, vertical, rotatory or a mixture of these. The amplitude of the nystagmus and its persistence should be noted. The direction of jerky nystagmus is defined by the direction of the fast phase by convention. Causes of nystagmus are shown in Table 2.5.

Trigeminal (fifth, V) nerve

Motor

The motor part of the trigeminal nerve is not often affected by the many pathologies that involve the surrounding structures.

Inspect for wasting of the temporalis muscles, which produces hollowing above the zygoma. Ask the patient to clench his or her teeth and palpate the masseters for contraction and relaxation. Assess the pterygoid muscles by resisting the patient's attempts to open the mouth. In unilateral trigeminal lesions, the lower jaw deviates to the paralytic side as the mouth is opened.

Jaw jerk

A jaw jerk is a brainstem stretch reflex. Ask the patient to open the mouth slightly. Rest your index finger on the apex of the jaw and tap it lightly with the patella hammer. The normal response is closure of the mouth, which is caused by reflex contraction of the pterygoid muscles. An absent reflex is not significant, but the reflex becomes pathologically brisk with bilateral damage to the UMNs to the motor fifth nucleus in the pons.

Sensory

The sensory aspect of the fifth nerve is often affected by local pathologies and loss of the corneal reflex is often one of the first clinical signs of a lesion at the cerebellopontine angle.

Test light touch, pin-prick and temperature over the forehead, the medial aspects of the cheeks and the chin. These

Table 2.5 Causes of nystagmus

Type	Description	Pathology
Pendular	Oscillations of equal velocity	Longstanding impaired macular vision (since early childhood), e.g., albinism, congenital cataracts, congenital nystagmus; lesions in upper brainstem, e.g., multiple sclerosis
Jerky	Fast phase towards the side of the lesion	Unilateral cerebellar lesions
	Fast phase to the opposite side of the lesion	Unilateral vestibular lesions or VIII lesions
	Direction of nystagmus varies with the direction of gaze	Brainstem pathology
	Upbeat nystagmus	Lesions at or around the superior colliculi (midbrain)
	Downbeat nystagmus	Lesions at or around the foramen magnum
Rotatory	Specific to one head position, and fatigues with repeated testing	Unilateral labyrinthine pathology
Mixed	Jerky and rotatory	Brainstem pathology

correspond to the ophthalmic, maxillarya and mandibular branches of the trigeminal nerve, respectively (see Chapter 9). It should be noted that the angle of the jaw is not innervated by the trigeminal nerve. A partial loss can be detected by comparing the response to the same stimulus on different areas of the face. The clinical pattern of sensory loss depends on the anatomical site of the lesion (Fig. 2.3).

The corneal reflex is elicited by lightly touching the cornea (not the conjunctiva) with a wisp of cotton wool. Synchronous blinking of both eyes should occur. An afferent defect (fifth cranial nerve lesion) results in depression or absence of the direct and consensual blinking reflex. An efferent defect (seventh cranial nerve lesion) results in an impairment or absence of the reflex on the side of the facial weakness.

Facial (seventh, VII) nerve

Motor

Inspect the patient's face, looking for asymmetry of the nasolabial folds and the position of the two angles of the mouth. Assess the movements of the upper part of the face by asking the patient to:

- Elevate the eyebrows.
- Close the eyes tightly and resist your attempt to open them. Look for Bell's phenomenon – this is a reflex upward deviation of the eyes in response to attempted but failed forced closure of the eyelids.

Movements of the lower part of the face are assessed by asking the patient to:

- Blow out the cheeks with air.

- Purse the lips tightly and resist your attempt to open them.
- Show the teeth.
- Whistle.
- Smile (observe any facial asymmetry).

If you detect any weakness or asymmetry, decide if the weakness is confined to the lower part of the face (UMN lesion) or both the upper and lower parts of the face (LMN lesion). Do not miss bilateral facial weakness. In this case, the face appears to sag, with a lack of facial expression even though it is symmetrical.

Hyperacusis (oversensitivity to noise) is suggestive of a lesion affecting the nerve to the stapedius, which comes off the facial nerve in the facial canal within the petrous bone.

HINTS AND TIPS

The upper face has bilateral innervation from the facial nerve. Therefore, a UMN facial nerve lesion just affects the lower part of the face (i.e., forehead spared) and a LMN facial nerve lesion affects both the upper and lower parts of the face.

Sensory

Taste (visceral afferent)

Examine taste by applying a solution of salt, sweet (sugar), sour (vinegar) or bitter (lemon) to the anterior two-thirds of the tongue and comparing the response on the two sides. The mouth should be rinsed with water between testing. Lesions of the chorda tympani will cause loss of taste.

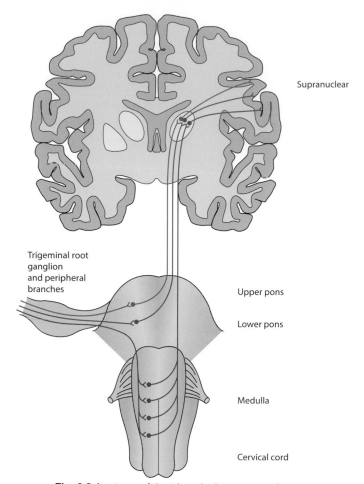

Supranuclear

Trigeminal root
ganglion
and peripheral
branches

Upper pons

Lower pons

Medulla

Cervical cord

Fig. 2.3 Anatomy of the trigeminal sensory pathways.

A few somatic afferent fibres from the seventh nerve subserve parts of the outer pinna. In Ramsay Hunt syndrome, there may be vesicles in this position with unilateral facial weakness associated with reactivation of herpes zoster in the geniculate ganglion.

Vestibulocochlear nerve (eighth, VIII)

Hearing

Clinical bedside assessment of hearing is not sensitive and can detect only gross hearing loss. Audiometry is usually required for detailed assessment.

Assess each ear separately while masking the hearing in the other ear by occluding the external meatus with your index finger. Test patients' hearing sensitivity by whispering numbers into their ears and asking them to repeat these.

Determine if the hearing loss is conductive or sensorineural by performing Rinne and Weber tests (see Chapter 10).

Vestibular function

Although not entirely satisfactory, bedside tests for vestibular function include examination of the patient's gait and eye movements for nystagmus. Hallpike manoeuvre (for positional vertigo) and head impulse test (for vestibular dysfunction) with associated findings are summarized in Chapter 10. A patient suspected of having vestibular dysfunction will sometimes require formal vestibular testing.

Glossopharyngeal (ninth, IX) and vagus (tenth, X) nerves

Motor

The motor component of the vagus nerve supplies the muscles of the palate, pharynx and larynx via the recurrent laryngeal nerve. Check the patient's speech quality and volume as well as strength of cough (see subsection 'Speech' in this chapter).

Palatal movement can be assessed by:

- Asking the patient to say 'ah' (voluntary activity).
- Touching the posterior pharyngeal wall with the end of an orange stick on both sides (the 'gag' reflex – unpleasant for patient).

Assess the afferent pathway of the 'gag' reflex (ninth cranial nerve) by asking the patient whether sensation is comparable on both sides. Assess the efferent pathway (tenth cranial nerve) by observing the normal response of a symmetrical rise of the soft palate and movement of the pharyngeal muscles; characteristically, a 'gagging' sound is made.

Supranuclear (UMN) innervation of the palatal and pharyngeal muscles is bilateral. Unilateral lesions will therefore not cause significant and prolonged dysfunction of swallowing and speech. In patients who have bilateral UMN lesions, the palate cannot be elevated voluntarily, but moves normally when testing the 'gag' reflex. This is part of a syndrome called a 'pseudobulbar palsy' and is associated with a brisk jaw jerk, spastic tongue and speech and emotional lability.

If the voluntary and reflex movements are bilaterally impaired, then the patient may have a bilateral bulbar palsy (i.e., damage to the LMNs or their nuclei in the brainstem on both sides). If the palate does not elevate on one side, the lesion almost always involves the LMN because the palate has bilateral UMN innervation. Therefore, in unilateral LMN lesions, the palate lies slightly lower on the affected side and deviates towards the unaffected side. Minor and inconsistent deviations of the uvula should be ignored.

Sensory

The posterior pharyngeal wall and tonsillar region are innervated by the glossopharyngeal (ninth cranial) nerve and sensation is tested by a wooden probe as described above. The ninth nerve also subserves sensation and taste to the posterior third of the tongue but taste is difficult to test in this location.

Accessory (eleventh, XI) nerve

The spinal part of the accessory nerve is a purely motor nerve that arises from the upper five segments of the cervical cord. It supplies the trapezius and sternocleidomastoid muscles and wasting, or weakness of these muscles should be noted on inspection.

The strength of the sternocleidomastoid muscles is assessed by asking the patient to turn his or her head to each side against the resistance of the examiner's hand. Turning of the head to the left involves contraction of the right sternocleidomastoid and vice versa. In a patient with a hemispheric stroke, it is the sternocleidomastoid muscle ipsilateral to the hemisphere that is affected. Therefore, there is weakness in head-turning towards the side of the hemiparesis.

Assess the strength of the trapezius muscles by asking the patient to shrug his or her shoulders upwards against resistance and note the bulk of the muscles on palpation.

Hypoglossal (twelfth, XII) nerve

The hypoglossal nerve is a purely motor nerve that supplies the muscles of the tongue. Inspect the tongue as it lies in the floor of the mouth for evidence of wasting (which may be unilateral or bilateral), fasciculations (wriggling movements at the tongue surface) or other involuntary movements. Then ask the patient to protrude the tongue.

THE MOTOR SYSTEM

The examination should start by simply observing the patient walk into the consultation room. Did the patient stand up from the chair with difficulty? Do they use a walking aid and what is their gait? This then proceeds to bedside examination of the motor system.

Inspection

- **Posture:** look for the characteristic posturing of a patient with a hemiparesis (see Chapter 16). Ask the patient to hold out both arms in front of the body with eyes closed. If the patient has a UMN lesion, he or she may demonstrate a drift of the arm downwards from the horizontal into a pronated and eventually flexed position. This is called 'pronator drift'. The fingers of the outstretched arm may move spontaneously, as if the patient was playing the piano. This is called 'pseudoathetosis' and is caused by loss of joint-position sense. In cerebellar disease, if the outstretched arms are rapidly displaced, they may oscillate about the horizontal rather than quickly returning to the initial position. This is called 'rebound'.
- **Muscle wasting:** look for the degree and distribution of muscle wasting. This is usually characteristic of LMN disorders (i.e., anterior horn cell, spinal nerve, plexus or peripheral nerve disorders as well as myopathies).
- **Fasciculations:** these are seen as brief, localized twitches or flickers of movement within the muscle at rest and are also a feature of LMN disorders. Each muscle should be carefully studied for up to several minutes if there is a strong suspicion of an LMN disorder.
- **Involuntary movements:** For example, a resting tremor may be evident in patients who have Parkinson's disease (see Chapter 13).
- **Atrophic skin changes:** This includes smooth hairless, purple oedematous skin may be a sign of associated sensory nerve damage in an LMN disorder or from disuse in a UMN disorder.
- **Scars:** These should be noted, particularly over the lateral aspect of the foot from a sural nerve biopsy or over the

vastus lateralis or triceps from a muscle biopsy. Some patients may have scars from orthopaedic surgery such as arthrodesis at the ankle in foot drop.

- **Walking sticks, ankle–foot orthoses and other orthotic devices:** These can often give an early clue as to the patient's main functional difficulty.

Tone

Tone refers to the activity of the stretch reflexes as assessed by the degree of resistance that occurs on stretching a muscle at different velocities.

Some patients have difficulty relaxing during an examination, which can artificially increase stiffness in their limbs. Distraction of the patient (e.g., with unrelated conversation) can relax the limbs.

Arm

Pyramidal hypertonia: spasticity

Take the patient's arm and flex and extend the elbow. Spasticity may be especially observed during extension. Then hold the patient's hand, with the elbow flexed, and rapidly pronate and supinate the forearm. If tone is increased, you may feel a 'supinator' or 'spastic catch', which is an interruption of the smooth movement on supination by increased tone of a spastic type. Alternatively, there may be increased tone on extending the elbow, which suddenly gives way to low tone. This is sometimes referred to as the 'clasp-knife' effect. These signs are suggestive of a UMN lesion.

Extrapyramidal rigidity

If there is increased tone throughout movement of a limb, this is called 'lead-pipe' rigidity. When the patient has a tremor, which may be subclinical, and lead-pipe rigidity, they may have 'cogwheel' rigidity. These two types of rigidity are typical of parkinsonism but can occur in many other extrapyramidal syndromes. All extrapyramidal types of increased tone can be enhanced by asking the patient to move the other arm up and down. If this brings out increased tone, then the rigidity is said to occur 'with synkinesis'.

> **COMMON PITFALLS**
>
> Increased tone may be due to an upper motor neurone or extrapyramidal disorder. Increased tone from spasticity is due to an upper motor neurone lesion—look for a supinator catch, clasp-knife phenomenon and clonus, brisk reflexes, and extensor plantar responses. Increased tone from an extrapyramidal disorder causes 'lead-pipe' rigidity or 'cogwheel' rigidity if there is a superimposed tremor. The reflexes are usually normal and plantar responses flexor.

Legs

- Rock each leg from side to side on the bed, holding it at the knee. Normally, the foot lags behind the leg. If tone is increased, the foot and leg move stiffly together. If tone is decreased, the foot moves limply from side to side with each movement.
- Passively flex and extend the knee at varying speeds, supporting both the upper leg and the foot.
- With the patient's legs extended on the couch, place your hand under the patient's knee and quickly lift the knee about 15 cm. The foot will normally stay on the bed as the knee is flexed. If tone is increased, the foot may jump up with the lower leg and if tone is decreased the limb will feel lax and slightly heavier than normal.

'Clonus' describes the rhythmic unidirectional contractions evoked by a sudden passive stretch of a muscle. This is elicited most easily at the ankle. A few beats may be normal but 'sustained clonus' is characteristic of a UMN lesion.

Power

Power is tested in each of the main muscle groups by the examiner stabilizing the limb proximal to the joint movement that is being tested. Power in each muscle is given a grade as defined by the Medical Research Council (MRC) scale (Table 2.6).

The scheme in Fig. 2.4 shows testing of the main muscle groups in the arms. The scheme in Fig. 2.5 shows testing of the main muscle groups of the legs. Table 2.7 summarizes the expected signs observed in lesions arising from different parts of the nervous system.

Reflexes

Tendon reflexes are most easily determined by briskly stretching the tendon. To perform this, the tendon hammer is held near the end of the shaft and the heavy end is swung onto the tendon directly or onto a finger placed over the tendon (biceps and supinator jerks). The tendon reflexes shown in Fig. 2.6A and B should be examined.

Table 2.6 The Medical Research Council scale for assessment of muscle power

Grade	Response
0	No movement
1	Flicker of muscle when patient tries to move
2	Moves but not against gravity
3	Moves against gravity but not against resistance
4	Moves against resistance but not to full strength
5	Full strength (you cannot overcome the movement)

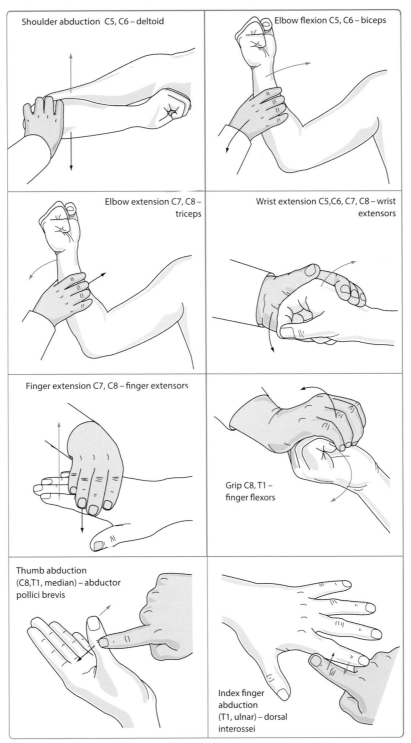

Shoulder abduction C5, C6 – deltoid

Elbow flexion C5, C6 – biceps

Elbow extension C7, C8 – triceps

Wrist extension C5,C6, C7, C8 – wrist extensors

Finger extension C7, C8 – finger extensors

Grip C8, T1 – finger flexors

Thumb abduction (C8,T1, median) – abductor pollici brevis

Index finger abduction (T1, ulnar) – dorsal interossei

Fig. 2.4 Testing muscle groups of the upper limb. The blue arrows indicate the direction of movement of the patient, and the black arrows the direction of resistance by the examiner. Each muscle group should be given a grade as defined by the Medical Research Council scale (see Table 2.6).

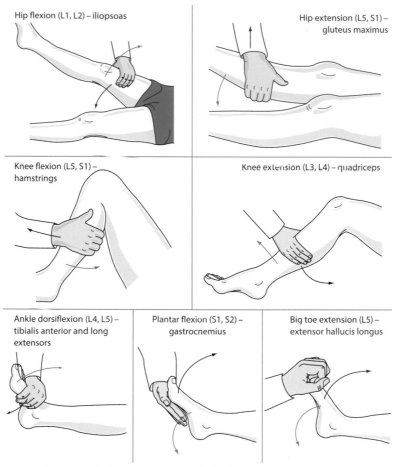

Hip flexion (L1, L2) – iliopsoas

Hip extension (L5, S1) – gluteus maximus

Knee flexion (L5, S1) – hamstrings

Knee extension (L3, L4) – quadriceps

Ankle dorsiflexion (L4, L5) – tibialis anterior and long extensors

Plantar flexion (S1, S2) – gastrocnemius

Big toe extension (L5) – extensor hallucis longus

Fig. 2.5 Testing muscle groups of the lower limb. The blue arrows indicate the direction of movement of the patient, and the black arrows the direction of movement of the examiner. Each muscle group should be given a grade as defined by the Medical Research Council scale (see Table 2.6).

Table 2.7 Clinical features of patients presenting with limb weakness

Site of lesion	Wasting	Tone	Pattern of weakness	Reflexes	Plantar response
Upper motor neurone	None	Increased	'Pyramidal' pattern weakness	Increased	Extensor
Lower motor neurone	Present	Decreased	Individual or groups of muscles	Decreased/absent	Flexor or absent
Neuromuscular junction	Uncommon	Usually normal, may be decreased	Bilateral and predominantly of the proximal limb girdle (fatigable)	Usually normal	Flexor
Muscle	From mild to severe	Decreased in proportion to wasting	Bilateral and predominantly of the proximal limb girdle	Decreased in proportion to wasting	Flexor

Note: Not every patient will have all the features of their syndrome.

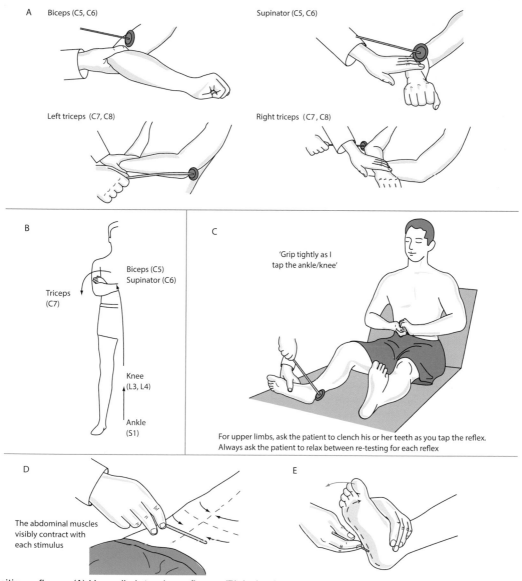

Fig. 2.6 Eliciting reflexes. (A) Upper limb tendon reflexes. (B) A simple way to remember root values of reflexes. (C) Testing jerk reinforcement. (D) Abdominal reflexes: test in the four quadrants shown. (E) Plantar reflex. The normal response is a downgoing hallux. In an upper motor neurone lesion, the hallux dorsiflexes and the other toes fan out (the Babinski response).

The tendon reflexes may be increased ('brisk'), decreased or absent. If they are absent, this should be confirmed by reinforcement (Fig. 2.6C). Abdominal reflexes can be tested as shown in Fig. 2.6D. The abdominal reflexes are lost in a UMN lesion, but may also be lost after abdominal injury or in an obese patient. The plantar response is elicited by scratching the sole as demonstrated in Fig. 2.6E.

Tendon reflexes are conventionally annotated as shown in Box 2.1.

Coordination

The ability of a patient to perform smooth and accurate movements is dependent on power, intact joint-position sense, and coordination. Weakness and loss of joint-position sense, may give rise to apparent clumsiness, which may be misinterpreted as incoordination. Cerebellar dysfunction can only be accurately detected if weakness and/or joint-position sense loss is mild or there is severe incoordination.

BOX 2.1 CONVENTIONAL ANNOTATION FOR REFLEXES

Reduced	+
Normal	++
Very brisk (with associated clonus)	+++
Absent	0
Present with reinforcement only	±

Gait

A wide-based, sometimes lurching gait is seen in cerebellar disease. Unsteadiness is made more obvious if the patient is asked to walk 'heel to toe'.

Cerebellum

Cerebellar dysfunction in the arms can be assessed as follows:

- **The finger–nose test:** the examiner places a finger 50 cm in front of the patient's nose and asks the patient to move his or her index finger between the nose and the examiner's finger; both index fingers are tested. In patients who have a cerebellar lesion, on approaching the examiner's finger, the patient's arm may coarsely oscillate. This is called an intention tremor. The inability to perform smooth, accurate, and targeted movements is called dysmetria. If the patient overshoots the intended target, this is called 'past pointing'.
- **Dysdiadochokinesis:** this is the inability to carry out rapid, alternating movements with regularity. It can be tested by asking the patient to alternately pronate and supinate his or her arm and correspondingly tap the palm and then dorsum of his or her hand on the examiner's palm. In cerebellar disease, the movements are irregular in amplitude and speed.
- **The 'rebound phenomenon':** if the wrists are gently tapped when the patient's arms are outstretched, then the arms should rapidly come to the resting horizontal position. In patients with cerebellar disease, the arms oscillate about the horizontal before coming to rest. This is called the rebound phenomenon.

Cerebellar dysfunction in the legs can be assessed as follows:

- **The heel–shin test:** Ask the patient to place one heel on the other knee and slowly slide the heel down the shin, then lift the heel off the shin and repeat the test. This test should be performed on each side in turn.
- **The tapping test:** The rapid tapping of the foot is impaired in cerebellar disease. This test should be performed on each side in turn.

The combination of these abnormalities in a patient is called cerebellar ataxia and may be associated with other signs of cerebellar disease such as horizontal jerky nystagmus and slurring dysarthria (see Chapter 12).

THE SENSORY SYSTEM

Patients use various terms to describe sensory disturbance, including numbness, tingling, 'pins and needles' and burning. Medical terms include paraesthesia (tingling), dysaesthesia (unpleasant awareness of touch or pressure), hyperaesthesia (exaggeration of any sensation) and hyperalgesia (exaggerated perception of painful stimuli).

To test the sensory modalities, ask the patient to close his or her eyes and, for all modalities except joint-position sense, apply the test to a reference point such as the skin over the sternum and ask the patient if he or she can feel the sensation normally. Subsequently, test each sensory modality distally to proximally in each limb and ask the patient if it feels the same as the reference point on the chest. Fig. 2.7 demonstrates the different dermatomes.

Sensory testing

It is not recommended to spend too much time doing sensory testing because you will exhaust the patient and yourself. It is best to tailor your examination to the patient's complaint. In coming to the sensory examination in the neurological evaluation, one should have a hypothesis as to the pattern of sensory loss that is expected. The sensory examination can be tailored towards that pattern. Patterns of sensory impairment are discussed in more detail in Chapter 15.

Sensory modalities

Pain

A specialized disposable device (e.g., 'neurotip'), and not a hypodermic needle, should be used to test pain sensation. The patient will either feel nothing, a blunt sensation (abnormal) or a sharp pain (normal). If an abnormal area is found, then its margins should be further defined by moving from the area of reduced sensation to the normal area.

Temperature

A cold object such as the flat surface of a nonvibrating tuning fork can be used to test perception of cold temperature.

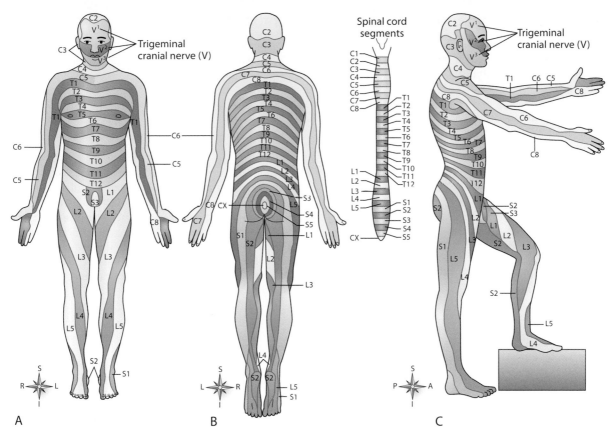

Fig. 2.7 Segmental innervation of the skin (dermatomes). (A) Ventral view. (B) Dorsal view. (From Patton KT, Thibodeau GA. *Anatomy and Physiology*. 9th ed. St. Louis: Mosby; 2015.)

Light touch

A wisp of cotton wool is used to test light touch with brief static stimuli. Remember that 'tickle' is carried by spinothalamic fibres.

Joint-position sense

Move the distal interphalangeal (DIP) joint of the index finger/big toe up and down while stabilizing the digit with your other hand. Ask the patient to indicate the direction in which the digit is being moved. If perception of joint position is abnormal, then test more proximal joints until the test is normal (e.g., DIP, wrist, elbow, shoulder).

Vibration

A 128-Hz tuning fork should be used to test vibration sense. Start the tuning fork vibrating and place it on the DIP joint of the finger/big toe and ask if the patient can feel it vibrating. If the patient cannot feel these vibrations, move the tuning fork proximally (e.g., lateral malleoli, tibial tuberosity, iliac crest, sternum). The tuning fork should always be touching bony elements under the skin. Vibration sense is often lost early in peripheral polyneuropathies.

Two-point discrimination

Test two-point discrimination with specific compasses. The pulp of the index finger (normal: 2–3 mm) and hallux (normal: 5 mm) are normally tested and the patient asked whether they feel one or two points.

GENERAL EXAMINATION

The conclusion of the neurological examination should include a more general examination of the other relevant body systems. In particular, where it is important, autonomic function should also be assessed. The easiest method of assessment is measurement of the blood pressure as the patient lies supine and again after standing for a couple of minutes. Orthostatic hypotension, defined as a fall in systolic blood pressure of >20 mm Hg and >10 mm Hg diastolic blood pressure, can be associated with autonomic dysfunction.

Ophthalmic examination

The ophthalmic examination involves many steps which are described above. An easy way to remember the ophthalmic examination is to use the acronym 'AFRO'.

Acuity
- Distant vision (visual acuity VA).
- Near vision.
- Colour vision.

Fields
- Visual inattention.
- Visual fields.
- Blind spots.

Reflexes
- Accommodation.
- Direct and consensual pupillary reflexes.
- Swinging light test.

Ophthalmoscopy

You should look at the:
- Red reflex.
- Optic disc (check the **3C's**)
  1. Cup
  2. Colour
  3. Contours
- Four quadrants: follow blood vessels from the optic disc.
- Macula.

This should be carried out in a darkened room; ask the patient to remove their glasses (if present) and consider giving mydriatic eye drops prior to carrying out fundoscopy. Then test for the extraocular muscles as described above. The extraocular muscles are supplied by the cranial nerves. Use this acronym to remember which cranial nerve supplies each extraocular muscle – $SO_4LR_6O_3$. **S**uperior **O**blique (CN4) and **L**ateral **R**ectus (CN6), **O**ther extraocular muscles supplied by CN3.

● Chapter summary

- The neurological examination involves assessing all parts of the nervous system from higher cerebral function to distal limb function.
- A good examination will direct any further investigations that need to be performed.
- Use the following acronym: **AFRO** – to remember the ophthalmic examination and $SO_4LR_6O_3$ to remember the ophthalmic examination – to remember cranial nerve supply of extraocular muscles.

ROUTINE INVESTIGATIONS

A number of routine tests are useful in neurology. These include:

- haematology (Table 3.1)
- biochemistry (Table 3.2)
- immunology (Table 3.3)
- microbiology (Table 3.4)
- cerebrospinal fluid findings

For each test, normal ranges are given, with neurological differential diagnoses for high and low values.

NEUROPHYSIOLOGICAL INVESTIGATIONS

Electroencephalography

Electroencephalography (EEG) measures electrical potentials generated by the neurones lying underneath an electrode on the scalp, and compares these with recordings from either a reference electrode or a neighbouring electrode. The normal trace is symmetrical; therefore asymmetries, as well as specific abnormalities, may indicate an underlying disorder.

EEG remains useful for detecting underlying abnormalities of cerebral function, especially for:

- epilepsy (see below)
- encephalitis (e.g., herpes simplex)
- encephalopathy (e.g., metabolic)
- coma

The main role of EEG is in the assessment of epilepsy. It can help in the following ways:

- Support of the diagnosis (although this is made primarily on the clinical history and the EEG may be normal in patients who have had witnessed seizures). An increased yield of abnormalities may be obtained if recording is made under conditions of sleep deprivation, with hyperventilation and with photic stimulation.
- Classification of seizure type, which may optimize therapy.
- Assessment for surgical intervention.

- Diagnosis of nonepileptic seizures (especially with simultaneous video recording, i.e., 'video telemetry').

'Invasive EEG monitoring' refers to prolonged recording from electrodes inserted directly into the brain, undertaken preoperatively, before a surgery to remove an epileptic focus.

Different normal rhythms are characteristically found over different regions of the brain (Fig. 3.1). Other than these rhythmic activities, other abnormal activity may be generated in certain conditions (Fig. 3.2).

Electromyography and nerve conduction studies

Electromyography (EMG) and nerve conduction studies (NCS), usually performed together, examine the electrical activity of muscle, neuromuscular junction and lower motor neurones. They are useful in:

- Identifying a cause of weakness (e.g., neuropathy, myopathy, anterior horn cell disease).
- Determining the distribution of the abnormality (e.g., length dependent, mononeuritis multiplex).
- Suggesting the type of myopathy (e.g., dystrophy, myositis or myotonia) or neuropathy (e.g., axonal or demyelinating and motor, sensory or sensorimotor).
- Diagnosing myasthenia gravis.
- Assessing baseline deficits before surgery (e.g., carpal tunnel syndrome).

Electromyography

EMG involves the insertion of a needle electrode into muscle.

Normal muscle at rest is electrically silent (apart from actually during needle insertion, 'insertional activity'). In abnormal muscles, either due to primary muscle disease or to denervation of the muscle, spontaneous activity may be seen at rest. The most common types of spontaneous activity include fibrillation potentials, positive sharp waves and fasciculations.

Fibrillation potentials and positive sharp waves are due to spontaneous contractions of individual muscle fibres, probably due to abnormal rhythmic fluctuations of membrane potential. They cannot be seen clinically through the skin. They are most commonly seen in denervation but may be found in some

Table 3.1 Possible clinical relevance of abnormalities in blood or serum levels of haematological indices (individual laboratories may have different normal ranges)

Test	Normal range	Abnormality	Possible clinical explanation
Full blood count			
Haemoglobin	13.5–18.0 g/dL male; 11.5–16.0 g/dL female	Low; anaemia	May cause nonspecific neurological symptoms (e.g., dizziness, weakness, faintness); may suggest an underlying chronic illness
		High; polycythaemia	Predisposes to stroke and chorea
Mean cell volume	76–96 fL	High; macrocytic	Vitamin B_{12} deficiency (peripheral neuropathy, dementia)
		Low; microcytic	May indicate an underlying chronic illness; associated with idiopathic intracranial hypertension
White cell count			
Neutrophils	$2–7.5 \times 10^9$/L	High: neutrophilia Low: neutropenia	Meningitis or other infection Leukaemia or lymphoma (infiltrative disease, space-occupying lesions, peripheral neuropathy) Multiple myeloma (neuropathy, vertebral collapse, hyperviscosity syndrome)
Lymphocytes	$1.5–3.5 \times 10^9$/L	High: lymphocytosis Low: lymphopenia	Viral infection (transverse myelitis, Guillain-Barré syndrome) Leukaemia or lymphoma, as above
Eosinophils	$0.04–0.44 \times 10^9$/L	High: eosinophilia	Hypereosinophilic syndrome (rare)
Platelet count	$150–400 \times 10^9$/L	High: thrombocythaemia Low: thrombocytopenia	Predisposes to stroke Intracranial bleeding
Erythrocyte sedimentation rate	20 mm/h	High	Vasculitis (e.g., PAN, SLE, giant-cell arteritis) may cause cerebral, cranial and peripheral nerve infarcts, confusion and fits
Coagulation tests			
Activated partial thromboplastin time (APT or PTTK)	35–45 s	High	SLE; antiphospholipid syndrome
Protein C, protein S	Varies with laboratory	Low: deficiency	Inherited predisposition to thrombosis (arterial and venous)
Factor 5 Leiden	Varies with laboratory	Present	Mutation causes a single amino acid substitution in factor 5, which results in activated protein C resistance and predisposition to thrombosis (arterial and venous)
Vitamin B_{12}	>150 ng/L	Low: deficiency	Peripheral neuropathy, myelopathy, confusion/dementia, optic neuropathy, SCDC, ataxia
Folate	4–18 µg/L	Low; deficiency	Peripheral neuropathy, dementia

APT, *Activated thromboplastin;* PAN, *polyarteritis nodosa;* PTTK, *partial thromboplastin time;* SCDC, *subacute combined degeneration of the cord;* SLE, *systemic lupus erythematosus.*

Table 3.2 Possible clinical relevance of abnormalities in blood or serum levels of biochemical indices (individual laboratories may have different normal ranges)

Test	Normal range	Abnormality	Possible clinical explanation
Urea and electrolytes			
Sodium	135–145 mmol/L	High: hypernatraemia Low: hyponatraemia	Both may cause weakness, confusion and fits
Potassium	3.5–5.5 mmol/L	High: hyperkalaemia Low: hypokalaemia	Hyper- or hypokalaemic periodic paralysis
Urea	2.5–6.7 mmol/L	High: renal failure	Confusion, peripheral neuropathy
Creatinine	<120 mmol/L	High: renal failure	Confusion, peripheral neuropathy
Glucose (fasting)	4–6 mmol/L	High: diabetes Low: hypoglycaemia	Neuropathy, coma Confusion, coma, focal signs
Calcium	2.2–2.6 mmol/L	Low: hypocalcaemia	Tetany, seizures
Liver function tests			
Bilirubin and liver enzymes	Bilirubin range: 3–17 mmol/L; enzyme levels vary between laboratories	High	Liver disease: confusion, tremor, neuropathy
Creatine kinase	24–195 U/L	High	Muscle disease: myositis, dystrophy
Thyroid function tests			
Thyroid-stimulating hormone	0.5–5.0 mU/L	High T_4 Low TSH: thyrotoxicosis	Tremor, confusion, hyperreflexia
Thyroxine (T_4)	10–24 pmol/L	Low T_4 High TSH: hypothyroidism	Apathy, confusion, hyporeflexia, neuropathy, dementia

Table 3.3 Immunology: selected autoantibodies and their associated syndromes (see Chapter 33 for further details)

Test	Associated disorder
Antinuclear factor	SLE: fits, confusion, neuropathy, aseptic meningitis Sjögren syndrome: gritty eyes, neuropathies, MCTD
Anti–double-stranded DNA (dsDNA) antibodies	SLE
Rheumatoid factor	Rheumatoid arthritis: cervical spine subluxation, neuropathies, vasculitis
Anti-Ro (SSA), anti-La (SSB) antibodies	Sjögren syndrome
Antiphospholipid antibodies (e.g., anticardiolipin)	Antiphospholipid syndrome
Antiribonucleoprotein antibodies	MCTD; myositis, trigeminal nerve palsies
ANCA	pANCA (peripheral): polyarteritis nodosa cANCA (classical): Wegener granulomatosis
Antiacetylcholine receptor antibodies	Myasthenia gravis

ANCA, *Antineutrophil cytoplasmic antibodies;* MCTD, *mixed connective tissue disease;* SLE, *systemic lupus erythematosus;* SSA, *Sjögren's-syndrome-related antigen A;* SSB, *Sjögren's-syndrome-related antigen B.*

Table 3.4 Microbiology: investigations that should be carried out if infections are implicated as the cause of neurological disease

Test	Associated disorder
Bacterial microscopy and culture (including blood, CSF, urine, stool, sputum and wounds)	Bacterial infections can cause a wide range of conditions – septicaemia, meningitis, pneumonia, urinary tract infections, cerebral abscess, etc. – or are implicated in their pathogenesis, e.g., Guillain–Barré syndrome (*Campylobacter pylori*)
	Do not forget atypical infections caused by *Listeria, Mycoplasma, Legionella*, etc.; diagnosis of tuberculosis requires special stains (Ziehl–Neelsen) and culture media (Lowenstein–Jensen)
Viral serology and culture (blood, CSF)	Viruses can cause a wide range of neurological infections, e.g., meningitis, encephalitis, shingles (herpes zoster)
VDRL (blood)	Primary syphilis (false positives in pregnancy, systemic lupus erythematosus, malaria)
TPHA (blood)	Syphilis, false positives in VDRL and other treponemal infections (yaws, pinta)
Borrelia serology (blood, CSF)	Lyme disease (see Chapter 32)
HIV (blood)	AIDS (see Chapter 32)
HTLV-1 (blood)	Myelopathy

CSF, *Cerebrospinal fluid*; HLTV-1, *human T-cell lymphotropic virus type 1*; TPHA, *Treponema pallidum haemagglutination assay*, VDRL, *venereal disease research laboratory.*

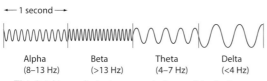

← 1 second →

| Alpha | Beta | Theta | Delta |
| (8–13 Hz) | (>13 Hz) | (4–7 Hz) | (<4 Hz) |

Fig. 3.1 Normal electroencephalographic rhythms.

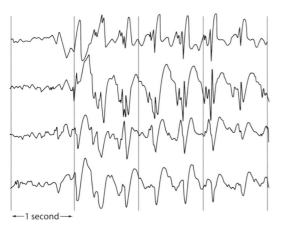

←1 second→

Fig. 3.2 Three-per-second (3/s) spike-and-wave activity, characteristic of typical absence seizure.

muscle diseases, especially inflammatory muscle disease (e.g., polymyositis).

Fasciculation potentials are much larger than fibrillations and represent the contractions of groups of muscle fibres supplied by a motor unit. They occur following denervation. They may be seen as a clinical fasciculation. They are common in motor neurone disease. Fasciculations may occur as a normal phenomenon, especially after excess caffeine or in thyrotoxicosis. However, in these situations, the firing rate is far more rapid than in diseases caused by denervation.

During voluntary movement, individual motor unit potentials (MUPs; the activity of a single anterior horn cell) can be seen on the EMG. Common abnormalities of EMG are shown in Table 3.5.

Nerve conduction studies

NCS involve stimulating a nerve with an electrical impulse via a surface electrode and recording further along the nerve (sensory studies) or recording the muscle action potential (motor studies).

The amplitude of the response, the latency to the beginning of the response and the conduction velocity are measured. As a general rule, a reduction in conduction velocity suggests demyelination whereas a reduction in amplitude suggests axonal loss (see Table 3.5).

Evoked potentials

Evoked potentials (EPs) use EEG electrodes to record responses centrally to peripheral stimuli:

- Visual EPs (VEPs): these are delayed in patients who have had an episode of optic neuritis (even if this was not clinically symptomatic); this is therefore a useful test to help in the diagnosis of multiple sclerosis.

Table 3.5 Common abnormalities found with electromyography and nerve conduction studies

Abnormality	Change in electromyographic trace
Denervation	Increased insertional activity; fibrillations, positive sharp waves and fasciculations; large amplitude, long duration, polyphasic MUPs
Myopathy	Small, short, polyphasic MUPs
Myasthenia gravis	Abnormal decrement of amplitude of response on repetitive stimulation using NCS; increased 'jitter' with single-fibre EMG (indicating variable neuromuscular transmission time)
Abnormality	**Change in nerve conduction**
Axonal neuropathy	Small action potential; normal nerve conduction velocity
Demyelinating neuropathy	Slow nerve conduction velocity; prolonged latency (time to travel from one point to the next); normal or slightly reduced action potential

EMG, *Electromyography*; MUPs, *motor unit potentials*; NCS, *nerve conduction studies*.

- Brainstem auditory EPs (BSAEPs): these assess the lower brainstem auditory pathways.
- Somatosensory EPs (SSEPs) and motor EPs (MEPs): mainly to assess spinal cord function.

Pure tone audiometry

This is a test of hearing sensitivity and assesses both peripheral and central auditory systems. Results are displayed as a function of noise frequency. PTA can aid in diagnosis of conductive, sensorineural and mixed hearing loss.

IMAGING OF THE NERVOUS SYSTEM

Plain radiography

Skull radiography has a limited role in current neurological practice. It is used in determining external cerebral shunt position. The three views are lateral, posteroanterior and Towne view (fronto-occipital). Spinal radiography is mainly seen in trauma and standard views are lateral and posteroanterior.

Computed tomography scanning

Using an X-ray source and a series of photon detectors housed in a gantry, computed tomography (CT) produces a series of consecutive two-dimensional axial brain digital images that show the X-ray density of the brain tissue.

The densities of different brain tissues vary according to their X-ray absorption properties, ranging from low (black: air, cerebrospinal fluid (CSF)) to high (white: bone, fresh blood).

The diagnostic yield of CT scanning is increased by injecting iodine-containing contrast agents. These enhance the distinction between the different brain tissues and outline areas of breakdown in the blood–brain barrier (around tumours, infarcts or abscesses).

Magnetic resonance imaging

The term 'nuclear magnetic resonance' describes the interaction between the hydrogen protons in the different body structures and strong external magnetic fields. As the patient lies in the scanner, the naturally spinning hydrogen protons align with the strong magnetic field of the scanner. When a further external magnetic field (radiofrequency pulse) of a specific frequency is applied at a right angle, the protons 'flip' out of the main external magnetic field.

As the protons 'relax' back to their original position, they emit a radiofrequency signal that can be digitally analysed and displayed as an image. This 'relaxation' time has two components, known as T1 and T2, which determine the magnetic resonance imaging (MRI) parameters of the different brain tissues. MRI is especially useful for looking at small detail of intracranial structures, especially in the posterior fossa and spinal column where the surrounding bone distorts the image on CT.

The paramagnetic agent gadolinium-labelled diethylene triamine penta-acetic acid (DTPA, or pentetic acid) is used as contrast agent. Modification of the field conditions can also produce good-quality images of the cervical or cerebral blood vessels (either arterial or venous). This is called magnetic resonance angiography or venography, respectively.

Despite the better resolution of MRI, CT is faster and has greater clinical availability, and is often better at examining fresh blood and bony structures.

Myelography

This procedure has now been largely supplanted by spinal MRI and reserved for patients in whom MRI is contraindicated.

Catheter arteriography

Serial cranial radiographs are taken after the injection of an iodine-containing contrast agent into a large artery (aorta, carotid, vertebral) to allow the identification of cerebral vessels. Simultaneous digital subtraction of the surrounding soft tissues and bony structures allows the use of more-dilute contrast and a shorter procedure time, although the spatial resolution of the images will be compromised.

The indications for traditional arteriography are:

- Detailed evaluation of aneurysms and arteriovenous malformations.
- Interventional angiography: therapeutic embolization of aneurysms and vascular malformations.
- Diagnosis of cerebral vasculitis and other rare angiopathies.
- Assessment of cerebral vessel anatomy and tumour blood supply before neurosurgery.

Duplex ultrasonography

Duplex ultrasonography offers a combination of real-time and Doppler-flow ultrasound scanning, allowing a noninvasive assessment of extracranial arteries. It is particularly helpful as a screening test for lesions at the carotid bifurcation, which avoids the need for angiography in many patients. The quality of this technique is dependent on the experience and skill of the operator.

LUMBAR PUNCTURE

Lumbar puncture is an important neurological investigation to aid in the diagnosis of infective, inflammatory and malignant CNS conditions, and in the diagnosis of subarachnoid haemorrhage. It also enables the measurement of intracranial pressure and can be used to administer intrathecal medications. It involves inserting a needle into the subarachnoid space in the lumbar intervertebral space, to obtain CSF (Fig 3.3). It is usually performed with the patient in the lateral position, which enables CSF opening pressure to be measured. It is carried out under sterile conditions, and the needle is inserted usually into the L3/4 interspace, which can be identified by the line connecting the highest point of the anterior iliac crests. CSF opening pressure can then be measured using a manometer. The normal CSF opening pressure ranges from 5 to 25 cm CSF. See Chapter 30 on Vascular diseases of the nervous system, Chapter 32 on Infections of the nervous system and Chapter 33 on Multiple sclerosis for relevant CSF investigations. The complications include infection, pain, bleeding and more commonly a postural headache (worse on sitting and standing and improved by lying flat), which can be treated by increased fluid and caffeine intake.

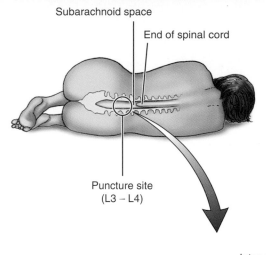

Subarachnoid space

End of spinal cord

Puncture site
(L3 – L4)

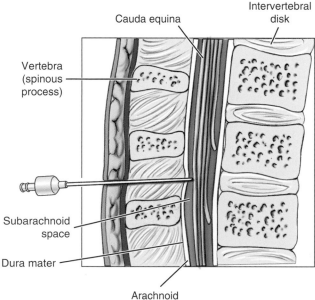

Cauda equina

Intervertebral
disk

Vertebra
(spinous
process)

Subarachnoid
space

Dura mater

Arachnoid

Fig. 3.3 Lumbar puncture. The patient lies on their side and the needle is typically inserted between the third and fourth (or fourth and fifth) lumbar vertebrae. Performing a lumbar puncture below the L3 level avoids injury to the spinal cord. (From Shiland B. *Medical Assistant: Nervous System, Law and Ethics, Psychology and Therapeutic Procedures—Module G*. 2nd ed. Elsevier Inc.; 2016.)

● Chapter Summary

- Analysis of cerebral spinal fluid can be very useful in the diagnosis of a number of neurological conditions including infective (viral/bacterial meningitis), inflammatory (Guillain-Barré syndrome) and malignancy (central nervous system lymphoma/paraneoplastic).
- Nerve conduction studies/electromyography can be used to investigate nerve, muscle and neuromuscular junction function. Electroencephalography can be used to investigate epilepsy and comatose states.
- MRI is usually the neuroimaging study of choice for visualizing the brain and spinal cord, as no ionizing radiation is used and image resolution is superior to CT especially around bony structures.

UKMLA Presentation
Fasciculations

The Patient Presents With

Neurological emergencies

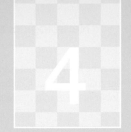

ACUTE ISCHAEMIC STROKE

See Chapter 30 for further information on stroke. The management of acute ischaemic stroke happens in the setting of an acute stroke unit (Fig. 4.1). When paramedics review a patient with a suspected acute stroke, they will transfer the patient urgently to the closest acute stroke unit. If a patient presents to an emergency department with a possible acute stroke, it is critical that the stroke team is involved as an emergency to initiate the management needed. The key aspect of management of acute ischaemic stroke is ensuring when a patient meets the criteria for thrombolysis and/or thrombectomy, that these are administered quickly and safely. For this, the 'Time is Brain' principle is applied – the quicker these treatments are given, the higher the chance of rescuing and preventing further neuronal loss due to cerebral ischaemia. For this reason, for patients eligible for thrombolysis, a door-to-needle time of less than 30 minutes is imperative, which is the time from when a patient arrives at the emergency stroke unit until the time the intravenous thrombolysis is administered.

Acute stroke management occurs as a multidisciplinary team, with stroke doctors and stroke nurses attending to the patient as an emergency, and with radiographers, radiologists and porters all involved in the acute pathway to ensure an urgent CT head and CT angiogram is obtained and reviewed. When the patient arrives at the stroke unit, a quick assessment of Airway, Breathing, Circulation, Disability and Exposure is needed. A brief history is taken, this may have already been obtained by the paramedics, and often a collateral history from a family member will be needed to establish time of onset of the stroke symptoms, especially if the patient is dysphasic. Any history of major comorbidities, including possible contraindications to thrombolysis, such as major recent surgery and previous intracranial haemorrhage, should also be obtained. A medication history, especially whether the patient is on any anticoagulation, should be checked. The doctor performs a rapid examination to assess the National Institutes of Health Stroke Scale score (NIHSS), which gives a score between 0 and 42 indicating the severity of any acute symptoms of stroke, including weakness, sensory loss, visual and sensory neglect, eye movements and speech. While this is happening, observations, an ECG and blood tests including a venous blood gas are obtained urgently and a large bore cannula is inserted. The patient is transported to the CT scanner, where a CT head and often a CT angiogram are obtained. This is rapidly reviewed by the stroke and radiology clinical teams, and if the findings are consistent with an acute ischaemic stroke and the patient meets criteria, intravenous thrombolysis can be administered. If the patient's blood pressure is severely elevated above the recommended range for thrombolysis, this needs to be reduced acutely with pharmacological treatment prior to administering thrombolysis.

After the thrombolysis, the patient must be closely monitored on an acute stroke unit, with regular neurological observations and review. There is a risk of cerebral haemorrhage post thrombolysis, therefore there is a low threshold to repeat any neuroimaging if there is a change in a patient's neurological symptoms or signs after the treatment. If the patient is eligible for mechanical thrombectomy, this is discussed with the local interventional neuroradiology team, and the patient will be closely reviewed on the acute stroke unit after thrombectomy.

SPONTANEOUS INTRACRANIAL HAEMORRHAGE

Also see Chapter 30 for further information on intracranial haemorrhage. The treatment of spontaneous intracranial haemorrhage in the first stages is similar to that for acute ischaemic stroke, as patients present with similar symptoms as they do for ischaemic stroke. Therefore, in the initial stages, the same pathway is followed as in Fig. 4.1; however, once a haemorrhage is diagnosed on the initial CT head scan, the patient will follow a different pathway. These patients are often also managed in acute stroke units.

Acutely, the patient with a spontaneous intracranial haemorrhage is managed by supportive care, with neurological observations including consciousness level with the Glasgow Coma Scale (GCS). If the patient is on any antiplatelets or anticoagulants these must be stopped. Anticoagulants should be reversed if possible. Hypertension must be closely and strictly managed to reduce the chance of an increase in the size of the haemorrhage and a worse clinical outcome. If a patient has a change in neurology, with a reduction in GCS or new focal neurology, then urgent repeat imaging must be obtained to assess for extension of the haemorrhage and cerebral oedema. It is important to seek an urgent neurosurgical opinion for all intracranial haemorrhages, as depending on the clinical assessment and neuroimaging findings, further neurosurgical intervention may be needed with clot evacuation, decompression and/or shunt insertion to relieve raised intracranial pressure. Assessing the underlying cause is also important to aid management and prevention of future haemorrhages, and possible causes may be hypertension, ruptured intracranial aneurysms and vascular malformations. Cerebral amyloid angiopathy causes superficial, lobar haematomas in older patients.

SUBARACHNOID HAEMORRHAGE

Also see Chapter 30 for further information on subarachnoid haemorrhage. As with all emergency care, an assessment of Airway, Breathing, Circulation, Disability and Exposure is required. Immediate investigations include an ECG, blood tests including clotting and a group and save, and once the patient is stabilized and a cannula is inserted, an urgent CT head is needed. If this shows evidence of subarachnoid haemorrhage, immediate management is centred on supportive care with regular neurological observations, bedrest and fluid replacement, analgesia for headache and prevention of hypotension and hypertension. Neurosurgical input is required for further investigations and management. Patients are usually managed on a neurosurgical unit. A CT angiogram is

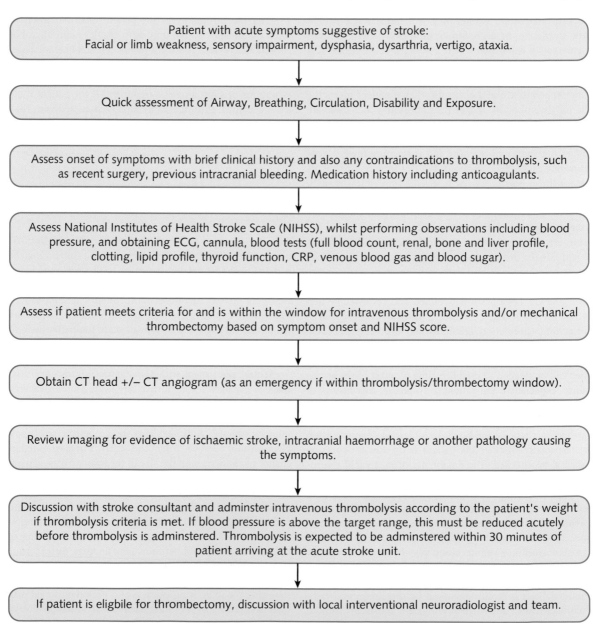

Fig. 4.1 Acute management of ischaemic stroke. CRP, *C-reactive protein*.

required, and sometimes digital subtraction angiography is also needed to establish the location of any aneurysms. Management of an aneurysm can be through clipping by neurosurgery, or endovascular coiling by interventional neuroradiology. Regular nimodipine (a calcium-channel blocker) should be started as this reduces the risk of delayed ischaemia secondary to vasospasm.

MENINGITIS

See Chapter 32 for further information on meningitis. The management plan starts with an assessment and stabilization of Airway, Breathing, Circulation, Disability and Exposure (Fig. 4.2). Immediate investigations to be performed are an ECG, CXR, blood tests including full blood count, C-reactive protein and blood cultures, a venous blood gas, a bacterial throat swab and an IV cannula must be inserted. A lumbar puncture should be performed immediately (within the first 30 minutes of presentation) if there are no contraindications. However in patients with signs of sepsis or a meningococcal rash, do not wait for a lumbar puncture and administer antibiotics immediately after blood cultures. The lumbar puncture should test for CSF opening pressure, MCS, glucose (and paired serum glucose), protein, viral PCR, TB culture and cytology. A CT head should be performed prior to lumbar puncture if there are focal neurological signs, papilloedema, seizures or

a reduced GCS, to exclude brain swelling which may predispose to cerebral herniation post lumbar puncture. Also perform a CT head in immunocompromised patients or those with a history of central neurological disease. If antibiotics have been administered, and if it is safe to do so, ensure the lumbar puncture is performed as soon as possible to enable the best chance of achieving a definitive diagnosis. The antibiotic choice for bacterial meningitis is the third-generation cephalosporins (IV ceftriaxone or cefotaxime), and IV amoxicillin or ampicillin should be used in addition in cases of suspected Listerial meningitis. If there is a suspicion of viral meningitis, IV aciclovir should be started in addition. An urgent discussion with microbiology should happen in complex cases, such as in a returning travelling, an immunocompromised patient, when tuberculosis is suspected, or after neurosurgery. The CSF results will then guide the ongoing treatment strategy with close liaison with microbiology. If patients develop complications from meningitis, management on Intensive Therapy Unit (ITU) may be required. Adjunctive dexamethasone should be started in all adult patients with suspected or proven pneumococcal meningitis (*Streptococcus pneumoniae*) and in those with tuberculous meningitis. For pneumococcal meningitis, this should only be continued if the CSF Gram stain reveals gram-positive diplococci, or if blood or CSF cultures are positive for *S. pneumoniae*. There is no evidence to recommend adjunctive dexamethasone in adults with meningitis caused by other bacterial pathogens.

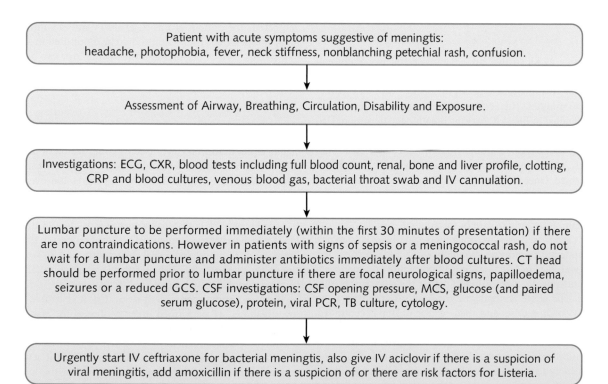

Fig. 4.2 Acute management of meningitis. CRP, *C-reactive protein;* CSF, *cerebrospinal fluid;* MCS, *microscopy, culture and sensitivities;* PCR, *polymerase chain reaction;* TB, *tuberculosis.*

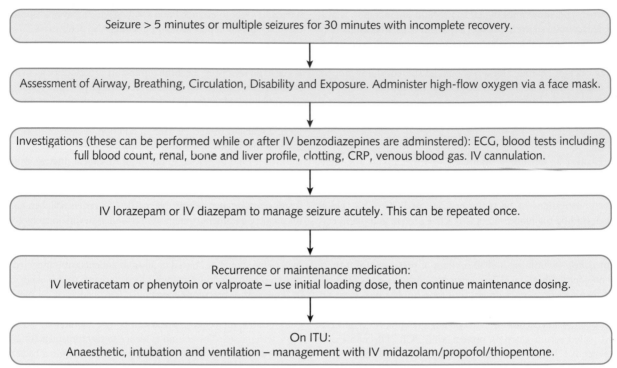

Fig. 4.3 Acute management of status epilepticus. CRP, *C-reactive protein*.

STATUS EPILEPTICUS

See Chapter 22 for further information on epilepsy. Status epilepticus is a seizure lasting longer than 5 minutes, necessitating emergency treatment, or a series of seizures without recovery lasting 30 minutes. The acute management in the hospital setting is detailed in Fig. 4.3. Airway, Breathing, Circulation, Disability and Exposure are assessed and breathing is stabilized with high-flow oxygen administered through a face mask. Subsequently, urgent blood tests are obtained and IV cannulation is performed. Once IV access is established, first-line treatment is with IV lorazepam or diazepam. If seizures are ongoing, a repeat dose can be given. In the out of hospital setting, buccal midazolam, rectal midazolam or intramuscular midazolam can also be used. If seizures are ongoing despite benzodiazepines, an antiepileptic medication should be given, and if seizures terminate with benzodiazepines, it is important to consider starting an antiepileptic medication to reduce the chance of further seizures. The acute antiepileptic medications are given as an initial IV loading dose, and then regular dosing is continued. The options are IV levetiracetam, phenytoin and valproate, and choice should be decided on an individual patient basis with consideration of each medication's side effect profile. If seizures continue despite this, the next step is an anaesthetic agent to be administered in an ITU setting, with the patient intubated and

ventilated. The options at this stage are IV midazolam, propofol or thiopentone. The patient should be monitored in an open bay, so that further seizures and their semiology can be documented closely, and further treatment instigated as needed.

CAUDA EQUINA SYNDROME

Cauda equina syndrome is caused by compression of the nerve roots which are caudal to the termination of the spinal cord. In most patients the onset is acute, with progression over hours or days. Patients may not have every single symptom of cauda equina syndrome. The symptoms and signs they may have include lower back pain, weakness or sensory loss in the lower limbs which may be asymmetrical, reduced reflexes in the lower limbs, bladder, bowel and sexual dysfunction, and loss of sensation in the perianal area. A digital rectal examination can reveal reduced perianal sensation and reduced anal tone.

If cauda equina syndrome is suspected, it is critical further investigations are performed urgently, due to the risk of permanent weakness, sensory loss and bladder, bowel and sexual dysfunction if treatment is delayed. A post-void bladder scan should be performed at the bedside to assess for a urinary residual. The patient requires an urgent MRI of the lumbosacral cord to assess for compression of the cauda equina from a herniated lumbar disc. Other possible causes are compression due to a tumour, trauma or an abscess. There should be urgent involvement of neurosurgery for further management, and spinal decompression may be needed.

NEUROMUSCULAR BULBAR/ RESPIRATORY CRISIS

Acute neuromuscular weakness causing bulbar and respiratory weakness can be caused by disorders of the nerve, muscle or neuromuscular junction. Common causes are Guillan–Barre syndrome and myasthenia gravis (see Chapters 27 and 28). These patients can progress rapidly. Other possible causes

are botulism and acute myelitis causing respiratory weakness. One of the most important bedside tests to perform in cases of suspected acute neuromuscular weakness is a forced vital capacity with spirometry. If this is below 20 mL/kg (around 1.5 L for the average adult), then this can indicate respiratory compromise and a high risk of respiratory arrest. Patients with acute neuromuscular weakness must have regular bedside spirometry, and if the forced vital capacity falls, ITU must be informed immediately, as these patients should be monitored in an ITU setting in case they require mechanical ventilation. By the time the pO_2 falls or the pCO_2 rises on an arterial blood gas, this is a late indicator of respiratory involvement. Further management is for the underlying neurological condition, which may include plasmapheresis and intravenous immunoglobulin.

● Chapter Summary

- Acute ischaemic stroke management is centred around a 'Time is Brain' approach, so that if a patient is eligible for the acute treatments of intravenous thrombolysis and thrombectomy, these are administered as quickly as possible, to prevent further cerebral ischaemia and neuronal death.
- Spontaneous intracranial haemorrhage is managed with supportive care, regular observations, strict management of hypertension and urgent neurosurgical involvement.
- Subarachnoid haemorrhage management involves supportive care with regular neurological observations, bedrest and fluid replacement, prevention of hypotension and hypertension and neurosurgical and interventional radiology input regarding clipping or coiling of an aneurysm.
- In cases of meningitis, it is critical to perform an urgent lumbar puncture, but administration of antibiotics must not be delayed for this.
- Management of status epilepticus involves step-wise escalation of pharmacological treatments for seizures.
- In suspected cauda equina, MRI imaging of the lumbosacral spine must be performed urgently, with neurosurgical input.
- In patients with acute neuromuscular bulbar and respiratory weakness, an urgent forced vital capacity is obtained, to help guide whether a patient will need ITU management with intubation and ventilation.

UKMLA Conditions
Epilepsy
Meningitis
Myasthenia gravis
Peripheral nerve injuries/palsies
Stroke
Subarachnoid haemorrhage

UKMLA Presentations
Altered sensation, numbness and tingling
Back pain
Facial weakness
Fits/seizures
Limb weakness
Urinary symptoms

Disturbances of consciousness

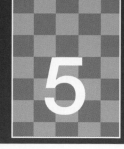

5

When consciousness is disturbed, patients usually exhibit an alteration in the awareness of their external environment. The ascending reticular activating system is a network of neurones originating in the brainstem that is modulated by external stimuli and projects to both cerebral cortices. The normal conscious state depends on the integrity of both the brainstem reticular activating system and the cerebral hemispheres. Impairment of consciousness clinically can range from either complete loss of awareness or 'unconsciousness' through varying degrees of impairment. The prodrome features during an event and the duration of impaired consciousness are also important in formulating a differential diagnosis. Impairment of consciousness can be transient with a return to normal function between attacks or ongoing, prolonged unconsciousness otherwise called 'coma'.

TRANSIENT LOSS OF CONSCIOUSNESS

Transient loss or disturbance of consciousness is a very common presenting problem. The patient usually has no ongoing symptoms or physical signs when seen, and subsequent investigations are often unhelpful in ascertaining the cause. The diagnosis depends on taking a careful history from the patient and from any available witness. The most common causes of transient loss of consciousness (TLoC) are (Table 5.1):

- syncope
- seizures
- psychogenic or 'nonepileptic' attacks

Uncommon causes include:

- hypoglycaemia
- narcolepsy/cataplexy
- hyperventilation
- vertebrobasilar ischaemia
- vertebrobasilar migraine

Syncope

Syncope is the TLoC and posture that results from a global reduction in blood flow to the brain. There are five common causes.

Table 5.1 Differentiating syncope from seizures

	Syncope	Seizures
Relationship to posture	Usually when standing	Unrelated
Prodrome	Hypotensive symptoms, e.g., light-headed/faint, blurred/dim vision, sounds seem distant, tinnitus, perception of weakness, nausea, hot/cold, sweating	None or symptoms of a focal seizure/aura, e.g., déjà vu, epigastric rising sensation, feeling of anxiety and fear, focal sensory symptoms, focal twitching
Skin colour	Pale	Blue or normal
Respiration	Shallow	Stertorous (noisy)
Tone	Floppy (may jerk)	Tonic–clonic in a generalized seizure
Convulsion	Rare	Common
Urinary incontinence	Rare (though it can occur)	Common
Tongue biting	Rare	Can occur
Recovery phase	Rapid. Usually no confusion. Pallor may persist	Often prolonged confusion is common and prominent
Focal neurological symptoms	No	Occasional
Clues to underlying aetiology	Situational, e.g., having blood taken. Cardiac arrhythmia. Aortic stenosis. Cardiomyopathy. Postural hypotension	History of known epileptic seizures. Structural lesion in brain, e.g., tumour. Severe head injury. Alcohol excess

Vasovagal syncope

Vasovagal syncope, or 'simple faint', is caused by a sudden drop in blood pressure resulting from peripheral vasodilatation. There is a subsequent reduction in cardiac output, which is followed by vagal stimulation and therefore bradycardia. Typical precipitating situations are strong emotion, sudden intense pain and prolonged standing in hot crowded situations (e.g., on a train).

The patient is usually upright or sitting up at the onset of syncope. Prodromal symptoms include feeling light-headed, gradual dimming of vision, ringing in the ears, salivation, sweating, nausea and sometimes vomiting. These symptoms can last from several seconds to a few minutes. The attack can be aborted if the patient lies flat, but a patient who remains standing will lose consciousness and fall. The patient is usually pale and clammy, the pulse is low volume and slow and the systolic blood pressure drops to approximately 60 mm Hg. If this state persists for a sufficient time to cause cerebral hypoxia, the eyes may roll upwards and there may be brief myoclonic movements, which can be mistaken for a seizure. This typically occurs if the patient is kept standing by unwitting onlookers, which prevents a return of blood flow to the brain. Sphincter control is usually maintained and a typical postictal state is not seen, although malaise may persist.

Situational syncope – micturition and cough syncope

Micturition syncope usually occurs in men who get up during the night to pass urine. It results from a combination of vasodilatation (which occurs with emptying of the bladder), a degree of postural hypotension on standing and bradycardia. The LOC is sudden with a rapid recovery.

Sustained coughing can elevate the intrathoracic pressure sufficiently to impair the venous return to the heart. Increase of the cerebrospinal fluid pressure, reduction in pCO_2 and resultant vasoconstriction may also be contributory. Unconsciousness may also be associated with the Valsalva manoeuvre (exhalation against a closed glottis) and is seen in syncope following breath-holding attacks in children and strenuous activity (e.g., heavy lifting or laughing). The mechanism here is probably similar to cough syncope.

Postural hypotension

In a number of clinical conditions, the upright posture is accompanied by an uncompensated fall in blood pressure and therefore also cerebral blood flow. Postural hypotension can occur in:

- normal individuals, especially adolescents;
- drugs (e.g., antihypertensives);
- debilitating illness with prolonged recumbency;
- autonomic neuropathy (e.g., diabetes, Guillain–Barré syndrome);
- hypovolaemia (e.g., loss of blood, sepsis, hypoadrenalism);
- neurodegenerative diseases (e.g., Parkinson's disease, multisystem atrophy).

Syncope due to primary cardiac dysfunction

Syncope of direct cardiac origin is usually abrupt and without prodrome. The upright position is not a prerequisite. It is classically accompanied by marked pallor with a rapid return of colour as cardiac output is restored. Brief tonic or clonic movements and urinary incontinence may occur but recovery is usually rapid. The history, examination and further investigations including 24-hour electrocardiogram (ECG) monitoring and an echocardiogram will further support a cardiac cause. Causes include:

- cardiac arrhythmias (usually profound bradycardia or heart block);
- left ventricular outflow obstruction: aortic stenosis, hypertrophic obstructive cardiomyopathy;
- right ventricular outflow obstruction: pulmonary stenosis, pulmonary hypertension, pulmonary embolism;
- ventricular failure (e.g., acute anterior myocardial infarction, dilated cardiomyopathy).

Carotid sinus disease

The carotid sinus responds to stretch by sending signals to the medullary cardiac centre. This produces a reflex bradycardia or drop in blood pressure. If a patient with a hypersensitive sinus, e.g., atheromatous disease, turns their head rapidly when wearing a tight collar, or if the carotid sinuses are massaged, then the patient can become hypotensive and lose consciousness.

Seizures

The most common diagnostic problem is distinguishing a syncopal attack from a seizure. Certain clinical features aid the differentiation as illustrated in Table 5.1.

COMMUNICATION

It is important to have a witness account of an episode of loss or disturbed consciousness. The witness may have also videoed the event, which is even more useful. A correct history is usually vital to make a diagnosis. If the relative or friend who witnessed the event does not come to clinic with the patient, then they should be contacted.

The different types of seizures are dealt with in more detail in Chapter 22.

Hypoglycaemia

Prodromal symptoms of hypoglycaemia include feeling tremulous and sweaty, palpitations, confusion and may result in LOC. Seizures can occur as a secondary phenomenon, usually when the blood glucose (BM) is ≤3. Causes of hypoglycaemia include overtreatment of diabetes, liver failure and, more rarely, hypopituitarism, Addison disease and insulinomas. Hypoglycaemia does not occur in a healthy subject who has not eaten.

Narcolepsy/cataplexy

Narcolepsy is a disorder associated with excessive sleepiness and sleep attacks at inappropriate times. It can be associated with cataplexy (attacks of sudden reduction in muscle tone, lasting several seconds to minutes, usually precipitated by emotion or laughing), hallucinations on going to sleep (hypnogogic) and hallucinations on waking (hypnopompic). There may be a positive family history.

Hyperventilation

Overbreathing results in a reduction of pCO_2, cerebral vasoconstriction, metabolic alkalosis and a reduction in ionized calcium. Characteristic features are:

- breathlessness and air hunger with rapid respiration
- light-headedness
- perioral and digital paraesthesia
- carpopedal spasm
- anxiety and fatigue

The attacks may occur in particular situations due to phobic anxiety, commonly in crowds or sometimes after physical exertion. Hyperventilation rarely causes complete LOC.

Vertebrobasilar ischaemia

The brainstem reticular formation is supplied by the vertebrobasilar system and, if this is compromised, LOC might occur. Symptoms of brainstem origin, such as vertigo, nausea and diplopia are often associated, and cerebrovascular risk factors may be present.

COMMON PIFALLS

Loss of consciousness due to a transient ischaemic attack is extremely rare and is usually associated with focal symptoms of brainstem ischaemia. This should therefore be a diagnosis of exclusion.

Nonepileptic attacks

This is a diagnosis that is based on the exclusion of other causes and features suggestive of nonepileptiform events. Patients should be assessed by a specialist before being given this diagnosis.

Investigating transient loss of consciousness

In patients presenting with episodes of transient LOC, the diagnosis is made primarily from the history and an eyewitness account.

If a seizure is suspected, electroencephalography (EEG) can provide information about the presence of abnormal activity but it is not a diagnostic test, since even in the presence of epilepsy, the EEG can be normal between seizures. Imaging with computed tomography (CT) or magnetic resonance imaging (MRI) may help to identify structural causes of epilepsy.

If the history and examination are more suggestive of syncope, then a 12-lead, 24-hour ECG monitoring and echocardiogram need to be considered. If the attacks have a postural component, then tilt table testing should also be considered. Twenty-four-hour ECG monitoring may detect arrhythmias if they occur every day. For less frequent attacks, longer recordings or an internal REVEAL device may need to be implanted to detect infrequent, but clinically important, arrhythmias.

Often, investigations are normal in both conditions and the diagnosis is made by the history alone.

ETHICS

DRIVING AND EPISODES OF DISTURBANCES OF CONSCIOUSNESS

Below are the Driver and Vehicle Licensing Agency (DVLA) guidelines for loss of consciousness.

Episode	DVLA recommendations
Vasovagal faint	No restriction
Cardiovascular with identified cause	4 weeks' restriction
Cardiovascular with no identified cause	6 months
Positive seizure markers	6 months
Dissociative seizures	Controlled for 3 months

Patients are legally required to notify the DVLA after an episode of loss of consciousness or altered awareness. Driving restrictions are more severe for those with group 2 licenses.

COMA

Coma is a state of impaired consciousness in which the patient is not rousable despite external stimuli. Confusion, delirium, obtundation and stupor are terms describing progressive states between full alertness and coma (see Chapter 2). However, they are not clearly defined and therefore interobserver interpretation is highly variable. The Glasgow Coma Scale (Table 5.2) provides a more objective and reproducible method by which conscious level can be assessed and documented. It is based on eye opening and verbal and motor responses. A patient with a normal conscious state will score 15 out of a total score of 15.

Classification of coma

The severity of the coma can be stratified as follows.

Minimally conscious state

Patients can show limited but reproducible signs of awareness; such as word/few words speech or purposeful behaviour. Functional MRI studies show reduced overall cerebral metabolism in patients with minimally conscious state compared with fully conscious individuals, but increased medial parietal lobe and posterior cingulate cortex activity compared with more severe coma states.

Persistent vegetative state

Patients have lost cognitive neurological function and awareness of the environment but retain noncognitive function and a preserved sleep–wake cycle. Respiration and circulation remain relatively intact. Spontaneous movements may occur and the eyes may open in response to external stimuli, but the patient does not speak or obey commands. Patients may occasionally grimace, cry or laugh. This condition usually represents diffuse damage to the cerebral cortex but intact brainstem.

Permanent vegetative state

If patients remain in a vegetative state for more than 6 months if caused by a nontraumatic brain injury, or more than 12 months if caused by a traumatic brain injury, it is termed permanent vegetative state.

Table 5.2 Glasgow Coma Scale

Eye opening		
1	None	
2	In response to pain	Patient responds to pressure on fingernail bed – if this does not elicit a response, supraorbital and sternal rub may be used
3	In response to speech	Not to be confused with an awakening of a sleeping person
4	Spontaneous	
Verbal responses		
1	None	
2	Incomprehensible sounds	Moaning but no words
3	Inappropriate words	Random or exclamatory articulated speech, but no conversational exchange
4	Disorientated speech	Patient responds to questions coherently but there is some disorientation and confusion
5	Orientated speech	Patients respond coherently and appropriately to questions such as their name and age, where they are and what year/month/time it is
Motor responses		
1	None	
2	Extensor response to pain	Decerebrate response (see Fig. 5.2)
3	Flexor response to pain	Decorticate response (see Fig. 5.2)
4	Flexion/withdrawal to pain	Flexion of elbow, supination of forearm, flexion of wrist when supraorbital pressure is applied; pulls part of body away when nail bed pinched
5	Localization of painful stimulus	Purposeful movements towards a painful stimuli, e.g., hand crosses midline and gets above clavicle when supraorbital pressure applied
6	Obeys commands	

Differential diagnosis of coma

There are a number of conditions that may resemble coma but are not true coma. The most important is nonconvulsive status epilepticus, which is potentially reversible.

Nonconvulsive status epilepticus

Nonconvulsive status epilepticus should be suspected in patients who do not regain consciousness after convulsive status epilepticus. It can also occur spontaneously and should be suspected in any patient with ongoing confusion/disturbance of consciousness. An EEG usually confirms ongoing nonconvulsive epileptic activity.

Locked-in syndrome

Locked-in syndrome results from an extensive lesion of the ventral pons, e.g., in stroke, which interrupts the corticobulbar and corticospinal pathways, with sparing of the reticular pathways and therefore sparing of consciousness. Patients are alert but unable to speak or move their face or limbs. The pathways for eye movement are relatively spared, so patients can communicate with vertical eye movements and blinking. This carries a grave prognosis and requires ventilatory support.

Akinetic mutism

Akinetic mutism (e.g., in prion disease) is caused by damage to the prefrontal or premotor areas responsible for initiating movements. Patients have preserved awareness, and can follow with their eyes, but are unable to initiate movements or obey commands.

Catatonia

A catatonic patient is silent and there is no volitional motor or emotional response to external stimuli. The patient may resist an examiner's attempt to move, for example, a limb, and if the limb is moved, the patient may keep it fixed in this position for some time. This may be seen in catatonic depressive and schizophrenic states.

Causes of persistent disturbance of consciousness

The causes of persistent loss or disturbance of consciousness may be structural or nonstructural (Table 5.3). Alteration in awareness is caused by damage to the ascending reticular activating system in the brainstem or damage to the cerebral hemispheres. In the latter case the damage is typically bilateral, or if unilateral, is large enough to exert remote effects on the brainstem or other hemisphere.

Clinical approach to the comatose patient

The first step is to resuscitate via an A, B, C approach:

- Airway: establish and clear the airway.
- Breathing: ensure the patient is adequately ventilated with oxygen.
- Circulation: ensure there is cardiac output; otherwise begin external cardiac massage.

If there is respiratory or circulatory failure, this must be corrected and the potential causes investigated. Once a stable cardiorespiratory status has been established, a history should be taken from a relative, friend or eyewitness, and a clinical examination and initial investigations must be performed to ascertain the cause of coma. Check if the patient is being treated with any medications which may affect consciousness (such as opiates).

Examination of the comatose patient

Examine the patient for:

- signs of head injury
- neck stiffness (if no evidence of cervical spine injury)
- respiratory pattern
- pupil responses
- resting position of the eyes
- ocular movements
- fundoscopic abnormalities
- corneal reflexes and gag reflex
- limb posture, tone and spontaneous movements
- reflexes and plantar responses
- Glasgow Coma Scale
- clinical signs of seizure activity
- signs of rash

Signs of head injury

Lacerations and bruising may be present and occur over an underlying fracture. A basal skull fracture may present with a normal skull X-ray. It is important to look for evidence of an anterior fossa fracture such as rhinorrhoea, bilateral periorbital haematoma and subconjunctival haemorrhage. A fracture of the petrous bone may produce cerebrospinal fluid (CSF) or blood otorrhoea and be associated with a Battle sign (swelling and bruising over the mastoid process).

Neck stiffness

Resistance to passive neck flexion may be present in meningism, which can be seen in meningitis and subarachnoid haemorrhage.

Table 5.3 Common causes of persistent loss (coma) or disturbance of consciousness

Symmetrical and nonstructural	Symmetric and structural	Asymmetric and structural
Toxins	**Supratentorial**	**Supratentorial**
Alcohol Carbon monoxide Methanol Ethylene glycol Cyanide Mushrooms	Bilateral internal carotid occlusion Sagittal sinus thrombosis Thalamic haemorrhage/infarct Trauma–contusion Hydrocephalus	Unilateral hemispheric mass (tumour, abscess, subarachnoid/subdural/extradural bleed) with herniation Intracerebral bleed Pituitary apoplexy Massive supratentorial infarction Subarachnoid haemorrhage Multifocal leucoencephalopathy Acute disseminated encephalomyelitis
Drugs	**Infratentorial**	**Infratentorial**
Opiates Sedatives Barbiturates Lithium Anticholinergics Salicylate	Basilar occlusion Midline brainstem tumour Pontine haemorrhage Central pontine myelinolysis	Brainstem infarction Brainstem haemorrhage
Metabolic		
Hypoxia Hypercapnia Hypoglycaemia Hypernatraemia Hypothermia Hypothyroidism Hypopituitarism Adrenal crisis Thiamine deficiency (Wernicke encephalopathy) Liver failure Renal failure		
Infections		
Bacterial meningitis Viral encephalitis Sepsis Malaria		
Other		
Seizures or postictal state Diffuse ischaemia (e.g., myocardial infarction, heart failure, arrhythmias) Hypotension Hypertensive encephalopathy		

Respiratory pattern

- Cheyne–Stokes respiration: alternate hyper- and hypoventilation; seen in metabolic and iatrogenic (opiate) disturbances, impaired cardiac output, bilateral deep hemisphere lesions (thalamus or internal capsule) and brainstem dysfunction.
- Central neurogenic hyperventilation: lesions of the lower midbrain and upper pons.
- Apneustic respiration: pauses of 2 to 3 s occur after inspiration; seen in pontine lesions.

Pupil responses

- Pinpoint pupils: pontine lesions, opiates, parasympathomimetics.
- Bilateral fixed midposition: midbrain lesion, severe sedative drug overdose or hypothermia.

- Bilateral fixed and dilated pupil: significant brainstem damage or overdose of anticholinergics or sympathomimetics.
- Unilateral fixed and dilated (associated with ipsilateral third nerve palsy): supratentorial mass with uncal herniation, posterior communicating artery aneurysm or primary brainstem lesion.
- Enlarged, slowly reactive pupils: metabolic or toxic.

Resting position of the eyes

- Conjugate lateral deviation: large cerebral lesions produce eye deviation towards a lesion (contralateral to limb paralysis), whereas seizures produce eye deviation away from the lesion.
- Lateral and downward deviation: usually due to an ipsilateral third cranial nerve palsy (often associated with a fixed and dilated pupil).
- Inward deviation: usually due to an ipsilateral sixth cranial nerve lesion.
- Conjugate depression of eyes: midbrain lesion or compression.

Ocular movements

- Oculocephalic reflex (Fig. 5.1): seen in patients with an intact brainstem. On rotating the head to the left and right, the eyes will maintain their position by conjugate movement in the opposite direction. This is called the 'doll's eye' reflex.
- Oculovestibular reflex: pouring cold water into the ear, or 'caloric stimulation', causes deviation of the eyes towards the side irrigated (Fig. 5.1).
- Lesions of the midbrain or pons may result in absent reflexes or dysconjugate movements of the eyes.

Fundoscopic abnormalities

Look for papilloedema suggestive of raised intracranial pressure, and subhyaloid haemorrhage associated with subarachnoid haemorrhage.

Corneal reflexes and gag reflex

Corneal reflexes may be suppressed (no blink with corneal stimulation) in large, contralateral acute cerebral lesions and intrinsic brainstem lesions. Ensure the patient is not wearing contact lenses. Assess if the patient has a gag reflex, which can help differentiate between coma and brainstem death.

Limb posture, tone and movement

- Look for asymmetry of muscle tone, movement and reflexes, which may indicate a lesion in the contralateral cerebral hemisphere or within the brainstem.
- Decerebrate posturing: extension at the elbow, pronation and flexion at the wrist, extension at knee and ankle, plantar

flexed feet (Fig. 5.2). Classically associated with lesions at the level of the upper brainstem, but can occur in association with massive hemispheric lesions, or in the setting of metabolic coma.
- Decorticate posturing: arms flexed at the elbow and wrist, legs extended at the knee and ankle (Fig. 5.2). Classically associated with lesions at or above level of the diencephalon.

Clinical signs of seizure activity

Observe closely for any motor activity in the face, arms and legs, to assess for any subtle signs of clinical seizures.

Investigations in the comatose patient

Immediate investigations include:

- temperature (hypothermia)
- blood glucose
- electrolytes, calcium, urea and creatinine
- full blood count and coagulation screen
- arterial blood gases
- blood culture and toxicology
- ECG and chest X-ray

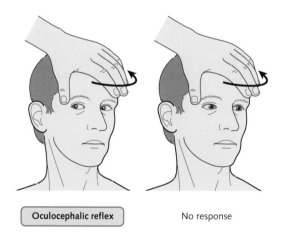

Oculocephalic reflex   No response

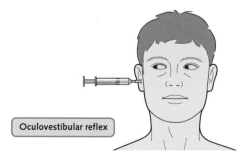

Oculovestibular reflex

Fig. 5.1 Oculocephalic and oculovestibular reflexes.

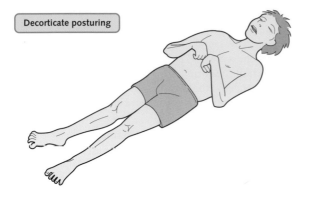

Decorticate posturing

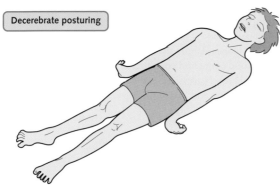

Decerebrate posturing

Fig. 5.2 Decerebrate and decorticate posturing.

Neurological investigations in selected cases include:

- brain imaging (CT or MRI)
- lumbar puncture for CSF examination
- EEG
- cerebral angiography

Prognosis of coma

In patients in whom a drug overdose or a reversible metabolic cause has caused coma and there has not been a prolonged period of unsupported cardiorespiratory failure, the prognosis can be excellent with appropriate critical care. Other causes have a poorer prognosis. In patients with a Glasgow Coma Scale score of 3 for more than 6 hours, there is a mortality rate of more than 50% and, of the remainder, only a small minority will return to independent existence.

HINTS AND TIPS

Two common causes of coma are head injury and postanoxic brain injury following cardiopulmonary resuscitation.

BRAINSTEM DEATH

Guidelines have been drawn up to diagnose brainstem death. Certain preconditions need to exist before testing can take place:

- The patient requires ventilatory support in the absence of depressant drugs.
- There is a known cause for the coma, capable of resulting in brainstem death.
- The patient's core temperature and any metabolic abnormality or effects of drugs must be normalized.
- The effects of any neuromuscular drugs must have worn off.

Specific clinical features on examination indicate brainstem death:

- Midposition, fully dilated, fixed and nonreactive pupils.
- Absent corneal reflexes.
- Absent oculocephalic and oculovestibular reflex.
- Absent gag reflex – no cough in response to pharyngeal or tracheal stimulation or suction.
- No grimace in response to facial pain (from firm supraorbital pressure).
- Absent ventilatory reflexes – no spontaneous respiration even when pCO_2 rises to >6.5 kPa.

It should be noted that the tendon reflexes might be intact because these occur at spinal level. There might also be limb posturing to painful stimuli in some cases. The examination should be repeated within 24 hours by a second experienced clinician to confirm that irreversible brainstem death has occurred. EEG is not a diagnostic investigation. It might show slight residual activity in some brain-dead subjects and, exceptionally, might be flat in reversible coma resulting from hypothermia, drug intoxication or recent cardiac arrest.

Chapter Summary

- Impairment of consciousness usually is either transient and self-resolves (e.g., in syncope or seizures) or persistent (e.g., in comatose states).
- Syncope and epilepsy are the most common causes of transient loss of consciousness. Although difficult, they can be differentiated by the clinical presentation, as investigations are usually unhelpful.
- Patients who present in a comatose state can be objectively assessed and monitored using scores such as the Glasgow Coma Scale.

UKMLA Condition
Epilepsy

UKMLA Presentations
Blackouts and faints
Confusion
Decreased/loss of consciousness
Driving advice
Fits/seizures
Head injury
Neck pain/stiffness
Sleep problems
Trauma

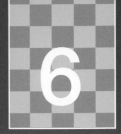

The term 'cognition' refers to our ability to perform complex intellectual behaviours such as attention, memory, communication, navigating our way around our environment and performing tasks.

Focal damage to the cerebral hemispheres usually results from vascular events (infarction or haemorrhage), tumours, trauma or localized inflammatory/infective lesions (e.g., abscess, tuberculoma). Generalized or multifocal cerebral dysfunction results from degenerative diseases (Alzheimer's disease, dementia with Lewy bodies), multiple infarcts, demyelination or diffuse infections (encephalitis, meningitis). For these reasons it is important to understand the basic functions of the different lobes and anatomical areas of the cerebral hemispheres. The left and right cerebral hemispheres each contain a frontal, parietal, temporal and occipital lobe (Fig. 6.1). The side of the brain that controls writing and speech is called the 'dominant' hemisphere and the other side is the 'nondominant' hemisphere. The left hemisphere is dominant in over 90% of right-handed people and in about 60% of left-handed people.

A summary of the symptoms arising from lesions to the major lobes of the brain is illustrated in Fig. 6.2.

FRONTAL LOBE

Normal functions

- Primary motor cortex: this is located in the precentral gyrus (see Fig 6.1) and is concerned with motor function of the opposite side of the body. The upper motor neurone cell bodies are topographically organized in the primary motor cortex in a 'homunculus' (Fig. 6.3). These neurones project axons in the corticospinal and corticobulbar tracts. The axons travel in the internal capsule to reach the brainstem and spinal cord to synapse with lower motor neurone cell bodies (see Chapter 15: Limb weakness).
- Supplementary motor and premotor cortices: these areas are concerned with coordinating and planning complex movements.
- Frontal eye field: this is involved in making conjugate eye movements to the contralateral side.
- Broca area (dominant hemisphere only): the motor or 'expressive' centre for the production of speech.
- Prefrontal cortex: the anterior and orbital parts of the frontal cortex govern personality, emotional expression, initiative and the ability to plan.

- Cortical micturition centre: this region lies in the paracentral lobule and is involved in the cortical inhibition of voiding of the bladder and bowel.

Blood supply

The blood supply to the frontal lobe is from the anterior cerebral artery (ACA) and middle cerebral artery (MCA). The ACA supplies the medial surface of the primary motor cortex, which controls the leg; the MCA supplies the lateral surface of the primary motor cortex, which controls the face and arm (see Chapter 27: Vascular diseases of the nervous system).

Symptoms from lesions of the frontal lobe

- Primary motor cortex: lesions here cause contralateral monoparesis or hemiparesis and facial weakness in an upper motor neurone pattern.
- Supplementary motor and premotor cortices: lesions here cause gait apraxia, which is the inability to walk normally despite preservation of normal power, coordination and sensory function, and no extrapyramidal dysfunction. The gait is slow and shuffling but upright and wide based, distinct from the flexed posture and narrow base of the Parkinsonian gait (see Chapter 16: Disorders of gait).
- Frontal eye field: lesions here (usually part of large MCA strokes) cause conjugate eye deviation. This is where both eyes look towards the side of the lesion and away from the side of weakness.
- Broca area: lesions here cause expressive dysphasia: nonfluent, hesitant speech with intact comprehension. The patient knows what he or she wants to say but has difficulty finding the correct words, often producing the wrong word. The ability to repeat words is better than spontaneous speech. Handwriting is also often poor.
- Prefrontal cortex: lesions here cause personality and behavioural change, including social disinhibition, loss of initiative and interest, inability to solve problems with loss of abstract thought and impaired concentration and attention without intellectual or memory decline. These symptoms usually occur with bilateral lesions resulting from head injury, small vessel disease, frontal degenerations (e.g., frontotemporal dementias) and acute hydrocephalus. Primitive (grasping, sucking, pouting, rooting and palmomental) reflexes may originate from the parietal

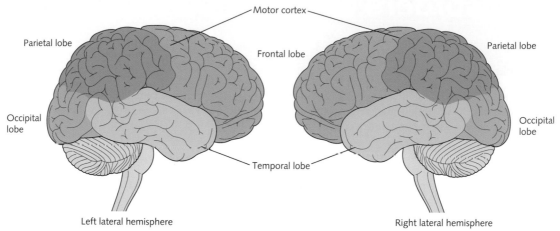

Fig. 6.1 Functional regions of the cerebral cortex.

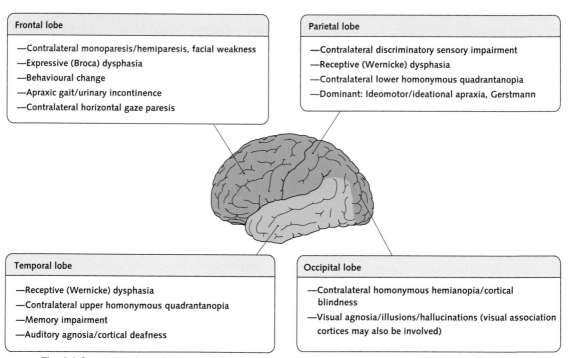

Frontal lobe

—Contralateral monoparesis/hemiparesis, facial weakness
—Expressive (Broca) dysphasia
—Behavioural change
—Apraxic gait/urinary incontinence
—Contralateral horizontal gaze paresis

Parietal lobe

—Contralateral discriminatory sensory impairment
—Receptive (Wernicke) dysphasia
—Contralateral lower homonymous quadrantanopia
—Dominant: Ideomotor/ideational apraxia, Gerstmann

Temporal lobe

—Receptive (Wernicke) dysphasia
—Contralateral upper homonymous quadrantanopia
—Memory impairment
—Auditory agnosia/cortical deafness

Occipital lobe

—Contralateral homonymous hemianopia/cortical blindness
—Visual agnosia/illusions/hallucinations (visual association cortices may also be involved)

Fig. 6.2 Summary of localization of symptoms arising from focal lesions of the cerebral hemispheres.

cortex but are usually inhibited by the prefrontal cortex, although the exact anatomical substrate is uncertain. They are essential in infancy and subsequently suppressed as the child grows.

- Anosmia: lesions of the inferior or 'orbital' frontal lobes can be accompanied by disturbances of the olfactory pathway and optic nerves as a result of the close proximity of these pathways to the orbital surfaces of the lobes.

- Cortical micturition centre: lesions here cause incontinence of urine and/or faeces. There is no desire to micturate. Milder symptoms are frequency and urgency of micturition.

Patients with frontal lobe disease often have poor insight into their cognitive problems. It is vital that a relative is interviewed to obtain a full history.

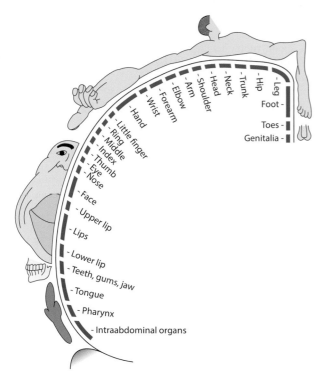

Fig. 6.3 Topographical distribution of the sensorimotor cortices or 'homunculus'.

HINTS AND TIPS

In Broca dysphasia, there is nonfluent speech but intact comprehension. In Wernicke dysphasia, there is fluent speech with errors but impaired comprehension.

PARIETAL LOBE

Function

- Primary somatosensory cortex: this is located in the postcentral gyrus and is concerned with perceiving complex somatosensory stimuli from the contralateral side of the face and body. It receives afferent (incoming) projections via the thalamus from the somatosensory pathways. The fibres are represented topographically, in a homunculus, similar to that of the primary motor cortex.
- Visual pathways: the upper part of the optic radiation (subserving the lower quadrant of the contralateral visual field) passes deep within the parietal lobe and might be affected in lesions of the deep white matter.

Dominant

- Language: pathways within the arcuate fasciculus connecting Broca area (frontal) with Wernicke area (posterior temporal) pass through the inferior parietal region.
- Calculation.

Nondominant

- Integration of somatosensory, visual and auditory information allows awareness of the body and its surroundings, appropriate movement of the body and constructional ability.

Blood supply

The blood supply to the parietal lobe is from the MCA.

Symptoms from lesions of the parietal lobe

- Primary somatosensory cortex: lesions here cause contralateral sensory loss. There is an inability to integrate sensory information, which manifests as impairment of joint position and two-point discrimination, an inability to recognize objects by form and texture, e.g., patient cannot recognize a key or coin in the hand with the eyes closed (astereognosis) or figures drawn on the hand (agraphaesthesia). Cortical damage alone (as opposed to deep hemispheric damage) does not impair the ability to be able to appreciate light touch, pain, temperature or vibration, but that information cannot be used to make sensory judgments.
- Visual pathways: lesions here cause a contralateral homonymous inferior quadrantanopia.

Dominant parietal lobe

- Language: lesions to the inferior parietal and superior temporal regions cause Wernicke receptive 'fluent' aphasia. There is impaired comprehension of speech and written language. The speech is fluent but words are replaced with partly correct words and an incorrect word related to the word intended (paraphasia) or newly created meaningless words (neologisms). The speech does not make sense and the patient has poor insight into the problem.
- Gerstmann syndrome: this consists of the inability to differentiate the right and left sides of the body, inability to distinguish the fingers of the hands (finger agnosia), and impairment of calculation (dyscalculia) and writing (dysgraphia). Difficulty with reading (dyslexia) may also occur; this is a function of the dominant parietooccipital cortex.

- Bilateral ideomotor and ideational apraxia: this is the inability to carry out a sequence of tasks when there is normal comprehension and intact motor and sensory function. Ideomotor apraxia occurs when a patient fails to mimic a meaningful or meaningless hand gesture by the examiner or cannot perform a movement to command such as sticking out their tongue, closing their eyes, whistling or pretending to brush their hair. Ideational or 'conceptual' apraxia is more profound and is due to disturbances in the temporal sequencing of motor actions, and a failure to understand the use of tools and objects at a basic level, e.g., squeezing toothpaste onto a toothbrush.

Nondominant parietal lobe

- Contralateral inattention: this is an inability to perceive a contralateral stimulus when two simultaneous sensory stimuli are applied with equal intensity to corresponding sites on opposite sides of the body. However, when the stimulus is applied unilaterally it is perceived. Inattention or neglect when severe can be motor, sensory, or visual. For example, a hemiplegic patient may ignore the paralysed side or there may be denial of the hemiplegia (anosognosia). Sensory and visual neglect are discussed in Chapter 16.
- Constructional apraxia (visuospatial dysfunction): there is difficulty in drawing simple objects (e.g., a house) and with construction (e.g., using building blocks). This also occurs to a lesser extent with dominant lesions.
- Topographical disorientation or topographagnosia: the patient cannot find his or her way around normally familiar spaces, e.g., the home.

TEMPORAL LOBE

Function

- Wernicke area (dominant hemisphere): this area, in the posterior part of the superior temporal gyrus, is concerned with comprehension of written and spoken language.
- Primary auditory cortex receives fibres arranged in order of tone frequency. The auditory pathways from each ear project to both auditory cortices. The dominant temporal lobe is important for the comprehension of spoken words, and the nondominant for the appreciation of sounds and music. Vestibular fibres terminate just posterior to the auditory cortex.
- Medial temporal lobe and limbic system: these areas are important in memory, learning and emotion. The olfactory and gustatory cortices lie in the medial temporal lobe.
- Visual pathways: the fibres of the lower part of the optic radiation (subserving the upper quadrant of the contralateral visual field) pass deep through the white matter of the temporal lobe.

Blood supply

The blood supply to the temporal lobe is from the posterior cerebral (medial part of the lobe) and middle cerebral (lateral part) arteries.

Symptoms from lesions of the temporal lobe

- Wernicke receptive dysphasia: associated with fluent speech but a loss of comprehension of speech.
- Visual pathways: a lesion involving the deeper fibres within the temporal lobe will cause a contralateral superior homonymous quadrantanopia (most commonly stroke or tumour).
- Medial temporal lobe and limbic system: lesions here involving the hippocampus and parahippocampal gyrus cause memory impairment (e.g., neurodegenerative conditions like Alzheimer's disease). Difficulty in learning verbal information occurs in dominant lesions and nonverbal information in nondominant lesions. Bilateral damage results in marked impairment of retention of new information. Emotional disturbances from damage to the limbic system can include aggression, rage, apathy, hyperorality and hypersexuality.
- Primary auditory cortex: lesions here cause auditory agnosia, i.e., the inability to recognize sounds, e.g., whistling of a kettle, a melody. It occurs in lesions of the nondominant hemisphere. Cortical deafness will occur only with bilateral lesions of the primary auditory cortices and is uncommon.

OCCIPITAL LOBE

Function

Primary visual cortex: this area receives input from the retina and is responsible for the perception and recognition of vision. It is closely related to a larger visual association cortex involving the inferior temporal cortex and posterior parietal cortex, which processes the information the primary visual cortex receives.

Blood supply

The blood supply is from the posterior cerebral artery but the occipital poles, subserving macular vision, have an additional supply from a branch of the MCA.

Symptoms from lesions of the occipital lobe

- Contralateral homonymous hemianopic field defect: this is caused by a lesion of the posterior cerebral artery. There will be sparing of the macular area leaving central vision intact with loss of peripheral vision.

- Cortical blindness: bilateral occipital lesions render the patient blind, with retention of the pupillary reflexes. The patient might deny the blindness (Anton syndrome).
- Visual agnosia: lesions of the visual association cortices cause impairment of perception or identification of faces and objects, even though visual acuity and fields are normal. Achromatopsia refers to an inability to distinguish different colours, whereas prosopagnosia refers to an inability to recognize human faces. A patient knows that they are looking at a face but cannot recognize who they are.
- Visual illusions: objects might appear larger (macropsia) or smaller (micropsia); there might be disturbances of shape, colour and number. This is more common with lesions of the nondominant hemisphere.

Chapter Summary

- There are four major lobes of the cerebral neocortex: frontal, temporal, parietal and occipital. Each lobe is responsible for specific functions and damage to the lobe is clinically characterized by how these functions are affected.
- Focal cortical dysfunction generally affects one or two lobes and common causes include stroke and tumour. Global cortical dysfunction will eventually affect the whole brain and is normally caused by a dementive process.

UKMLA Conditions
Dementias
Parkinson's disease

UKMLA Presentations
Anosmia
Behaviour/personality change
Memory loss
Speech and language problems

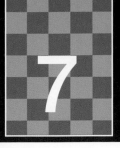

INCIDENCE

Headache is common and affects an estimated 40% of people in the United Kingdom at some point in their lives. Through absence days at work, headache is estimated to cost the economy £1.5 billion a year.

The most important role of the general physician is to determine whether the headache is primary (i.e., symptoms caused by the disease itself) or secondary (i.e., the headache is caused by another pathological process).

The most common primary headache syndrome is migraine. Although secondary headache can be caused by serious intracranial diseases such as a brain tumour and meningitis, the most common cause of secondary headache is systemic infection.

The diagnosis in these cases is made entirely from the history because there are few physical signs. The approach to assessing a patient with headache should be based on the temporal pattern of symptoms, especially the mode of onset and subsequent course (Fig. 7.1). This may be:

- Acute onset and progressive over hours;
- Subacute onset and progressive over days to weeks;
- New daily persistent headache;
- Recurrent and episodic with acute or subacute onset;
- Chronic and daily with fluctuations in severity over months or years.

HISTORY

A good history is essential to differentiate the type of headache. Determine:

- Age at onset (including childhood).
- Presence or absence of an aura and prodrome.
- Mode of onset: acute, subacute, chronic or recurrent and episodic.
- Site: unilateral or bilateral; frontal, temporal or occipital; radiation to neck, arm or shoulder.
- Character of pain: constant, throbbing, stabbing or dull ache; pressure-like; a tight band.
- Frequency and duration: constant or intermittent with pain lasting seconds, hours or days.
- Accompanying features: neck stiffness, autonomic symptoms (conjunctival injection, lacrimation, rhinorrhoea, nasal congestion, ptosis, pupillary changes, facial or eyelid swelling), aura-like symptoms (visual, motor, sensory or speech).
- Exacerbating factors: movement, light, noise, smell, coughing, sneezing, bending.
- Precipitating factors: alcohol (cluster headache, migraine), menstruation (migraine), stress (all headache types), postural change (high or low cerebrospinal fluid (CSF) volume headache), head injury (subdural haemorrhage or posttraumatic migraine).
- Particular time of onset: mornings (raised intracranial pressure, sleep apnoea syndrome) or awoken at night (cluster headache).
- Past history of headache and response to any previous treatment.
- Family history: migraine, intracranial haemorrhage.
- General health: systemic ill health, existing medical conditions, overweight (sleep apnoea), stress, low mood and depression.
- Drug history: analgesic overuse, the oral contraceptive pill, recreational drugs, anticoagulants, vasodilators, e.g., nitrates, nifedipine.

EXAMINATION

When examining a patient with headache, look for:

- Level of consciousness including Glasgow Coma Scale.
- Focal neurological signs including performing fundoscopy for papilloedema.
- Signs of local disease of the ears, eyes or sinuses; restriction of neck movements and pain; temporomandibular joint dysfunction; thickening of the superficial temporal arteries and an absence of pulsation; tenderness of the scalp and neck muscles.
- Signs of systemic disease, and if overweight measure the body mass index (for risk of sleep apnoea).
- Abnormal blood pressure.

HINTS AND TIPS

The clinical examination is often entirely normal in patients with headache. The history is therefore vital, especially with regard to migrainous symptoms and overuse of analgesics, particularly codeine.

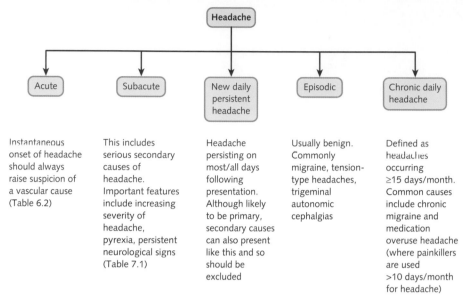

Fig. 7.1 Temporal organization of headache syndromes.

PRIMARY HEADACHE

Tension type headache

Primary tension type headache is usually featureless, although photophobia and aggravation with movement are common to a number of headache subtypes. It is increasingly recognized that patients who develop persistent daily headache actually have migraine mislabelled as a primary tension headache syndrome, often in the context of overuse of analgesics.

The patient often complains of a diffuse, 'bandlike', dull headache, which may be accompanied by scalp tenderness. The headache can last up to several hours and occurs either episodically or chronically. There are no abnormal physical signs.

True episodic (headache on <15 days per month) tension type headache should be managed with physical treatments (massage, relaxation therapy) and simple analgesics such as paracetamol, aspirin or other nonsteroidal antiinflammatory drugs (NSAIDs). When chronic (headache on >15 days per month), the only proven effective treatment is with amitriptyline. Chronic opiate and analgesic use should be avoided to prevent overuse headache.

Migraine

Migraine affects 15% of the UK adult population, affecting women more than men (3:1). Migraine is characterized by an episodic unilateral throbbing headache typically lasting up to 4 to 72 hours. The headache is often preceded by a visual aura with fortification spectra or flashing lights or, less commonly, a sensory aura with numbness and tingling in the fingers and/or face. Auras last between 5 and 60 minutes and may extend into the headache phase.

The patient often complains of photophobia, phonophobia and occasionally osmophobia, as well as nausea and sometimes vomiting. Patients with migraine often cannot bear to do anything apart from lying quietly in a dark room until their headache subsides. Exacerbation of pain by movement is a prominent feature of migraine. Patients may also have a history of motion sickness/sensitivity. Patients may also have autonomic symptoms associated with the headache.

Table 7.1 Common causes of subacute-onset headache

Cause	Clinical features
Intracranial tumour	Features associated with raised intracranial pressure – headache exacerbated by coughing, sneezing, bending over or straining; blurring of vision on bending over; papilloedema; associated nausea and vomiting; may be associated focal neurological symptoms and signs including seizures
Idiopathic intracranial hypertension	Most common in young, overweight women with hypertension. Features associated with raised intracranial pressure (as above) CT or MRI/MRV is normal
Meningitis/encephalitis	Fever, neck stiffness, positive Kernig sign, inflammatory (infective) CSF
Venous sinus thrombosis	Nausea, vomiting, drowsiness, seizures, focal signs; usually female gender, pregnancy and puerperium are risk factors
Subdural haematoma	History of head injury (falls in elderly and alcoholics), fluctuating level of consciousness, confusion, focal neurological signs
Intracranial abscess	Direct extension from local disease (e.g., frontal, sinusitis) or metastatic spread (e.g., lung abscess), fever, systemically unwell, focal neurological signs
Giant-cell arteritis	Patients usually older than 50 years of age Visual disturbance – acute monocular loss of vision – signs include papillitis with normal blind spot Associated polymyalgia rheumatica Elevated erythrocyte sedimentation rate and CRP Tender thickened superficial temporal artery ± absent pulsation
Acute hydrocephalus	Nausea, vomiting, diplopia (sixth nerve palsy – false localizing sign), fluctuating conscious level, papilloedema, diagnosis confirmed on CT head scan
Acute glaucoma	Pain typically frontal, orbital or ocular, accompanied by persisting visual impairment, fixed oval pupil and conjunctival injection This is an ophthalmological emergency
Posttraumatic headache	Posttraumatic headache syndromes include several subtypes, the most common being migrainous headaches
Low CSF volume/ pressure headache	Orthostatic headache occurs following lumbar puncture or a spontaneous or traumatic chronic leakage of CSF – headache better with recumbency

CRP, C-reactive protein; CSF, cerebrospinal fluid; CT, computed tomography; MRI, magnetic resonance imaging; MRI/V, magnetic resonance imaging/venography.

Table 7.2 Common causes of acute-onset headache

Cause	Clinical features
Subarachnoid haemorrhage	Explosive and instantaneous 'thunderclap' headache, neck stiffness, photophobia. CT head scan – subarachnoid blood (within 48 hours) CSF – xanthochromia (12 hours to 1 week) CT or formal angiography may show aneurysm, seizures and focal neurological signs if there has been intracerebral extension of blood
Haemorrhagic stroke	Note history of hypertension, stroke, smoking, diabetes, anticoagulation Focal neurological signs depending on site of bleed
Arterial dissection	This presents with head and neck pain; can be spontaneous or secondary to rapid deceleration or high/low-velocity rotation of the head and neck
Migraine	Migraine can present with an explosive 'thunderclap' headache; the diagnosis of a migrainous aetiology is one of exclusion
Coital/exertional headache	Can occur with an explosive onset before or during orgasm. At initial presentation this is a diagnosis of exclusion

CSF, Cerebrospinal fluid; CT, computed tomography.

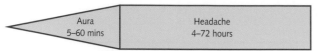

Fig. 7.2 Temporal nature of migraine.

Pathophysiology: The familial nature of migraine is very suggestive of a genetic component. Rare forms of migraine like familial hemiplegic migraine (below) are caused by specific mutations. The aura is thought to be caused by abnormal electrical activity within the cortex termed 'cortical spreading depression'. Surrounding large cerebral vessels are nerves arising from the trigeminal ganglion. Calcitonin gene-related peptide is released when the trigeminal ganglion is stimulated in a scenario such as migraine, likely causing the pain element.

There are various subdivisions of migraine, although migraine with aura (classical) and without aura (common) are the most frequently encountered forms (Fig. 7.2).

Basilar migraine

In basilar migraine, the brainstem aura causes symptoms that arise from dysfunction in the territory of the posterior cerebral circulation, which supplies the brainstem, cerebellum and most of the occipital cortices. The aura can consist of bilateral visual symptoms, ataxia, dysarthria, vertigo, limb paraesthesia and weakness. There may be loss of consciousness before, during or after the onset of headache, which often causes diagnostic confusion.

Hemiplegic migraine

Hemiplegic migraine is rare and causes additional one-sided limb weakness that can persist for days after the headache has settled. In some cases, there is an autosomal dominant transmission and in 50% of these, it is associated with defects in genes that encode calcium, sodium and potassium channels. Hemiplegic migraine must be differentiated from stroke or transient ischaemic attacks (TIAs). In a patient who presents for the first time with hemiplegia and headache, it must be initially assumed that the patient has had a stroke or TIA unless there is a family history of hemiplegic migraine.

Management

The patient needs to be reassured that there are no secondary causes of the headache, and that migraine is essentially an inherited tendency to headache caused by a patient's genes, that cannot be cured, but can be modified and controlled. The avoidance of any precipitating lifestyle factors (e.g., particular food types, stress, sleep deprivation, dehydration, too much sleep)

may be helpful. For patients using oral contraceptives/hormone replacement therapy and who have migraine with aura, there is an increased incidence of stroke. The risk is especially high in smokers with aura. In these patients the hormone treatment should be stopped, and in the case of contraceptives, an alternative contraception should be used.

During an attack

In the stepped model of migraine care, assuming there are no contraindications, patients use simple analgesia such as soluble aspirin 900 mg or paracetamol 1000 mg with antiemetics (e.g., domperidone) to allow ingestion of the other drugs. NSAIDs can also be useful, but adequate doses must be given. Gastrointestinal side effects such as dyspepsia may be limiting. Patients should avoid the regular use of codeine because of the risk of induction of a chronic 'analgesic' headache. More severe, or refractory, attacks may be terminated by the use of 5-HT agonists (sumatriptan, naratriptan, zolmitriptan, rizatriptan, eletriptan). There are now preparations that can be given subcutaneously or nasally that bypass the need for gastric absorption. They may have different rapidity and duration of action, which should dictate choice in individual patients. Ergotamine is still used for acute attacks, but relatively infrequently because of liability to side effects.

Prophylaxis

For frequent and severe attacks that occur more than four times per month, daily treatment for 6 months or more may be required to prevent headaches. Medications include:

- propranolol (beta-adrenergic receptor blocker)
- tricyclic agents, e.g., amitriptyline, dothiepin
- pizotifen (5-HT antagonist)
- topiramate or sodium valproate (anticonvulsants)
- candesartan (angiotensin II inhibitor)
- methysergide (5-HT antagonist): rarely used now because it can cause retroperitoneal fibrosis

Neurology centres may also provide procedures such as greater occipital nerve injections, botulinum toxin injections and calcitonin gene-related peptide monoclonal antibodies for refractory cases.

HINTS AND TIPS

In patients with 'medication overuse' headache, preventative medications are unlikely to be effective until the regular analgesic use has been curtailed.

Cluster headache

Cluster headache is a rare, primary headache syndrome with a prevalence of approximately 0.1%. It occurs more commonly in men (male:female is 6:1), with an onset in early middle life. Cluster headache is so called as the headaches that typically last for 6 to 12 weeks on a yearly basis, often at the same time each year.

Features of cluster headache comprise severe unilateral pain localized around the eye with ipsilateral autonomic features such as conjunctival injection, lacrimation, rhinorrhoea and sometimes a transient Horner syndrome. The headache and associated features last between 15 minutes and 3 hours. The onset of an attack typically has circadian periodicity, often being in the early hours of the morning, waking the patient from sleep. There may be migrainous features, but movement sensitivity is not typical and in fact patients with cluster headache often want to pace around, rather than lie still in bed. Patients with cluster headache should have brain neuroimaging as they can sometimes be associated with underlying pituitary pathology.

Treatment

Cluster headaches peak rapidly, and therefore the acute attack should be treated promptly.

Rapid treatment
- Inhalation of 100% oxygen at 10 to 15 L/min for 15 to 20 minutes.
- Sumatriptan injections or sumatriptan/zolmitriptan nasal sprays.

Preventative treatment
- Verapamil – regular electrocardiograms should be carried out as the drug is titrated to high doses (above 240 mg) and can cause bradycardia and heart block.
- Lithium – requires careful monitoring.
- Topiramate.
- Short course steroids (e.g., 60 mg of prednisolone tapering over 10–20 days) during a bout.
- Methysergide – for resistant cases and should be prescribed under hospital supervision because it can lead to retroperitoneal fibrosis.

In patients with medically intractable, chronic (a bout of attacks lasting 1 year with <1-month remission) cluster headaches, neuromodulation may have a role to play and include occipital nerve stimulation and deep brain stimulation.

OTHER NEUROLOGICAL CAUSES OF HEADACHE AND CRANIOFACIAL PAIN

Headache of raised intracranial pressure

The headache of raised intracranial pressure has certain characteristic features:

- There is a generalized ache.
- It is aggravated by bending, coughing or straining, which all raise intracranial pressure.
- It is worse in the morning or after prolonged recumbency.
- It may awaken the patient from sleep.
- The severity gradually progresses.

It is often accompanied by:

- vomiting;
- visual obscurations (transient loss of vision with sudden changes in intracranial pressure);
- progressive focal neurological signs;
- papilloedema, enlarged blind spots and decrement in visual acuity.

Investigation: Urgent imaging of the brain with computed tomography or magnetic resonance imaging is essential with venography, as a differential is a cerebral venous sinus thrombosis. Contrast may be required to visualize any lesions. See Chapter 31 for further management of intracranial masses.

COMMON PITFALLS

A worsening or a change in patients with a chronic primary headache disorder must be independently assessed because these patients can develop a new pathology causing secondary headache in addition to their original condition.

Low cerebrospinal fluid volume headache

This type of headache typically arises after a lumbar puncture. Patients report no pain while recumbent, but develop a headache when they sit or stand up. The headache may

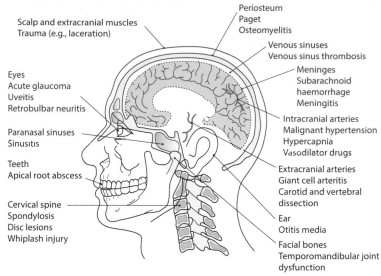

Fig. 7.3 The pain-sensitive structures in the head and neck, and disorders that may give rise to secondary headache.

worsen as the day progresses. Symptoms improve within minutes with recumbency and typically worsen again within minutes to an hour on standing or with vigorous Valsalva (e.g., straining or coughing). The underlying cause can also include an epidural or a spontaneous CSF leak. Magnetic resonance imaging of the brain with contrast may show diffuse meningeal enhancement. Treatment options include bed rest, intravenous caffeine or autologous blood patches around the lumbar puncture site.

Headache referred from facial structures

Pain in the head and neck may be referred from the ears, eyes, nasal passages, teeth, sinuses, facial bones and cervical spine (Fig. 7.3). It is conveyed predominantly by the trigeminal nerve (fifth cranial nerve), and also by the seventh, ninth and tenth cranial nerves, and the upper three cervical roots. Structures of the anterior and middle cranial fossa generally refer pain to the anterior two-thirds of the head through the branches of the trigeminal nerve and structures of the posterior fossa refer pain to the back of the head and neck via the upper cervical roots.

Other neurological causes of headache include:

- stroke, especially intracranial haemorrhage (see Chapter 30);
- meningitis (see Chapter 32);
- trigeminal and postherpetic neuralgia (see Chapter 9).

NONNEUROLOGICAL

Giant cell arteritis (temporal arteritis)

Giant cell arteritis is a granulomatous inflammation that usually affects the branches of the external carotid artery, including the superficial temporal artery, in those older than 60 years of age. The majority of patients experience pain over thickened, tender, often nonpulsatile, temporal arteries. The headache is accompanied by:

- A raised erythrocyte sedimentation rate (ESR): often highly elevated (60–100 mm/h).
- Visual loss (25% of untreated cases): amaurosis fugax (a TIA involving the retinal vessels) or permanent visual loss due to inflammation or occlusion of the posterior ciliary vessels. Once infarction has occurred in one eye, there is a severe risk that the second eye may also be affected without prompt treatment with steroids.
- Jaw claudication and scalp tenderness.
- Systemic features include proximal muscle pain in the form of polymyalgia rheumatica in up to 50% of cases, weight loss and fatigue.
- Rarer complications: brainstem ischaemia, cortical blindness, cranial nerve palsies, aortitis, involvement of coronary and mesenteric arteries.

Diagnosis

The diagnosis is made from the history and a raised ESR, and cases should be confirmed by a biopsy of the temporal artery or an ultrasound of the temporal and axillary arteries, or both. At least 1 cm of the artery needs to be excised as the disease process may be patchy and may be missed by smaller biopsy samples.

Treatment

Treatment is with high-dose corticosteroids (e.g., prednisolone 60 mg/day). There is a risk of blindness if treatment is delayed, and therefore the steroids should be started immediately and not be delayed until after the biopsy. The dose of steroids is gradually reduced as the ESR falls. It is usually possible to withdraw steroids slowly after several months to years.

Sleep apnoea syndrome

Patients with obstructive sleep apnoea (OSA) can have a headache on waking in the morning. Sleep apnoea headaches are associated with bilateral pain, short duration (<30 min) and a frequency greater than 15 days/month. The main risk factor for OSA is a high body mass index. OSA can be diagnosed by overnight pulse oximetry testing. In a number of patients nighttime continuous positive airway pressure can improve the headaches.

● Chapter Summary

- Headache is a very common neurological disorder. Although the clinical presentation can be extremely diverse, headache can be divided into temporal categories (acute, subacute, episodic, chronic daily) to aid diagnosis.
- There are a number of pain-sensitive structures in the head and neck, e.g., sinus, temporomandibular joint, that need to be excluded before primary headache is diagnosed.
- There is a set of important red flag symptoms to consider when investigating a new onset headache as their presence suggest potentially sinister causes, e.g., tumour, meningitis.

UKMLA Conditions
Migraine
Raised intracranial pressure
Tension headache
Trigeminal neuralgia
Vertigo

UKMLA Presentations
Acute and chronic pain management
Dizziness
Eye pain/discomfort
Facial pain
Headache

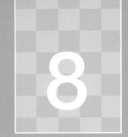

Alteration of the sense of smell is not a common presenting symptom and often not important in making a neurological diagnosis. Consequently, smell is not always tested during a routine clinical examination. However, anosmia, or the loss of sense of smell, is a significant problem after some head injuries and, rarely, it can be the only physical sign of a serious structural lesion involving the frontal lobes.

Odours enter the nose and sinuses where they stimulate olfactory receptors on cells of the nasal mucosa. These cells are bipolar neurones that have peripheral and central processes. The peripheral processes contain many cilia, which carry the olfactory receptors. The unmyelinated central processes enter into the cranial cavity through the cribriform plate of the ethmoid bone to synapse with dendrites of the mitral cells in the olfactory bulb. Axons from mitral cells, in the olfactory bulb, form the olfactory tract and run in the olfactory groove of the cribriform plate beneath the frontal lobes and above the optic nerve and chiasm. Some of these axons synapse within the anterior perforated substance but most continue into the brain and ultimately terminate in the primary olfactory cortex (in the anterior aspect of the parahippocampal gyrus and the uncus of the temporal lobe) and nuclei of the amygdaloid complex (Fig. 8.1).

DIFFERENTIAL DIAGNOSIS

Anosmia and hyposmia

Anosmia is loss of the sense of smell. Hyposmia is impairment of the sense of smell. Anosmia or hyposmia may be due to:

- inability of odours to reach the olfactory receptors (hypertrophy or oedema of the nasal mucosa);
- destruction of the receptor cells and their central connections;
- central lesions including neurodegeneration.

The patient will not notice unilaterally impaired olfaction. Olfaction tends to naturally deteriorate with age. The following causes should be considered:

- Upper respiratory tract infection: chronic rhinitis, sinusitis (allergic, vasomotor or infective).
- Heavy smoking causes metaplastic changes in the nasal epithelium.

- Viral infections, such as influenza, herpes simplex and SARS-CoV2 may cause permanent destruction of the receptor cells.
- Drugs, such as antibiotics, antihistamines and penicillamine.
- Local trauma to the olfactory epithelium.
- Head injury: unmyelinated fibres from the receptor cells are damaged along their vulnerable course through the cribriform plate, particularly if there is an associated fracture. If the dura is torn, there may be cerebrospinal fluid rhinorrhoea; this can be differentiated from mucous secretion by its higher glucose concentration. This is the most common neurological cause of anosmia.
- Tumours: meningioma of the dura in the olfactory groove may extend posteriorly to involve the optic nerve. Rarely, frontal lobe gliomas and pituitary tumours can cause anosmia.
- Aneurysm of the anterior cerebral or anterior communicating artery.
- Raised intracranial pressure: olfaction may be impaired without evidence of damage to the olfactory structures.
- Frontal lobe abscess.
- Degenerative disorders such as Alzheimer's disease and Parkinson's disease (PD) can be associated with anosmia. Anosmia usually predates the motor symptoms of PD by several years.

Ageusia and dysgeusia

Ageusia is the perception of loss of taste. Dysgeusia is the perception of an impaired sense of taste. Many patients with bilateral anosmia complain of loss or impairment of taste. This is because the appreciation of food and drink is by olfaction rather than by elemental taste. Taste itself is normal if tested formally in anosmic subjects.

Hyperosmia

Hyperosmia is an abnormally increased sensitivity to odours and may be seen in the following conditions:

- Anxious patients may complain of hypersensitivity to various odours.
- Migraine attacks with and without aura may be accompanied by hypersensitivity to light, sound and smell (osmophobia).

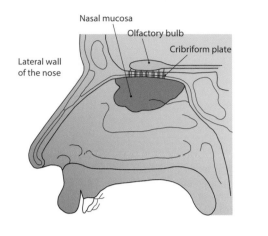
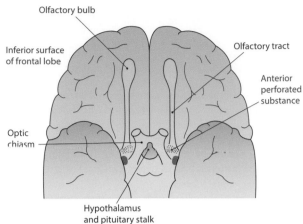

Fig. 8.1 The anatomical relations of the olfactory nerve.

Olfactory hallucinations

- Focal seizures of the temporal lobe origin can give rise to brief olfactory hallucinations, which are part of the aura.
- Olfactory hallucinations may occur following alcohol withdrawal.
- Olfactory hallucinations and delusions of unpleasant nature can be due to a psychotic illness, e.g., depression or schizophrenia.
- Hallucinations and delusions may also occur in patients with some forms of dementia.
- A persistent unpleasant smell may occur from local disease of the nasopharynx such as purulent sinusitis.

HINTS AND TIPS

DISORDERS OF SMELL

- Anosmia: The patient will only notice this if the impairment is bilateral. It is most often caused by disease of the nasopharynx and alterations of the nasal epithelium in smokers but head injury is the most common neurological cause.
- Ageusia/dysgeusia is an apparent alteration in taste perception in individuals with bilateral anosmia.
- Hyperosmia is a hypersensitivity to odours and is usually seen in anxious patients or migraine.
- Olfactory hallucinations may occur with temporal lobe seizures, following alcohol withdrawal, as a manifestation of psychosis or in patients with some dementias.

EXAMINATION

A stimulus for smell (e.g., peppermint, clove oil) is held under each nostril in turn while the other is occluded and the patient keeps the eyes closed. An individual with intact olfaction will be able to detect the smell and name it. The recommended special testing bottles are rarely available when needed and most clinicians perform preliminary assessment with nearby objects such as fruit, a coffee jar or cigarette packet. When examining patients with anosmia, it is important to look carefully for frontal lobe signs and evidence of optic nerve or chiasmal damage.

Pathology in the nasal passages or sinuses is a more common cause of anosmia than any neurological condition.

INVESTIGATIONS

Unexplained anosmia may require referral for more expert ear, nose and throat (ENT) examination if there is no suspicion of a neurological cause or obvious ENT cause.

If the patient has any evidence in the history or examination of frontal lobe or visual field defects in combination with anosmia, then it is appropriate to image the brain with computed tomography or magnetic resonance imaging to look for a structural lesion such as a tumour or abscess. Established posttraumatic anosmia requires no investigation unless there are also features to suggest a cerebrospinal fluid fistula or intracranial infection. The prognosis for a return of smell in posttraumatic patients is often poor, but late recovery can occur.

Chapter Summary

- The neurological pathway responsible for the sense of smell begins with olfactory receptors in the nasal mucosa and ends at the primary olfactory cortex.
- Reduced sense of smell can be caused by various pathologies affecting this neurological pathway, but the most common causes are peripheral.
- Rarely anosmia can be caused by serious pathologies such as tumour, e.g., meningioma.

UKMLA Presentations
Altered sensation, numbness and tingling
Anosmia

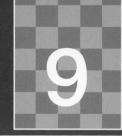
Facial sensory disturbance may result from disorders affecting the trigeminal (fifth cranial) nerve or its central connections within the brainstem, high cervical cord, thalamus, internal capsule and sensory cortex. Facial weakness may result from lesions involving the seventh cranial nerve and its central connections in the brainstem, internal capsule and motor cortex, as well as from disease of the neuromuscular junction (myasthenia) or of muscle (myopathies).

THE TRIGEMINAL NERVE

The trigeminal or fifth cranial nerve is the largest cranial nerve and is a mixed motor and sensory nerve. It arises from the lateral aspect of the pons and passes forwards across the subarachnoid space to form a large ganglion over the tip of the petrous bone where it divides into three parts:

1. Ophthalmic branch (V_1): this traverses the lateral wall of the cavernous sinus and enters the orbit through the superior orbital fissure. Its cutaneous distribution is shown in Fig. 9.1; it also supplies the cornea (supplying most of the afferent limb of the corneal reflex), mucosae of the nasal cavity and frontal sinuses, dura mater of the falx and the superior surface of the tentorium.
2. Maxillary branch (V_2): this traverses the lower lateral wall of the cavernous sinus and exits the skull in the foramen rotundum. It enters the floor of the orbit via the inferior orbital fissure. In addition to supplying the skin (see Fig. 9.1), it supplies the floor of the middle cranial fossa, the upper teeth and gums and the adjacent palate. It contributes secretomotor parasympathetic fibres to the lacrimal gland.
3. Mandibular branch (V_3): this carries the motor component of the nerve that supplies the muscles of mastication (chewing) including masseter and temporalis. It exits the skull via the foramen ovale. Its sensory supply is to the lower face (see Fig. 9.1), mucosa of the cheek, lower lip, jaw, incisor and canine teeth, floor of the mouth, lower gums and anterior two-thirds of the tongue.

The proximal axons of the somatic sensory Gasserian ganglion cells divide in the pons into short ascending and long descending branches. The short fibres carry light touch and deep pressure to the main sensory nucleus, and proprioception to the mesencephalic nucleus in the mid pons. The long descending fibres form the spinal trigeminal tract and carry information about pain and temperature. The nucleus of the spinal trigeminal tract extends from the junction of the pons and medulla to C2 of the spinal cord and fibres cross to the opposite side and ascend to the thalamus in the trigeminothalamic tract (see Fig. 2.3).

The motor nucleus of the fifth nerve is in the mid pons. The fibres from the motor root pass below the Gasserian ganglion to join the sensory fibres in the mandibular nerve (V_3) and innervate the muscles of mastication.

DIFFERENTIAL DIAGNOSIS OF FACIAL SENSORY LOSS

The wide anatomical distribution of the fifth nerve means that complete motor and sensory lesions of the fifth nerve are uncommon. The sensory component is mostly affected and the motor component is often spared.

On examination look for:

- Sensory deficit in the distribution of the three branches of the fifth nerve: loss of the corneal reflex is an early sign of damage to the ophthalmic branch. Lesions of the lower pons, medulla or upper cervical cord produce dissociated sensory loss of pain and temperature, with normal light touch, vibration and proprioception in a 'Balaclava' distribution (Fig. 9.2). As the lesion extends up the brainstem, the sensory deficit spreads towards the nose.
- Motor involvement: this may be manifested by weakness of the muscles of mastication and deviation of the jaw towards the side of the lesion because of weakness of the pterygoid muscles.
- The jaw jerk (a trigeminal pontine reflex): this is brisk in upper motor neurone lesions above the motor nucleus of the fifth nerve.
- A supranuclear lesion is contralateral to the facial sensory loss because the sensory fibres cross the midline after they synapse in the brainstem. Lesions at all other sites are therefore ipsilateral to the facial sensory loss.

Supranuclear lesions

These include lesions to the primary sensory cortex, internal capsule, thalamus and upper brainstem. There may be associated:

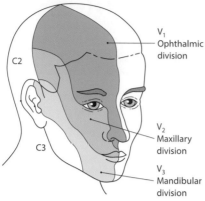

Fig. 9.1 The cutaneous distribution of the trigeminal nerve. Note that the upper cervical dermatomes (C2, C3) extend onto the face, above the angle of the jaw and onto the back of the head to the vertex.

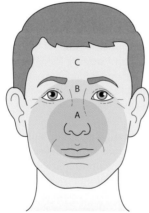

Fig. 9.2 (A) Low pontine, (B) medullary and (C) cervical lesions produce an 'onion skin' distribution of pin-prick (pain) and temperature loss due to lesions in the descending trigeminal tract and nucleus.

- contralateral 'pyramidal' weakness
- contralateral lower facial weakness (upper motor neurone)
- other cortical signs such as dysphasia, inattention, apraxia and hemianopia

  Causes:

- cerebral infarction/haemorrhage
- demyelination, e.g., multiple sclerosis
- neoplasms (glioma, metastatic deposits)

Brainstem lesions

These include lesions of the pons for all sensory modalities and the medulla/upper cervical cord for pain and temperature sensation only. There may be:

- contralateral 'pyramidal' weakness
- ipsilateral cranial nerve lesions in close proximity to the fifth nerve nuclei
- horizontal conjugate gaze palsies if the pons is involved
- lesions of the lower pons, medulla or upper cervical cord can produce dissociated sensory loss due to involvement of the descending trigeminal spinal tract and/or nucleus. There is ipsilateral loss of pain and temperature in an 'onion skin' distribution with preservation of light touch, vibration and proprioception

  Causes:

- infarction
- demyelination
- neoplasia (glioma, metastatic disease)
- syringobulbia and syringomyelia

Cerebellopontine angle lesions

Lesions at the cerebellopontine angle (CPA) are often associated with a disturbance in ipsilateral facial sensation and a reduced corneal reflex early in the disease before the onset of facial weakness. There may be:

- damage of the ipsilateral seventh and eighth cranial nerves with late involvement of the sixth, ninth and tenth nerves
- ipsilateral cerebellar signs in the limbs

  Causes:

- vestibular schwannoma (acoustic neuroma)
- meningioma
- metastatic deposits
- trigeminal neuroma
- arteriovenous malformation
- basilar artery aneurysm

Cavernous sinus lesions

Patients with pathology in the cavernous sinus may have signs of third, fourth and sixth cranial nerve palsies, as well as the ophthalmic branch, and occasionally the maxillary branch, of the fifth nerve (Fig. 9.3). Proptosis, eyelid and conjunctival oedema and papilloedema may be present if there is venous obstruction or a caroticocavernous fistula (also pulsating exophthalmos and orbital bruit).

Causes can be divided into several groups:
Vascular:

- aneurysm of the intracavernous portion of the internal carotid artery
- caroticocavernous fistula

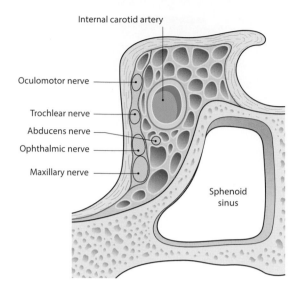

Internal carotid artery

Oculomotor nerve

Trochlear nerve

Abducens nerve

Ophthalmic nerve

Maxillary nerve

Sphenoid sinus

Fig. 9.3 A coronal section through the cavernous sinus.

- cavernous sinus thrombosis

  Inflammation:

- sarcoidosis
- meningitis (acute and chronic)

  Neoplasms:

- meningioma of sphenoid wing
- metastatic infiltration
- extension of a pituitary tumour

Lesions of the trigeminal root, ganglion and peripheral branches of the nerve

These lesions include:

- Skull fractures affecting the superficial branches of the trigeminal nerve (cutaneous deficit) or at the skull base (additional cranial nerve palsies).
- Herpes zoster: this manifests as a vesicular rash in the cutaneous distribution of the nerve (usually the ophthalmic division).
- Guillain–Barré syndrome and other peripheral neuropathies.
- Granulomatous disease: tuberculosis, sarcoidosis.
- Connective tissue disease: Sjögren syndrome, scleroderma and systemic lupus erythematosus.
- Neoplastic infiltration or compression: from tumours of the sinuses, cholesteatoma, fifth nerve neuroma, nasopharyngeal carcinoma at the skull base or lesion of the superior orbital fissure (third, fourth and sixth nerve palsies).

- Malignant and infective infiltration of the meninges affecting the skull base.
- Trigeminal neuralgia.
- Isolated trigeminal sensory neuropathy.

Trigeminal neuralgia

Trigeminal neuralgia typically presents with recurrent brief episodes of unilateral electric shock-like pain in the distribution of the trigeminal nerve. The pain is paroxysmal and comes on suddenly, lasting for seconds and up to a couple of minutes. Touching the face, chewing, brushing teeth and cold air can precipitate the pain. There may also be autonomic symptoms associated with the pain. Trigeminal neuralgia can be caused by vascular compression of the trigeminal nerve root, or brainstem lesions, such as in multiple sclerosis, affecting the trigeminal nerve pathways. Neuroimaging with MRI is performed to assess for vascular compression of the trigeminal nerve root. First-line management is medical, and carbamazepine is used as the first agent and is usually very effective. Other pharmacological options are oxcarbazepine, gabapentin or lamotrigine. Surgical options for the patient are refractory to medical treatment with vascular compression of the trigeminal nerve root and include microvascular decompression via a craniotomy, rhizotomy (a percutaneous surgical technique using fluoroscopic or computed tomographic guidance to lesion the trigeminal ganglion or root) or gamma knife radiosurgery.

FACIAL NERVE

Facial nerve anatomy

This can be divided into:

- brainstem – internal auditory meatus (IAM)
- geniculate ganglion – stylomastoid foramen
- extracranial

Brainstem – internal auditory meatus

- The seventh cranial nerve is composed of motor fibres, which innervate the muscles of facial expression, and the nervus intermedius, which carries taste fibres from the anterior two-thirds of the tongue, sensory fibres from the external auditory meatus and parasympathetic fibres to the salivary glands and stapedius.
- The motor nucleus of the facial nerve lies in the lateral pons and its intrapontine fibres hook around the nucleus of the sixth nerve (abducens) before exiting the pons at the CPA.
- The facial nerve enters the IAM with the nervus intermedius and the eighth nerve.

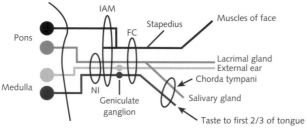

Fig. 9.4 The anatomy of the facial nerve and its branches. The chorda tympani supplies taste sensation to the anterior two-thirds of the tongue. FC, *Facial canal; IAM, internal auditory meatus; NI, nervus intermedius.*

Geniculate ganglion – stylomastoid foramen

- The eighth nerve subsequently dives deep within the petrous bone to the middle ear and the nervus intermedius and facial nerve enter the geniculate ganglion. This contains the cell bodies of taste fibres subserving the anterior two-thirds of the tongue.
- The greater petrosal nerve comes off the geniculate ganglion and carries parasympathetic fibres to the lacrimal gland.
- The seventh nerve then courses through the facial canal in the petrous temporal bone and gives off two important branches within the canal. The first is a small branch to the stapedius muscle, which is involved in controlling the sensitivity of the ossicles to sound. If it is damaged then sounds become louder (hyperacusis). The second branch is the chorda tympani, which subserves taste to the anterior two-thirds of the tongue as well as parasympathetic fibres to the submandibular and sublingual glands.

Extracranial

- The main facial nerve continues in the facial canal and leaves the skull through the stylomastoid foramen. It enters the parotid gland and divides into branches that supply the muscles of facial expression (Fig. 9.4).

Upper and lower motor neurone facial weakness

- The facial motor nucleus is supplied by upper motor neurones from both primary motor cortices, which travel in the corticobulbar pathway in the internal capsule to synapse on the lower motor neurones in the facial nerve nucleus in the pons.
- The lower facial muscles receive input from the contralateral hemisphere only, whereas the upper facial muscles receive input from both cortices. Consequently, a supranuclear (upper motor neurone) lesion will cause contralateral weakness of only the lower facial muscles, because the upper facial muscles remain innervated by the intact ipsilateral pathway. In contrast, a lower motor neurone lesion will

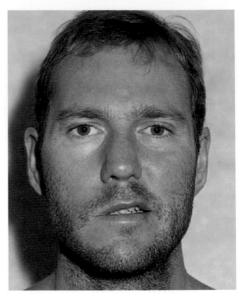

Fig. 9.5 Image of right-sided Bell's palsy. (From Swartz MH. *Textbook of Physical Diagnosis.* 5th ed. Philadelphia: WB Saunders; 2006.)

cause ipsilateral weakness involving both the upper and lower facial muscles.

Differential diagnosis of facial weakness

Facial weakness arises from a lesion anywhere from the motor cortex to the seventh cranial nerve and its distal connections (including the neuromuscular junction and muscle).

To differentiate the site of the lesion, the first step is to determine whether the weakness involves the upper and lower or only the lower part of the face, and then whether it involves one side or both. Lesions of the neuromuscular junction and muscle itself cause weakness of the upper and lower face as in a lower motor neurone lesion, but it is bilateral and usually symmetrical. A summary of the differential diagnosis of facial weakness is shown in Table 9.1.

COMMUNICATION

When a patient presents with unilateral lower motor neurone facial weakness it is important to ask about associated neurological symptoms such as loss of taste, perception of loud sounds and a dry eye. If these symptoms are absent, then be suspicious that the lesion may be distal to the facial canal, e.g., tumour within the parotid gland.

Table 9.1 Differential diagnosis of facial weakness

Syndrome	Clinical features and causes
Unilateral upper motor neurone facial weakness	**Unilateral weakness of the lower face** Unilateral weakness of the lower face is due to a contralateral supranuclear (upper motor neurone) lesion. It is usually caused by a contralateral stroke or tumour. Associated symptoms may include ipsilateral hemiparesis, hemisensory loss, hemineglect or hemianopia.
Unilateral lower motor neurone facial weakness	**Unilateral weakness of the upper and lower face** Unilateral weakness of the upper and lower face is due to disorder of the nucleus of the seventh nerve, the geniculate ganglion or the peripheral nerve; additional clinical features aid lesion localization; lesions may occur at the following sites: • Pons–ipsilateral sixth nerve lesion, contralateral 'pyramidal' weakness (recall that the intrapontine fibres hook around the nucleus of the sixth nerve), ipsilateral limb ataxia, facial numbness, gaze palsy to the side of the facial weakness, e.g., infarction, demyelination, tumour deposits • Cerebellopontine angle: ipsilateral facial sensory loss, loss of corneal reflex, ataxia and sensorineural hearing loss, e.g., cerebellopontine angle tumours • Facial canal–hyperacusis (denervation of nerve to stapedius) and loss of taste in the anterior two-thirds of the tongue (involvement of the chorda tympani), e.g., middle ear infection, Bell's palsy (Fig. 9.5), tumour deposits, fracture of the skull base, (carcinomatous) basal meningitis; lacrimation is often spared • Geniculate ganglion, e.g., herpes zoster infection of the ganglion; look for pain and vesicles in the auditory canal • Peripheral branches of the nerve, e.g., parotid gland lesions (tumour, infection), trauma • Facial mononeuropathy, e.g., small vessel disease (vasculitis), sarcoidosis, Behçet or Sjögren syndrome, syphilis, Lyme disease

Bilateral lower motor neurone facial weakness	**Bilateral weakness of the upper and lower face**
	If a patient presents with bilateral upper and lower facial weakness (i.e., bilateral lower motor neurone facial weakness), the following differential diagnoses should be borne in mind:
	• Guillain–Barré syndrome
	• Myasthenia gravis
	• Myopathies – dystrophia myotonica, rarer differentials include:
	  • Lyme disease
	  • sarcoidosis
	  • (carcinomatous) basal meningitis

● Chapter Summary

- The trigeminal nerve is the largest cranial nerve and composed of three branches: ophthalmic (V_1), maxillary (V_2) and mandibular (V_3).
- The trigeminal nerve can be compromised at any point in its pathway, from supranuclear lesions (e.g., primary sensory cortex) to peripheral nerve branches (shingles). The clinical findings (especially associated signs such as pyramidal weakness, other cranial nerve palsies) should point to the level of the lesion.
- The facial nerve is commonly affected and can present as unilateral lower face weakness (e.g., stroke), unilateral upper and lower face weakness (e.g., Bell's palsy) or bilateral face weakness (e.g., Guillain–Barré syndrome).

UKMLA Conditions
Acoustic neuroma
Bell's palsy
Trigeminal neuralgia

UKMLA Presentations
Altered sensation, numbness and tingling
Facial pain

Deafness, tinnitus, dizziness and vertigo 10

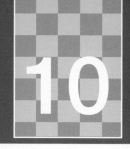

DEAFNESS AND TINNITUS

Deafness and tinnitus usually result from diseases of the cochlea and patients are generally seen by ear, nose and throat (ENT) surgeons. A vestibular schwannoma (previously referred to as an acoustic neuroma) is a rare but important 'neurological' cause of deafness, and the eighth (vestibulocochlear) cranial nerve may be involved in other conditions affecting the brainstem or multiple cranial nerves.

The eighth cranial nerve comprises the cochlear nerve, which subserves hearing, and the vestibular nerve, which is concerned with maintenance of balance (Fig. 10.1). Deafness and tinnitus arise from damage to the auditory apparatus and its central connections via the eighth nerve.

THE AUDITORY SYSTEM

Sound waves channelled through the external auditory meatus make the tympanic membrane and ossicles (malleus, incus and stapes) vibrate. These vibrations are received by the cochlea.

Cochlea

- The cochlea is a spiral tunnel containing a fluid called perilymph. Vibrations of the oval window are transmitted through the perilymph to the hair cells of the organ of Corti (which rests on the cochlear basement membrane; see Fig. 10.1).
- Hair cells have upward projections called stereocilia that are fixed to an immobile tectorial membrane. When the basement membrane vibrates, the stereocilia sway with the same frequency, and attached hair cell membrane changes structure. This causes ion channel opening and changes in membrane potential producing nerve impulses (Fig. 10.2).

Auditory pathway

- These nerve impulses travel in the cochlear nerve, which, together with the vestibular and facial nerves, passes through the internal auditory canal within the temporal bone to enter the posterior fossa. It then synapses in the cochlear nuclei in the lower pons.
- Fibres from the cochlear nuclei project to the superior olives bilaterally (important in sound localization) from where fibres ascend in the lateral lemniscus to the inferior colliculus (midbrain) on both sides (Fig. 10.3).

- These fibres project to the medial geniculate nucleus of the thalamus.
- Fibres then pass from the thalamus through the internal capsule to the auditory cortex in the superior temporal gyrus.
- The bilateral nature of the connections ensures that unilateral central lesions do not cause lateralized hearing loss.

DIFFERENTIAL DIAGNOSIS OF DEAFNESS

There are two types of deafness:

1. Conductive: there is failure of transmission of sound from the outer or middle ear to the cochlea.
2. Sensorineural: this is due to disease of the cochlea, cochlear nerve, cochlear nuclei and their supranuclear connections.

Clinically, conductive and sensorineural deafness can be distinguished by the Rinne and Weber tests.

Rinne test

The base of a vibrating 512 Hz tuning fork is held first against the mastoid process, and then, when the tone has disappeared, in front of the external auditory meatus. Normally the transmission of sound through the outer and middle ear to the cochlea is better than transmission through bone to the cochlea, which bypasses the middle ear apparatus. Thus, in normal ears, air conduction is better than bone conduction.

In conductive deafness, this ability is impaired due to disease of the outer or middle ear and bone conduction is better. In sensorineural deafness, there is impairment of sound perception whether transmitted through air or bone. However, with the latter, the sound may be transmitted through bone to the normal contralateral ear, giving a false positive result.

Weber test

When a vibrating tuning fork is placed in the middle of the forehead, sound is normally heard equally in both ears. In conductive deafness, the sound localizes to the affected ear (due to lack of competitive sounds that would normally be heard on that

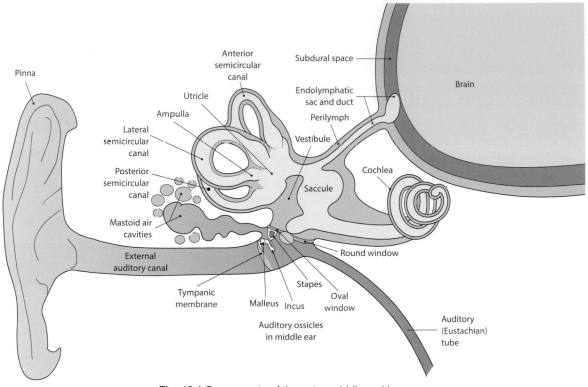

Fig. 10.1 Components of the outer, middle and inner ear.

side). By contrast, in sensorineural deafness, the sound lateralizes to the normal ear.

Conductive deafness

In conductive deafness, there is impaired perception, especially of low-pitched sounds.

Conductive deafness can be caused by:

- Disorders of the outer ear: the build-up of wax in the external auditory canal is the commonest cause.
- Disorders of the middle ear: otitis media, cholesteatoma, otosclerosis, rupture of the tympanic membrane.

Sensorineural deafness

In sensorineural deafness, there is often preferential impairment of perception of high-pitched sounds. Sensorineural deafness can be caused by a variety of disorders.

Disorders of the cochlear apparatus

- Congenital disorders: from rubella or syphilis in the pregnant mother.

- Infection: basal meningitis, spread of infection from the middle to the inner ear, mumps or measles.
- Medication: aminoglycosides, diuretics, salicylates, quinine (deafness is transient with the last two but can be permanent with aminoglycosides).
- Presbycusis: neuronal degeneration in the elderly causing high-frequency hearing loss.
- Noise-induced disorders: high-frequency hearing loss from, e.g., gun blasts or industrial machinery.
- Ménière's disease: vertigo, fluctuating tinnitus and deafness.
- Head injury: fractures through the base of the skull and petrous temporal bone can lead to damage to the cochlea and eighth nerve.

Disorders of the cochlear nerve

- Lesions of the cerebellopontine angle (CPA), e.g., vestibular schwannoma, other tumours, granulomatous disease, arteriovenous malformation, stroke (anterior inferior cerebellar artery).
- Lesions of the base of the skull, e.g., infective (meningitis), inflammatory (sarcoidosis), carcinomatous meningeal seeding such as nasopharyngeal carcinoma.

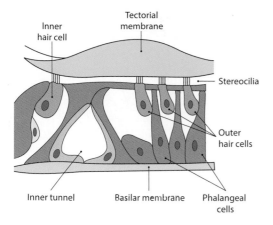

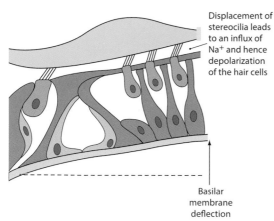

Fig. 10.2 Vibration of the organ of Corti causes bending of hair cell stereocilia, resulting in an oscillating depolarization/ hyperpolarization.

Disorders of the brainstem

- Multiple sclerosis: plaques of demyelination involving the cochlear nuclei
- Infarction
- Neoplastic infiltration

Disorders of the supranuclear connections

Unilateral lesions of the supranuclear pathways will not cause deafness as the cochlear nuclei on each side have bilateral connections projecting to the temporal cortices.

Investigations for deafness

Several audiometric procedures can distinguish deafness caused by cochlear lesions from those caused by lesions of the eighth nerve. Auditory evoked potentials test the integrity of the pathway from the cochlea to the auditory cortex in the temporal lobe; this does not need the cooperation of the patient (i.e., it can be done in a comatose patient).

Differential diagnosis of tinnitus

Tinnitus is the sensation of ringing, buzzing, hissing, chirping or whistling in the ear. It is a manifestation of disease of the middle ear, inner ear or cochlear component of the eighth nerve, and is usually accompanied by some degree of deafness. Conductive deafness is associated with low-pitched tinnitus, and sensorineural deafness with high-pitched tinnitus (except Ménière's disease, where the tinnitus is low-pitched). Vibratory mechanical noises in the head can be mistaken for tinnitus. The most common is a bruit from turbulent blood flow in the great vessels of the neck. This may occur as a result of high cardiac output (e.g., febrile or anaemic state) or mechanical obstruction within the lumen of an artery (e.g., arteriovenous malformation or carotid artery stenosis), when the noise heard is in time with the pulse.

THE VESTIBULAR SYSTEM

The sensory feedback from the vestibular, visual and proprioceptive systems is required to maintain balance. The labyrinthine–vestibular apparatus lies in each inner ear. It consists of the utricle, saccule and semicircular canals. There are three semicircular canals (lateral, anterior and posterior), each positioned perpendicularly with respect to one another (see Fig. 10.1). They respond to rotational acceleration of the head. The utricle and saccule respond to linear acceleration, including gravity.

Afferent information from the labyrinth is relayed by the vestibular component of eighth cranial nerve, the vestibular nerve. The vestibular and cochlear nerves follow the same route from the inner ear through the internal auditory meatus to the CPA before entering the brainstem at the lower pons. The vestibular fibres synapse in the four vestibular nuclei located at the junction of the pons and medulla. From here there are connections to the:

- Anterior horn cells of the spinal cord, via the vestibulospinal tract;
- Flocculonodular lobe of the cerebellum;
- Third, fourth and sixth ocular motor nuclei, via the medial longitudinal fasciculus;
- Pontine reticular formation;
- Temporal cortex.

Differential diagnosis of dizziness and vertigo

Dizziness is a very common symptom but is nonspecific. It can be used by patients to refer to vertigo but also to feelings of

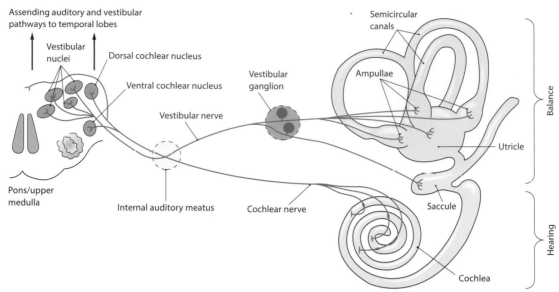

Fig. 10.3 The auditory and vestibular system.

faintness, disorientation, drowsiness, visual disturbance or even unsteadiness in the legs (imbalance).

It is important to separate all of these from the phenomenon of vertigo, which is best defined as an illusion of movement. This perceived movement may be described as to-and-fro, up-and-down or spinning, but often it has a swaying, rocking or heaving quality. It is often associated with nausea and vomiting. The patient might veer to one side when walking and the gait is more unsteady in the dark or with the eyes closed. Nystagmus usually accompanies vertigo. Vertigo may arise from a lesion of the labyrinth, vestibular nerve, CPA, brainstem, cerebellum or, rarely, the supranuclear connections (Table 10.1).

Examples of labyrinthine failure

Ménière's disease

Ménière's disease is characterized by recurrent attacks of vertigo, deafness, tinnitus and a feeling of pressure or fullness in the ears. It occurs in middle age and the vertigo is usually self-limiting. It is thought to arise from excessive accumulation of endolymphatic fluid and degeneration of the organ of Corti. Permanent deafness may occur after repeated attacks.

Benign paroxysmal positional vertigo

Benign paroxysmal positional vertigo arises from dislocation of particulate material from the otoliths, usually into the posterior semicircular canals. Sudden paroxysms of vertigo occur with movements of the head, particularly lying down, rolling over in bed, bending forward, straightening up and extending the neck. The vertigo lasts less than a minute and is fatigable with recurrent movements. The accompanying nystagmus is torsional and similarly fatigable. Symptoms may be present for several days or months at a time. Some cases follow head trauma or a viral infection of the labyrinth. The Hallpike manoeuvre (see later) can make the diagnosis and a similar manoeuvre can sometimes be therapeutic (Epley manoeuvre; Fig. 10.4).

Other causes

Other causes of labyrinthine dysfunction include purulent labyrinthitis following meningitis, motion sickness and toxic effects from alcohol, quinine and aminoglycosides.

Vestibular nerve lesions

The vestibular nerve may be damaged in the petrous temporal bone or the CPA. The latter is dealt with below. Trauma or infection of the petrous temporal bone may involve the seventh and fifth cranial nerves, as may occur with a herpes zoster infection of the nerve or ganglion. Purely vestibular dysfunction occurs in vestibular neuronitis.

Vestibular neuronitis

Vestibular neuronitis manifests as a single severe paroxysm of vertigo without deafness and tinnitus, usually in young or middle-aged adults. Symptoms usually subside within several days, but may persist for weeks. An inflammatory aetiology is presumptive rather than proven, but the condition frequently follows an upper respiratory tract infection, thus a viral cause has been postulated.

Table 10.1 Differential diagnosis of vertigo and dizziness

		Peripheral		Central	
	Labyrinthine failure	**Vestibular nerve lesion**	**Cerebellopontine angle lesion**	**Brainstem lesions**	**Cerebellar lesions**
Vertigo	Common short attacks which may be triggered or worsened by head movements	May be short or prolonged	Rare	May be prolonged	Brainstem connections involved
Nystagmus	Horizontal and/or rotary and suppressed with visual fixation	Horizontal and/or rotary and suppressed with visual fixation	Horizontal	Vertical/horizontal and may persist despite visual fixation	Horizontal and may persist despite visual fixation
Fast phase	Opposite to lesion	Opposite to lesion	Towards lesion	Towards lesion	Towards lesion
Gait	Veers towards lesion	Veers towards lesion	Ataxia towards lesion; hemiparetic	Hemiparetic	Ataxia towards lesion
Hearing	Conductive or sensorineural loss	Sensorineural loss	Sensorineural high-frequency loss early	Unaffected	Unaffected
Other neurological signs	May have positive Hallpike test	± 7th, 5th nerve lesions Ipsilateral cerebellar signs Contralateral 'pyramidal' signs	5th, 7th, 9th, 10th nerve lesions Contralateral 'pyramidal' weakness Ipsilateral ataxia	Ipsilateral cranial nerve palsies	Unilateral cerebellar signs from an ipsilateral cerebellar hemisphere lesion

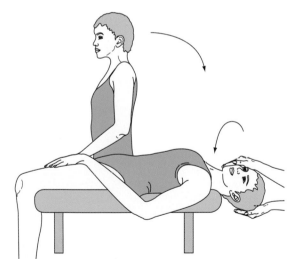

Fig. 10.4 Technique for exhibiting positional nystagmus (Hallpike manoeuvre).

Cerebellopontine angle lesions

The CPA is the junction between the pons and cerebellum where the seventh and eighth nerves exit the brainstem. Both brainstem and cranial nerve involvement occur. Causes to consider are vestibular schwannoma, other tumours, granulomatous disease and vascular lesions.

Brainstem lesions

Causes include infarction, demyelination, primary brainstem tumour or metastatic infiltration. Episodes of vertigo may arise from transient vertebrobasilar ischaemia, but it is rarely the only manifestation of brainstem transient ischaemic attacks.

Cerebellar lesions

Causes of cerebellar dysfunction are considered in Chapter 12.

Other types of dizziness

Patients use the word 'dizziness' to describe a wide range of symptoms such as light-headedness, a feeling of being on a ship and faintness. Other causes must be considered in the history and examination:

- anxiety with hyperventilation–'light-headed'
- anaemia
- postural hypotension: in the elderly, due to drugs, usually antihypertensives, or as part of an autonomic neuropathy
- cardiac: low-output cardiac failure and arrhythmias
- vasovagal presyncope/syncope
- iatrogenic: with or without hypotension

Investigations for vertigo

Hallpike manoeuvre

The Hallpike manoeuvre is performed with the patient sitting on a bed. The patient's head is positioned 30 degrees to the affected side and taken to 30 degrees below bed level. After a latent period of a few seconds, vertigo is experienced. There is accompanying torsional nystagmus beating towards the floor; the direction of vertigo and nystagmus are reversed on sitting up again. With peripheral (labyrinthine) lesions, symptoms and signs last for about 30 s and fatigues with repetition such that they cannot then be reproduced (see Fig. 10.4).

Caloric test

The caloric test is a test of vestibular function. With the patient lying supine, the head is raised 30 degrees from horizontal so that the horizontal canals are vertical. Each external meatus is irrigated for 30 s with water, first at 30°C, and then, about 5 minutes later, at 44°C. The normal response is summarized by the acronym 'COWS': *c*old water results in nystagmus, with the fast phase *o*pposite to the side irrigated; *w*arm water results in nystagmus, with the fast phase to the *s*ame side irrigated.

Two pieces of information can be obtained from the caloric test:

1. Canal paresis: there is no response to irrigation of the external meatus with either cold or warm water; this occurs in peripheral lesions, i.e., the labyrinth, or vestibular ganglion or nerve.
2. Directional preponderance: cold water in the left ear and warm in the right will both result in nystagmus to the right. If this response is greater than left-sided nystagmus produced by cold water in the right ear and warm in the left, a right directional preponderance exists. This usually implies a lesion of the brainstem vestibular nuclei on the left.

COMMON PITFALLS

When assessing a patient with vertigo, the main differentiation is whether there is a peripheral (labyrinth/vestibular nerve) or central (brainstem) cause. Central causes usually have associated neurological findings such as ataxia or other cranial nerve palsies, whereas peripheral causes usually have associated symptoms such as nausea.

● Chapter Summary

- Hearing (auditory) and balance (vestibular) are subserved by distinct systems. Auditory input is ultimately transmitted by the cochlear nerve and vestibular input by the vestibular nerve.
- Conductive and sensorineural hearing loss can be differentiated clinically by the Rinne and Weber test using a 512 Hz tuning fork.
- The cause of vertigo can be localized by assessing accompanying signs such as the nature and direction of nystagmus, presence/absence of hearing loss and direction of gait disturbance.

UKMLA Conditions
Acoustic neuroma
Ménière's disease

UKMLA Presentations
Dizziness
Unsteadiness
Vertigo

Dysarthria, dysphonia and dysphagia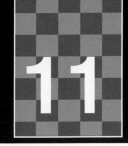

DEFINITIONS

- Dysarthria is a disorder of articulation of speech; there is no difficulty in comprehension or expression of language.
- Dysphonia is a disorder of vocalization, i.e., strength or quality of spoken words.
- Dysphagia is difficulty with swallowing.

Dysarthria, dysphonia and dysphagia may result from lesions at all levels from the motor cortex down to the numerous muscles involved in articulation, phonation and swallowing. The intervening pathways include the basal ganglia, cerebellum, brainstem, cranial nerves and the neuromuscular junctions (Fig. 11.1).

Non-neurological local pathology can account for these symptoms (e.g., dysarthria due to absence of dentures,

dysphagia due to oesophageal stricture, dysphonia due to lesions of the vocal cords).

DYSARTHRIA

Aulation involves the use of the respiratory musculature, larynx, pharynx, palate, tongue and lips. When a word is heard, signals from the primary auditory cortex are received by Wernicke area (comprehension of speech), from where the signal is transmitted to Broca area (expression of speech) and thence to the motor area of the precentral gyrus (primary motor cortex), which controls the speech muscles. The motor pathways for articulation arise from the left (dominant

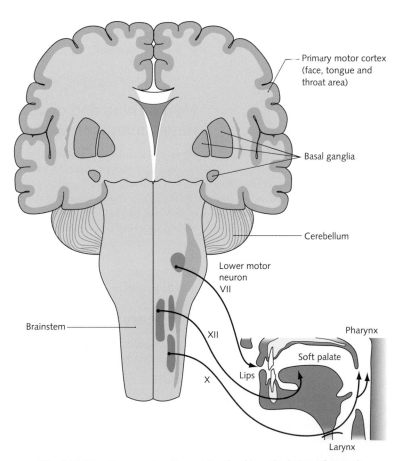

Fig. 11.1 Structures and pathways involved in articulation of speech.

81

hemisphere in most people) precentral gyrus and cross to the opposite motor cortex as well, then descend in both corticobulbar tracts to the nuclei of the seventh (motor fibres to the facial muscles, including those of the lips), tenth (nucleus ambiguus: motor fibres to the pharynx, larynx and soft palate) and twelfth (motor fibres to the tongue) cranial nerves and in the corticospinal tracts to the diaphragm and intercostal muscles. The nuclei of the seventh, tenth and twelfth cranial nerves receive corticobulbar fibres from both the ipsilateral and contralateral hemispheres. As with all movements, articulation is modulated by the cerebellum and by the basal ganglia (see Fig. 11.1).

Dysarthria can be caused by a lesion at any level in these pathways.

Upper motor neurone lesions

The muscles of articulation are bilaterally innervated and a unilateral lesion may be asymptomatic. A lesion may interrupt the corticobulbar tract at the level of the motor cortex, internal capsule, midbrain or pons before the fibres synapse in the cranial nerve nuclei with the lower motor neurones. Examination findings are discussed in Chapter 2. Causes of bilateral upper motor neurone lesions include:

- multiple sclerosis
- motor neurone disease
- bilateral subcortical ischaemic lesions/stroke
- rare neurodegenerative disorders, e.g., progressive supranuclear palsy
- central pontine myelinolysis

Lower motor neurone lesions

Lower motor neurone lesions result from damage to the motor nuclei of the seventh, tenth and twelfth cranial nerves, or their peripheral extensions (the corresponding cranial nerves) and give rise to a 'bulbar palsy'. Examination findings are discussed in Chapter 2. Causes of bilateral lower motor neurone lesions include:

- motor neurone disease
- Guillain–Barré syndrome
- medullary tumours
- syringobulbia
- subacute/chronic infective, inflammatory or malignant meningitis
- poliomyelitis

Basal ganglia lesions

Parkinson's disease

The speech in Parkinson's disease is often low volume and monotonous; it often trails off at the end of sentences. There

may be alternating acceleration and stuttering pauses in the speech analogous to the 'festinating' gait.

Chorea

The speech in chorea (e.g., Huntington's disease) is hyperkinetic. It is loud, harsh, intonation is variable and there is poor coordination of the diaphragm and respiratory muscles. This results in short, breathless sentences.

With the above syndromes, the diagnosis is often made by the accompanying characteristic movement abnormalities.

Cerebellar lesions

Cerebellar lesions cause ataxic dysarthria. The speech is slow and slurred with abnormally long pauses between syllables. This arises from impaired coordination of articulation, which is evident on attempted rapid side-to-side movements of the tongue. Other cerebellar signs are usually present. If there is also involvement of the corticobulbar tracts, the speech may be 'scanning', with words broken up into syllables, which are spoken with varying force.

Causes of cerebellar lesions include:

- multiple sclerosis
- vascular lesions, e.g., infarcts and haemorrhages
- alcoholic cerebellar degeneration
- tumours
- inherited ataxias, e.g., spinocerebellar ataxia

Myopathies and disorders of the neuromuscular junction

Myopathies and disorders of the neuromuscular junction give rise to a dysarthria similar to that of a bulbar palsy.

In a neuromuscular junction problem there may be evidence of fatigability, characterized by deterioration of the dysarthria at the end of the day and subsequent improvement the following morning (e.g., myasthenia gravis). If the patient has a myopathic dysarthria there may be a family history of a muscle disorder. There is often prominent wasting and weakness of the facial muscles, involvement of the proximal limbs and myotonia may be present (e.g., dystrophia myotonica).

Oropharyngeal lesions

Local lesions of the oropharynx can cause difficulty with articulation. Examples include:

- multiple mouth ulcers, e.g., following chemotherapy
- oral candidiasis
- quinsy
- dental abscess
- loose dentures

DYSPHAGIA

The descending motor pathways for swallowing closely follow those for articulation. Dysarthria is therefore often accompanied by dysphagia. Corticobulbar fibres travel bilaterally to the nuclei of both ninth and tenth cranial nerves. Motor fibres from the tenth nucleus (nucleus ambiguus) supply the soft palate and pharynx, which are required for swallowing. The adjacent ninth nucleus (also the nucleus ambiguus) sends motor fibres to the middle constrictor of the pharynx and stylopharyngeus but the ninth nerve is mostly involved in the sensory component of the swallowing reflex and supplies the sensation to the back of the tongue and oropharynx as part of the gag reflex.

HINTS AND TIPS

Dysfunction of the swallowing mechanism can be confirmed by videofluoroscopy, when a radio-opaque dye is swallowed and real-time radiographs are taken at each step of swallowing.

Sites of lesions causing dysphagia

Dysphagia can be caused by lesions of:

- both cerebral hemispheres (vascular, trauma, neurodegeneration, e.g., Alzheimer's disease)
- brainstem (multiple sclerosis, vascular, tumours, syringobulbia)
- cranial nerves (ninth and tenth, e.g., motor neurone disease, Guillain-Barré syndrome)
- neuromuscular junction (myasthenia)

- muscle (polymyositis)
- pharynx and oesophagus (local pathology)

DYSPHONIA

Dysphonia is alteration of the volume or quality of vocal sound. Phonation is a function of the larynx and the vocal cords. Sound is produced by air passing over the vocal cords. The pitch is altered by changes in tension of the membranous part of the vocal cords. This is performed by the intrinsic laryngeal muscles, which are supplied by the laryngeal branches of the tenth cranial nerve, which arise from the nucleus ambiguus in the medulla. Lesions in this pathway will cause dysphonia (the voice having a husky quality) or aphonia (the inability to produce any sound). There may be impairment of coughing, which requires normal vocal cord function. Paralysis or a local lesion of the vocal cord can be visualized by indirect laryngoscopy. The paralyzed cord fails to abduct and adduct during attempted phonation.

Causes of dysphonia include:

- Medullary lesions involving the nucleus ambiguus: infarction, tumour, demyelination.
- Recurrent laryngeal nerve palsy: following thyroid surgery, bronchial carcinoma, aortic aneurysm.
- Vocal cord lesions: polyps, tumour.
- Functional (psychogenic aphonia).

The proximity of the motor pathways controlling articulation, swallowing and phonation often leads to impairment of one or more of these functions at the same time (e.g., a patient with a bulbar palsy may present with dysarthria and nasal intonation, drooling due to difficulty swallowing and a hoarse voice with poor cough).

● Chapter Summary

- Dysarthria, dysphonia and dysphagia may result from lesions at all levels from the motor cortex down to the numerous muscles involved in articulation, phonation and swallowing. The intervening pathways include the basal ganglia, cerebellum, brainstem, cranial nerves and the neuromuscular junctions.
- Dysarthria is a disorder of the articulation of speech; dysphagia is a disorder of swallowing. The descending motor pathway is common to both and consequently both usually occur together. Dysphonia is a disorder of vocal sound quality; common causes include local vocal cord damage and recurrent laryngeal nerve palsy.

UKMLA Condition
Myasthenia gravis

UKMLA Presentations
Speech and language problems
Swallowing problems

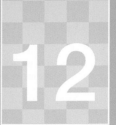
The cerebellum and its connections are responsible for the coordination of skilled voluntary movement, posture and gait.

The cerebellum can be divided into three functional units (Figs. 12.1 and 12.2):

1. The flocculonodular lobe (vestibulocerebellum) and inferior vermis, which are mainly involved in controlling information from the vestibular system.
2. The small anterior lobe and the anterior superior vermis (spinocerebellum), which are mainly involved in receiving proprioceptive information from the limbs.
3. The large posterior lobe and the middle part of the vermis (neocerebellum), which are mainly involved in receiving inputs from the contralateral cerebral cortex via pontine nuclei. They are involved in fine motor control, e.g., finger movements.

Efferent pathways pass from the cerebellum to the deep cerebellar and brainstem nuclei and enable coordination of skilled movements.

BLOOD SUPPLY

This is provided by three arteries: the superior cerebellar artery (SCA), which supplies the majority of the cerebellar cortex; the anterior inferior cerebellar artery (AICA) and the posterior inferior cerebellar artery (PICA).

CLINICAL FEATURES OF CEREBELLAR DYSFUNCTION

HINTS AND TIPS

Cerebellar dysfunction is characterized by:
- ataxia of limbs and gait
- dysarthria
- nystagmus
- dysdiadochokinesis (impaired rapid alternating movements)
- pendular reflexes and the rebound phenomenon may also be present (secondary to hypotonia)

Incoordination of movement

Cerebellar dysfunction causes impairment of the process of controlling movements once they have been initiated. This gives rise to ataxia (incoordination) as manifested by the following signs:

- Intention tremor: there is no tremor at rest. When the patient moves a limb towards a target a tremor develops, e.g., abnormal finger–nose test.
- Dysdiadochokinesia: the inability to carry out rapid alternating movements with regularity.

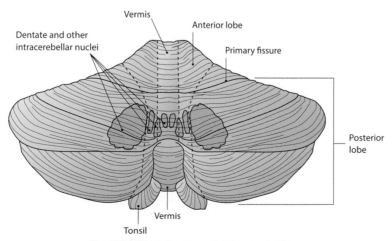

Vermis
Anterior lobe
Dentate and other intracerebellar nuclei
Primary fissure
Posterior lobe
Vermis
Tonsil

Fig. 12.1 Posterior aspect of the cerebellum.

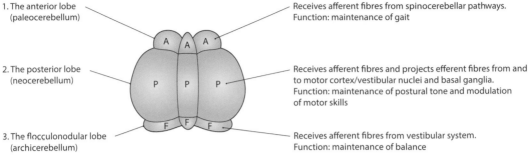

1. The anterior lobe (paleocerebellum) — Receives afferent fibres from spinocerebellar pathways. Function: maintenance of gait

2. The posterior lobe (neocerebellum) — Receives afferent fibres and projects efferent fibres from and to motor cortex/vestibular nuclei and basal ganglia. Function: maintenance of postural tone and modulation of motor skills

3. The flocculonodular lobe (archicerebellum) — Receives afferent fibres from vestibular system. Function: maintenance of balance

Fig. 12.2 The major phylogenetic subdivisions of the cerebellum.

- Dysmetria: the inability to control smooth and accurate targeted movements. The movements are jerky, with overshooting of the target as manifested in the finger–nose and heel–shin tests.

Ataxic gait

The patient walks with a staggering gait and may later develop a wide-based gait to improve stability. In mild cases, the unsteadiness may be apparent only when walking heel-to-toe (tandem walking). In a unilateral cerebellar hemisphere lesion, there is unsteadiness towards the side of the lesion. In truncal ataxia, there is difficulty sitting or standing without support.

Ataxic dysarthric speech

Speech can be slow, slurred and scanning in quality. In scanning speech, there is loss of variation of intonation and the words may be broken up into syllables.

Abnormal eye movements

- Jerky pursuits: pursuit movements are slow, with catch-up saccadic movements on attempting to maintain fixation on the moving target or 'saccadic intrusions'.
- Dysmetria of saccades: when trying to fixate on a target, the eyes overshoot and oscillate several times before fixation is achieved.
- Nystagmus: this is maximal on gaze towards the side of the lesion. Nystagmus results from damage of the vestibular connections of the cerebellum.

Hypotonia

Hypotonia is a relatively minor feature of cerebellar disease, resulting from depression of alpha and gamma motor neurone activity. Hypotonia can sometimes be demonstrated clinically by decreased resistance to passive movement (e.g., extension of a limb), by 'pendular' reflexes or by the rebound phenomenon. This occurs when the patient's outstretched arms are pressed down for a few seconds and then abruptly released by the examiner. The arms rebound upwards much further than would be expected in the presence of cerebellar hypotonia. When testing reflexes, e.g., patellar reflex, the activated leg may move to and fro (like a pendulum).

The causes of cerebellar dysfunction are listed in Table 12.1.

Titubation

Nodding tremor of the head may occur. This is mainly in the anterior-posterior plane.

Altered posture

A unilateral cerebellar lesion may cause the head and – when the lesion is recent and severe – the body to tilt towards the side of the lesion. Head tilt may also be due to a fourth nerve palsy.

LOCALIZATION OF A CEREBELLAR LESION

Cerebellar hemisphere

A lesion of the cerebellar hemisphere causes ataxia in the limbs ipsilateral to the lesion. The gait is ataxic, with a tendency to fall towards the affected side. There may be nystagmus maximal towards the side of the lesion and the speech may be slurred.

Cerebellar vermis

Lesions of the midline vermis cause truncal ataxia (imbalance of gait and stance) typically without the classic triad of limb ataxia, dysarthria and nystagmus.

Lesions of the flocculonodular lobe cause truncal ataxia, vertigo (damage to the vestibular reflex pathways), vomiting (involvement of the floor of the fourth ventricle) and nystagmus.

Space-occupying lesions at midline sites can cause early obstruction of the cerebral aqueduct in the midbrain or the fourth ventricle. This results in hydrocephalus with dilated third and lateral ventricles as well as headache, vomiting and eventually papilloedema.

Table 12.1 Causes of cerebellar dysfunction

Cause	Additional clinical characteristics
Tumours	Type of tumour – metastatic disease, meningioma, acoustic neuroma, medulloblastoma, haemangioblastoma, paraneoplastic syndrome with bronchial, ovarian, uterine carcinomas and lymphomas
Multiple sclerosis	See Chapter 33
Vascular Haemorrhage	History of hypertension, bleeding disorder, on anticoagulants
Infarction	History of hypertension, ischaemic heart disease, atrial fibrillation, diabetes, hyperlipidaemia
Infections Abscess	Systemic infection, fever, intravenous drug user or immunocompromised
Viral encephalitis	Notably chickenpox within 3 weeks of initial infection
Toxins Anticonvulsants	Especially with long-term phenytoin use
Alcohol	Acute intoxication; history of chronic abuse, signs of alcoholic liver disease
Metabolic Myxoedema Vitamin deficiency (B_1, B_{12}, E)	Myxoedematous facies, increased weight, cold intolerance, bradycardia (see Chapter 34)
Trauma	Head injury
Neurodegenerative conditions Multiple system atrophy	Atypical parkinsonism (see Chapter 23)
Developmental deformities Arnold–Chiari malformation	Pyramidal signs, lower cranial nerve palsies, occipital headache, ± signs associated with a syrinx
Congenital aqueduct stenosis	Sixth nerve palsies, deafness, papilloedema, intellectual decline
Dandy–Walker syndrome	Large cystic fourth ventricle resulting in hydrocephalus
Inherited cerebellar ataxias	Early onset (<25 years of age) – tend to be autosomal recessive: • Friedreich ataxias, ataxia telangiectasia (see Chapter 36), ataxia with oculomotor apraxia, metabolic ataxias including vitamin E deficiency and mitochondrial disorders, progressive myoclonic ataxias Late onset (>25 years of age) – tend to be autosomal dominant: • Spinocerebellar ataxias (see Chapter 36), episodic ataxias, dentatorubropallidoluysian atrophy

● **Chapter Summary**

- The cerebellum is responsible for the coordination of skilled voluntary movement, posture and gait. It is divided into three lobes: the vestibulocerebellum, anterior spinocerebellum and posterior neocerebellum.
- Clinical features associated with dysfunction of the cerebellum include incoordination of movement, ataxia, a scanning dysarthria and nystagmus.

UKMLA Presentations
Abnormal involuntary movements
Tremor
Unsteadiness

Movement disorders 13

ANATOMICAL BASIS AND CLASSIFICATION OF MOVEMENT DISORDERS

The basal ganglia are symmetrical groups of grey matter or 'nuclei' deep within the cerebral hemispheres and brainstem. The main components are the caudate nucleus, globus pallidus, putamen, substantia nigra and subthalamus. It is thought that these structures coordinate movement and voluntary action via two pathways: the direct and indirect pathways (Fig. 13.1).

Movement disorders can be classified into two main categories: akinetic/hypokinetic disorders, i.e., loss of or decreased movement and hyperkinetic disorders, i.e., increased movement. Parkinson's disease is the most common hypokinetic movement disorder (see Chapter 23). Hyperkinetic disorders have additional or excessive movements and these can be subdivided into non-jerky (tremor or dystonia) and jerky hyperkinetic movements (chorea, tics or myoclonus). This chapter will focus on the hyperkinetic movement disorders.

THE HYPERKINETIC MOVEMENT DISORDERS: TREMOR AND DYSTONIA

The non-jerky hyperkinetic movement disorders include tremor and dystonia.

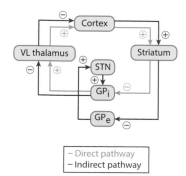

Fig. 13.1 Schematic of direct and indirect pathway. *GPe*, External globus pallidus; *GPi*, internal globus pallidus; *STN*, subthalamic nucleus; *VL*, ventrolateral.

Tremor

Tremor is an involuntary and oscillatory movement of one or more body parts. All tremors should disappear during sleep. Tremors may be normal (physiological) or abnormal (pathological) and are described as 'fine' if they are low amplitude and 'coarse' if they are high amplitude. A physiological tremor affects all muscle groups, although it is most commonly noted in the hands. The tremor is present during waking. It is usually bilateral, worse on maintaining a posture, fine in character and fast in rate (8–14 Hz).

A pathological tremor often occurs at rest or with movement, is slower (4–7 Hz), coarse in character, proximal as well as distal and often asymmetrical. This tremor often interferes with everyday activities.

The positions in which a tremor can occur are at rest, on posture (e.g., holding the arms outstretched) or during movement (kinetic tremor). Tremors should therefore be assessed by observing the patient at rest, during maintenance of a posture (e.g., holding the arms outstretched) and during volitional, kinetic movements of the limbs. The term intention tremor refers to a tremor that increases throughout the movement, whereas terminal tremor refers to a tremor that occurs at the end of the movement. Both are forms of a kinetic tremor (Fig. 13.2). Some people also use the term action tremor, which refers to all tremors that do not occur at rest, but for simplicity this term is best avoided.

Resting tremor

The most common cause of a resting tremor is Parkinson's disease. The parkinsonian tremor is a coarse 'pill-rolling' tremor and disappears during voluntary movement. It is usually observed in the hands and arms and is asymmetrical, being worse on one side than the other (see Chapter 23). The tremor may affect other parts of the body, including the jaw and feet. The patient may have other signs of Parkinson's disease (e.g., rigidity and bradykinesia). The tremor may respond to anticholinergic or dopaminergic medication.

Postural tremor

A postural tremor occurs when a body part assumes a position against gravity and is usually physiological but can occur in essential, dystonic and neuropathic tremor.

Physiological tremor

Physiological tremor may be exaggerated by:

- anxiety

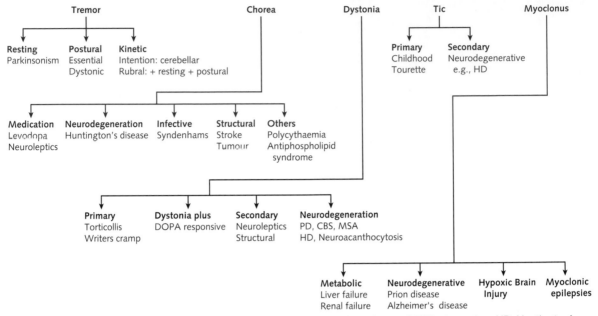

Fig. 13.2 Summary of hyperkinetic movement disorders. *CBS*, Corticobasal syndrome; *DOPA*, dopamine; *HD*, Huntington's disease; *MSA*, multiple system atrophy; *PD*, Parkinson's disease.

- metabolic disturbances: hyperthyroidism, phaeochromocytoma
- alcohol withdrawal
- drugs: lithium, sodium valproate, sympathomimetics, tea and coffee

β-blockers may diminish a physiological tremor.

Essential tremor

Essential tremor may be difficult to distinguish from an exaggerated physiological tremor. It is coarser and slower (8 Hz), affecting the upper limbs, and can spread to the head, trunk and legs. It can be inherited in an autosomal dominant manner in about 50% of patients, in which case it presents in childhood or early adulthood, otherwise its incidence increases with age. On movement (finger–nose testing) the tremor may worsen terminally (terminal tremor), but does not progressively worsen throughout the movement. The tremor can progress to be disabling and there is often temporary improvement with alcohol intake. This can be used as a diagnostic and therapeutic manoeuvre. Essential tremor may partially respond to β-blockers, anticholinergics (e.g., trihexyphenidyl) and primidone, and sometimes to barbiturates or benzodiazepines.

Neuropathic tremor

Peripheral neuropathies can cause a postural tremor, which is distinct from pseudo-athetoid movements that can be seen with proprioceptive loss. Signs of the underlying neuropathy are typically present when the tremor presents, and treatment of the neuropathy may improve the tremor.

Dystonic tremor

A tremor that involves a body part affected with dystonia is called a dystonic tremor. Dystonic tremor can mimic the tremor seen in Parkinson's disease and many cases of true dystonic tremor are misdiagnosed as essential tremor. Dystonic tremor is often position and task specific and is typically asymmetrical and of large amplitude when compared to essential tremor.

Cerebellar tremor (intention tremor)

Cerebellar dysfunction (see Chapter 12) gives rise to a coarse, often slow (4–6 Hz), action or 'intention' tremor. It is absent at rest and becomes apparent on movement. On performing the finger–nose test, the finger oscillates with increasing amplitude on approaching the target. Rhythmic oscillation of the head and trunk (titubation) may occur and there may be other signs of cerebellar dysfunction such as nystagmus, dysarthria, dysdiadochokinesis and an ataxic gait.

Red nuclear 'rubral' tremor

This tremor is present at rest and deteriorates with posture, but is worse during movement. It is caused by damage to the cerebellar–brainstem connections, typically from multiple sclerosis, but also from vascular lesions and tumours. It is an unusually coarse and often violent tremor. Slight movement of the arm may precipitate a wide-amplitude tremor of the limb.

Stereotactic surgical lesions of the contralateral ventrolateral thalamus may abolish pathological tremors.

Mixed tremors

Combinations of rest, postural and kinetic tremor may be present in severe essential tremor, dystonic tremor and rubral tremor.

Dystonia

Dystonia is a hyperkinetic movement disorder characterized by involuntary and repetitive contractions of opposing muscles, causing twisting movements and abnormal postures. Dystonias can affect one or more parts of the body. In addition, tremor often occurs with dystonia and tends to affect the same body part. Dystonias can be classified in a variety of ways. They may affect only one part of the body (focal dystonia), two or more contiguous body parts such as the head and neck (segmental dystonia), noncontiguous body regions such as laryngeal with limb dystonia (multifocal), one-half of the body (hemidystonia) or the whole of the body (generalized dystonia). The focal dystonias tend to be idiopathic or secondary to lesions often within the basal ganglia, whereas generalized dystonia tends to have a genetic basis. Adult-onset dystonia affects those older than 25 years of age, and young-onset dystonia affects those younger than 25 years of age. Dystonia can also be classified according to aetiology (see Fig. 13.2).

Primary dystonia

Patients have no features of neurodegeneration or secondary causes of dystonia. Dystonia is the only clinical feature except for perhaps a dystonic tremor. There may be a genetic aetiology. The most common primary forms are the late-onset, focal dystonias, accounting for 90% of all cases. Late-onset dystonia usually starts in mid-adulthood and often has a focal onset without a tendency to spread to other body parts (cervical dystonia such as torticollis, writer's cramp, blepharospasm or isolated laryngeal dystonia). The most effective treatment for focal dystonia is botulinum toxin injections into the affected muscles at approximately 3-monthly intervals:

- **Focal dystonia:** typically late in onset and sporadic:
  Cervical dystonia ('spasmodic torticollis'): usually occurs in the fifth decade of life. There are involuntary movements of the neck: laterally towards one side (laterocollis) or rotating around to one side (torticollis) and in extension (retrocollis) or flexion (anterocollis). The overactive muscles such as sternomastoid, trapezius and splenius are most affected, can be painful and may eventually hypertrophy. Women are affected more than men. Patients often demonstrate a 'geste antagonist', which is a manoeuvre that stops the involuntary movement (e.g.,

gentle pressure with the hand on the side of the jaw). Cervical dystonia may be complicated by a jerky postural and kinetic tremor referred to as a 'dystonic tremor'. Response to anticholinergics is often poor. Botulinum toxin injections to overactive muscles can provide good relief.
  Blepharospasm: involuntary contractions of the eyelid muscles where the eyes screw up and remain closed with a 'shampoo in the eyes' effect.
  Oromandibular dystonia: involuntary dystonic movements of the mouth, tongue and jaw can affect women in the sixth decade of life. Speech and swallowing may also be affected. It may also occur in patients on long-term neuroleptic therapy and the elderly.
  Writer's cramp: attempts at writing trigger a task-specific, focal hand dystonia which may be painful but resolves on cessation of writing. The symptoms can spread to the forearm and shoulders. It usually occurs in middle or late life and does not typically progress to involve other parts of the body. Other skilled functions of the hands are usually normal. Some patients respond to anticholinergics or to selective botulinum injections to affected muscles. Other focal, occupational, task-specific dystonias occur in musicians and athletes.
- **Early-onset generalized dystonia**: typically early in onset and genetic. It is rare but is the most common hereditary dystonia is caused by mutations in the gene *DYT1*. There is an autosomal dominant pattern of inheritance with incomplete penetrance as only 40% of patients with a mutation develop the disease. At its onset there appears to be focal dystonia that often starts in the legs and usually spreads over months to years, resulting in generalized dystonia, often with sparing of the head and neck. Treatment consists of the anticholinergics clonazepam and baclofen. Surgery is confined to patients who are severely affected and consists of deep brain stimulation to the globus pallidus.

Dystonia-plus syndromes – DOPA-responsive dystonia

Patients have no features of neurodegeneration or secondary causes of dystonia. However, other signs may occur with the dystonia. DOPA-responsive dystonia is the main example in this group. This is a rare disorder in which there is progressive dystonia that initially affects the lower limbs in early childhood. There is marked diurnal variation, with symptoms worsening as the day progresses but improving with rest and sleep. Patients also have parkinsonism and spasticity. There is a striking response to small doses of L-DOPA, which treats many of the symptoms of the disease. This disease is also familial and inherited in an autosomal dominant manner with incomplete penetrance.

Secondary dystonia

There is a clear secondary cause of the dystonia and other signs may be apparent. The most common cause of secondary dystonia is due to the side effects of medication. The dopamine-receptor-blocking-drugs, particularly the neuroleptics, cause acute transient dystonic reactions or a persistent dystonic disorder referred to as tardive dystonia. Tardive dystonia can persist despite discontinuing medication and often occurs after several years of treatment with neuroleptics. It typically manifests as axial dystonia with hyperextension of the spine and neck, referred to as retrocollis. Treatment can have limited success and prevention is the most important method of avoiding all of the tardive movement disorders. Dystonia can also present in patients on treatment for Parkinson's disease when the dopaminergic medication is wearing off (so-called off-state).

Other causes of secondary dystonia include focal brain lesions, e.g., from stroke, tumour or brain injury.

Neurodegenerative diseases

Conditions with diverse neurological symptoms that include dystonia are:

- Parkinson's disease, corticobasal degeneration, progressive supranuclear palsy, multiple system atrophy, Wilson disease
- Huntington's disease, neuroacanthocytosis, neuronal brain iron accumulation

Paroxysmal dystonia

These are a group of familial conditions which consist of brief attacks of dystonic posturing provoked by sudden noise, movement, emotional stimuli or exercise. There may be no clinical signs between attacks.

The most effective treatment for focal dystonias is botulinum toxin injections into the affected muscles at approximately 3-monthly intervals.

HYPERKINETIC MOVEMENT DISORDERS: CHOREA, TICS AND MYOCLONUS

Chorea

Chorea, from the Greek word for 'a dance', consists of involuntary movements that are nonrhythmic, abrupt and jerky and that randomly move from one body part to another. It can affect the face, trunk and limbs or be generalized. The causes of chorea are wide ranging:

- Medications: L-DOPA, neuroleptics (e.g., phenothiazines, butyrophenones), oral contraceptives, anticonvulsants and calcium antagonists.

- Inherited/degenerative disorders: Huntington's disease, Wilson disease.
- Autoimmune/postinfectious: systemic lupus erythematosus, antiphospholipid syndrome, vasculitis, Hashimoto thyroiditis and Sydenham chorea (poststreptococcal infection).
- Infections: HIV, Creutzfeldt–Jakob disease.
- Metabolic disorders: disorders of thyroid, parathyroid, glucose, sodium, calcium and magnesium.
- Haematological disorders: polycythaemia rubra vera.
- Structural disorders: vascular, demyelination, tumour.

Huntington's disease

Huntington's disease is clinically characterized by progressive personality/behavioural changes, generalized chorea and eventually dementia. Towards the end of the disease, chorea diminishes and parkinsonism and dystonia dominate the clinical picture. It typically manifests in the fourth decade of life and progresses to death within 12 to 15 years. Huntington's disease is a hereditary condition caused by an expanded trinucleotide repeat (CAG) in the *HTT* gene on chromosome 4. It shows genetic anticipation, such that with each generation the repeat increases in length, manifesting with a younger age of onset. About 6% of cases start before 21 years of age and are dominated by an akinetic rigid syndrome (Westphal variant). There is neuronal loss initially in the caudate nucleus and putamen, as well as other areas such as the cerebral cortex. There is no effective treatment, although dopamine-blocking or -depleting drugs may reduce the chorea by causing parkinsonism. Patients often have tic disorder that may also require treatment.

ETHICS

It is essential to counsel patients prior to performing genetic tests. The patients should understand what the implications of a positive and negative test are on other relatives, including those who may have inherited the mutation but have not shown the signs (asymptomatic carriers). Many relatives decide not to undergo presymptomatic testing.

Ballism

Ballism, which is derived from the Greek word 'to throw', is an additional term that describes chorea when it is severe, proximal and of large amplitude. In these cases it can appear as a violent flinging movement of the proximal limb. Hemiballism, the commonest presentation, affecting an arm and ipsilateral leg, is due to a stroke in the contralateral subthalamic nucleus. If the amplitude of limb movements is small, it is referred to as hemichorea, and if a single limb is affected, it is called monoballism.

Tics

A tic is an involuntary, stereotyped movement or vocalization, which can be suppressed for periods of time by patients, but at the cost of mounting inner tension. Tics can be motor or vocal, and simple (e.g., one discrete movement or unarticulated sounds) or complex (e.g., combination of movements or words or phrases). Tics can be primary (e.g., simple tics of childhood or Giles de la Tourette syndrome) or secondary to a variety of neurodegenerative, structural, developmental (e.g., Down syndrome), infective (e.g., streptococcal infection) or pharmacological causes.

Gilles de la Tourette syndrome is a rare disease in which multiple motor and, in particular, vocal tics develop before the age of 18 years. There may be psychiatric and behavioural disorders including attention-deficit hyperactivity disorder, depression or obsessive-compulsive disorder. The caudate nucleus has been implicated in the pathology of the condition and treatment is symptomatic. The syndrome is characterized by involuntary snorting, grunting, shouting of verbal obscenities, and aggressive and sexual impulses. It may respond to dopamine-blocking neuroleptic drugs (e.g., sulpiride).

Myoclonus

Myoclonus are sudden, brief and shock-like involuntary movements. It can be a normal experience in healthy individuals. For example, the jerks that can occur on falling asleep and hiccups are both forms of myoclonus. Pathophysiological myoclonus can occur in the same muscle (focal myoclonus) or affect many different parts at different times (multifocal myoclonus) or affect all of the body (generalized myoclonus). Myoclonus may also be sensitive to a variety of stimuli (e.g., a sudden noise, light, touch or voluntary movement). Generalized myoclonus arises from the cerebral cortex, whereas focal myoclonus can arise from cerebral cortex, brainstem, spinal cord or even peripheral nerves and roots.

Myoclonus can be classified according to the underlying cause.

Myoclonic epilepsy

Myoclonus may be a feature of many different forms of epilepsy (e.g., juvenile myoclonic epilepsy, Lennox–Gastaut syndrome). Myoclonus may be combined with epilepsy and progressive dementia in several rare inherited metabolic diseases, e.g., Lafora body disease and lipid -storage diseases (Gaucher disease).

Symptomatic myoclonus

Myoclonus can occur in the context of conditions causing encephalopathy. It can therefore be seen in patients with liver failure, renal failure, drug intoxication (alcohol lithium) and posthypoxia. Asterixis is the sporadic 'flapping tremor' of the hands observed with arms outstretched and hands dorsiflexed. These brief, nonrhythmic movements are not actually a tremor. It is actually a form of 'negative' myoclonus (sudden involuntary relaxation of a muscle group) and is seen in metabolic encephalopathies. Postanoxic action myoclonus occurs following severe cerebral anoxia (e.g., after cardiorespiratory arrest) and is known as 'Lance Adams syndrome'. Prognosis is usually poor in this event.

Symptomatic myoclonus can also be seen in neurodegenerative diseases. This includes those that cause dementia (e.g., Alzheimer's disease, Creutzfeldt–Jakob disease) or atypical parkinsonism (e.g., corticobasal degeneration, multiple system atrophy). Focal myoclonus can be seen in spinal cord/root/plexus injuries. Myoclonus may respond to benzodiazepines such as clonazepam.

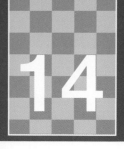

Weakness in the limbs can result from pathology at any level of the motor pathway:

- Pathology anywhere along the upper motor neurone (UMN) pathway (from motor cortex to the spinal cord)
- A lesion of the lower motor neurone (LMN) pathway (from the anterior horn cell to the peripheral nerve)
- Disorders of the neuromuscular junction
- Muscular disorders

The distribution and pattern of weakness, together with associated physical signs, usually allows determination of the level of the motor pathway affected, and therefore possible differential diagnoses.

NEUROANATOMY

Upper motor neurone pathway

UMN cell bodies are arranged in a homuncular distribution in the primary motor cortex, at the posterior limit of the frontal lobe (Fig. 14.1):

- The axons of the UMNs descend through the subcortical white matter (corona radiata and then internal capsule).
- The axons descend in the midbrain as the cerebral peduncles and then in the anterior pons and medulla, where they cross as the pyramidal decussation.
- During their brainstem course, some of the UMN axons synapse in motor nuclei (cranial nerve nuclei III, IV, V, VI, VII, X, XI, XII). These axons are called the corticobulbar fibres because the motor nuclei in the brainstem are known as the 'bulbar nuclei'.
- The remaining axons form the corticospinal tracts and descend in the lateral white matter of the spinal cord.

Lower motor neurone pathway

- At each spinal level, some of the corticospinal fibres enter the anterior horn of the grey matter and synapse with cell bodies of the LMN, the anterior horn cells or motor neurones.
- When these cell bodies are damaged, the syndrome is referred to as an anterior horn cell disorder.
- Each LMN sends out an axon in the ventral (motor) root which joins a dorsal (sensory) root at each spinal level in the intervertebral foramen to form a spinal segmental or mixed

nerve. When this nerve is damaged, it is called a radiculopathy.
- The spinal nerve in the cervical and lumbosacral regions joins other adjacent spinal nerves in a junctional network referred to as a plexus. If these structures are damaged, the clinical syndrome is a plexopathy.
- From the plexi emerge peripheral nerves and, when these are damaged, the patient develops a neuropathy.
- The axons in the peripheral nerves split into many fibres just before synapsing with muscle fibres.

Neuromuscular junction and muscle pathway

- One axon innervates from 10 to 10,000 muscle fibres, depending on whether fine motor control or a coarser antigravity use of the muscle is required. The group of muscle fibres innervated by one axon is called a motor unit. When the synapses are damaged, the condition is called a neuromuscular junction disorder.
- Finally, the muscle itself can be damaged and this is termed a myopathy.

Any disorder affecting the UMN, LMN, neuromuscular junction or the muscle can give rise to the symptom of weakness and/or the sign of loss of power (Table 14.1).

Terminology

Paralysis is the complete loss of voluntary movement. The words 'plegia', 'palsy' and 'paresis' are sometimes used interchangeably to describe weakness, although 'paresis' is the correct term to describe incomplete paralysis. 'Plegia' means complete paralysis, and the word 'palsy' is used when the paralysis affects cranial motor nerves (e.g., Bell palsy, pseudobulbar palsy) or when one is referring to a static weakness (e.g., cerebral palsy). There are several specific terms used to describe the anatomical distribution of weakness:

- **Pyramidal weakness:** loss of power is most marked in the extensor muscles in the arms and the flexors in the legs. This is characteristic of UMN lesions involving the pyramidal tract within the brain or spinal cord.
- **Proximal weakness**: affecting the shoulders, hips, trunk, neck and sometimes face. This is characteristic of muscle disease (myopathy) and also a common pattern in myasthenia gravis (neuromuscular junction).

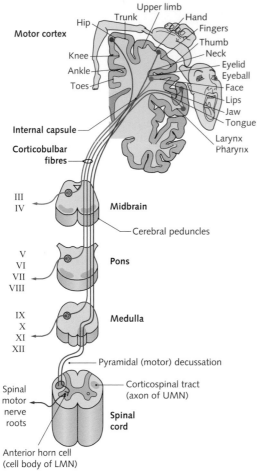

Fig. 14.1 Descending motor pathways from the cortex to the brainstem, cranial nerves and spinal cord. *LMN,* Lower motor neurone; *UMN,* upper motor neurone.

- **Distal weakness**: affecting the hands and feet. This is typical of peripheral motor neuropathy, often affecting the lower limbs first and more severely.

UPPER MOTOR NEURONE WEAKNESS

UMN weakness results from damage of the corticospinal tract at any point from the motor cortex to the spinal cord (see Fig. 14.1). If the lesion occurs above the pyramidal decussation at the level of the lower medulla, the weakness is contralateral to the site of the lesion. If it occurs below this level, the weakness is ipsilateral to the lesion.

The following clinical features characterize a UMN lesion.

Increased tone (spasticity)

Initially, UMN weakness may be flaccid, with absent or diminished deep tendon reflexes. Increased tone of a UMN type is called spasticity. It may develop several hours, days or even weeks after the initial lesion has occurred. Spasticity is manifested by:

- 'Spastic catch': mild spasticity may be detected as a resistance to passive movement or 'catch' in the pronators on passive supination of the forearm and in the flexors of the hand/forearm on extension of the wrist/elbow.
- The 'clasp-knife' phenomenon: in more severe lesions, following strong resistance to passive flexion of the knee or extension of the elbow, there is a sudden relaxation of the extensor muscles of the leg and flexor muscles in the arm.
- Clonus: rhythmic involuntary muscular contractions follow an abruptly applied and sustained stretch stimulus, e.g., at the ankle following sudden passive dorsiflexion of the foot.

Table 14.1 Anatomical sites of weakness

	Site of pathology	Clinical syndrome
UMN pathway	Motor cortex, corona radiata, internal capsule, brainstem Spinal cord (corticospinal tract)	Hemisphere or brainstem (pyramidal weakness) Myelopathy (pyramidal weakness)
LMN pathway	Anterior horn or motor neurone cell body Spinal nerve root Brachial or lumbosacral plexus Peripheral nerve	Motor neuronopathy or 'anterior horn cell disease' Radiculopathy Plexopathy Neuropathy
Neuromuscular junction	Synapse	Neuromuscular junction disorder
Muscle	Muscle	Myopathy

LMN, *Lower motor neurone;* UMN, *upper motor neurone.*

'Pyramidal-pattern' weakness

The antigravity muscles are preferentially spared and stronger (i.e., the flexors of the upper limbs and the extensors of the lower limbs). The patient can develop a characteristic posture of flexed and pronated arms with clenched fingers, and extended and adducted legs with plantar flexion of the feet.

Absence of muscle wasting and fasciculations

Focal muscle wasting and fasciculations are features of an LMN lesion. With chronic disuse, some loss of muscle bulk can occur after a UMN lesion, but this is rarely focal.

Brisk tendon reflexes and extensor plantar responses

The tendon reflexes are brisk. The cremasteric and abdominal or 'cutaneous' reflexes are depressed or absent. The plantar responses are extensor ('upgoing toes' or 'positive Babinski sign').

UPPER MOTOR NEURONE SYNDROMES

The common UMN syndromes are hemiparesis and paraparesis; tetraparesis and monoparesis are less common.

Hemiparesis – unilateral arm and leg weakness

Hemiparesis results from unilateral lesions of the contralateral cerebral hemisphere or brainstem (when the face is usually also affected) or from an ipsilateral lesion below the pyramidal decussation in the lower medulla or high cervical cord (when the face is spared; Fig. 14.2).

The clinical features associated with hemiparesis usually enable a more accurate localization of the site of the pathology. The most common cause of hemiparesis is a stroke involving the contralateral cerebral cortex or internal capsule (see Fig. 14.2).

Tetraparesis – weakness in all four limbs

Pyramidal (UMN) weakness of all four limbs may result from lesions in the brainstem or high cervical cord. When the UMNs are damaged, the condition is called a 'spastic' tetraparesis (or sometimes quadraparesis). Tetraparesis caused by spinal cord pathology is most commonly due to external compression (cervical spondylosis, secondary malignancy in the spine), inflammation of the cord (multiple sclerosis, neuromyelitis optica) and traumatic cord lesions. Less frequent causes include intradural neoplasms, arteriovenous malformations (AVMs) or spinal cord infarct. Cervical spondylotic myelopathy is usually associated

with a cervical radiculopathy affecting one or more spinal nerves, usually C6 and/or C7. The patient will therefore have UMN signs in the legs and predominantly LMN signs in the arms, a syndrome referred to as a myeloradiculopathy. Extensive bilateral pathology in the cerebral hemispheres can occasionally cause tetraparesis. Brainstem pathology is usually associated with additional cranial nerve symptoms such as diplopia, facial numbness, vertigo, dysarthria, dysphagia and signs such as ocular, facial or bulbar weakness. The most common brainstem pathologies to cause tetraparesis include stroke, neoplasms and multiple sclerosis.

Paraparesis – weakness in both legs

Paraparesis is usually due to spinal cord disease and is consequently a UMN syndrome, characterized by spasticity, pyramidal weakness, brisk reflexes and extensor plantar responses in the legs. This syndrome is called 'spastic paraparesis'. The most common causes are inflammation of the cord (e.g., multiple sclerosis) or extrinsic compression in the lower cervical or thoracic region of the cord. This is usually due to degenerative osteoarthritis and disc prolapse, which causes cord compression (Table 14.2).

Paraparesis can also be associated with decreased tone in the legs when it is called 'flaccid paraparesis'. This usually results from lesions in the cauda equina such as central lumbar disc prolapse or infiltrating neoplasms. A cauda equina syndrome is usually associated with severe and early sphincter dysfunction and sensory impairment over sacral and lower lumbar dermatomes or 'saddle anaesthesia' (see Fig. 14.2). Lower back pain accompanied by pain radiating into one or both legs may also be present in a cauda equina syndrome. The radicular pain reflects involvement of the dorsal nerve roots. The cauda equina is made up of the spinal nerves that exit at the inferior pole of the spinal cord called the conus medullaris. The conus is a highly compacted region of the spinal cord containing many spinal levels. The clinical signs of a conus lesion are therefore often mixed between UMN and LMN, such as brisk knee jerks and extensor plantar responses, but with flaccid tone and absent ankle jerks. Other causes of a flaccid paraparesis include a polyradiculopathy or a peripheral neuropathy (e.g., Guillain–Barré syndrome).

HINTS AND TIPS

Spastic paraparesis is often encountered in clinical examinations as well as in the clinic setting, and a systematic approach to the numerous causes is important.

A much rarer cause of bilateral UMN symptoms and signs in the legs, resembling a spinal cord syndrome, is a cerebral lesion involving both cortical leg areas in the parasagittal region of the brain. A parasagittal meningioma classically causes

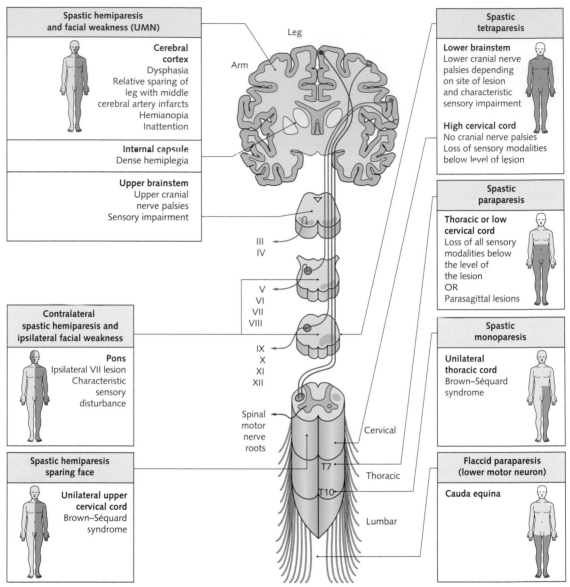

Fig. 14.2 Patterns of motor weakness. Note that these are all upper motor neurone (UMN) lesions except for pathology in the cauda equina, which damages multiple lumbar and sacral nerve roots.

this syndrome, but sagittal sinus thrombosis with subsequent venous infarction, the 'spastic diplegia' form of cerebral palsy and hereditary spastic paraplegias are other rare causes.

Monoparesis – weakness of a single limb

A stroke in one of the distal branches of the middle cerebral artery (MCA) is the most common cause of an isolated upper limb monoparesis. Usually the MCA is blocked more proximally and there is weakness in the contralateral upper limb with some UMN facial weakness and relative sparing of the leg. This is in contrast to anterior cerebral artery occlusion, which often spares the face and arm and causes contralateral leg weakness.

Other localized cerebral cortical lesions may cause weakness confined to one contralateral limb, such as cortical tumours, multiple sclerosis lesions, abscesses and granulomas.

Table 14.2 Causes of spastic paraparesis

Spinal cord compression	Cervical spondylosis Cervical or thoracic disc herniation Metastatic tumour Primary tumour (e.g., meningioma, neurofibroma) Infective (e.g., epidural abscess, spinal TB) Epidural haematoma
Inflammatory disorders	Multiple sclerosis Idiopathic transverse myelitis Sarcoidosis Infections (e.g., Lyme, zoster, TB, HIV, syphilis, HTLV-1)
Degenerative disorders	Motor neurone disease Syringomyelia
Vascular	Spinal cord infarction Vasculitis, systemic lupus erythematosus Spinal arteriovenous malformation
Trauma	Cord contusion, laceration or transection Displaced vertebral fracture or disc Traumatic epidural haematoma
Metabolic/nutritional	Vitamin B12 deficiency (subacute combined degeneration)
Rare hereditary conditions	Friedreich ataxia Hereditary spastic paraparesis
Parasagittal brain lesions	Meningioma Cerebral venous sinus thrombosis Congenital spastic diplegia (cerebral palsy)

HIV, *Human immunodeficiency virus;* HTLV-1, *human T-lymphotropic virus;* TB, *tuberculosis.*

A unilateral thoracic cord lesion may also occasionally present with monoparesis of the leg (see Fig. 14.2). There will usually be reflex and sensory findings of a Brown–Séquard syndrome to clarify the diagnosis. This is usually caused by a demyelinating plaque in multiple sclerosis.

COMMON PITFALLS

Many patients use the word 'weakness' to describe other deficits that are not actually characterized by a lack of power, such as stiffness, slowness, ataxia, fatigue and clumsiness due to sensory loss.

LOWER MOTOR NEURONE WEAKNESS

LMNs extend from the anterior horn cell in the spinal cord to the neuromuscular junction in the muscles. Lesions to the LMNs are characterized by a constellation of typical clinical signs, which vary in their presence and degree by the anatomical site of damage to the LMN in its course from the spinal cord to the muscles. There are typically four different types of LMN lesion (anterior horn cell, spinal nerve, plexus and peripheral nerve – see later). Although the neuromuscular junction and muscle are not strictly a part of the LMN, disorders of these structures are also considered in the differential diagnosis of LMN syndromes because they produce similar signs and symptoms.

LMN syndromes are characterized by the following features.

Decreased tone

Tone is typically reduced, particularly when muscle wasting has occurred.

Focal pattern of weakness and wasting

LMN weakness can occur in individual muscles and in groups of muscles if more than one level of LMN is involved. The denervated muscle becomes atrophied and wasting is evident within days to weeks after the onset. The pattern of weakness and wasting depends on the site of the lesion:

- **Anterior horn cell disease** (see Chapter 25): eventually causes generalized weakness and wasting; however, it can begin distally in either a hand or foot and it may mimic a peripheral nerve lesion, e.g., an ulnar neuropathy, common peroneal nerve palsy (foot drop).
- **Radiculopathies** (see Chapter 26): result in weakness and wasting in the respective myotomes, i.e., the group of muscles innervated by a single spinal nerve root.
- **Plexopathies** (see Chapter 26): cause weakness and wasting in the distribution of more than one spinal nerve root (see Fig. 14.3)
- **Peripheral neuropathies** (see Chapter 27): a single or several single peripheral nerves are affected, e.g., ulnar mononeuropathy
- **Neuromuscular junction disorders**, such as myasthenia gravis: typically cause weakness in muscles of the head and neck as well as proximal upper limbs. The weakness is characteristically fatigable, i.e., worsens quickly with exercise and there is little or no muscle wasting (see Chapter 28).
- **Myopathies:** usually cause symmetrical wasting and weakness in the proximal limb girdles (shoulders, hips and thighs), although distal muscles can be involved, depending on the cause of the myopathy (see Chapter 29).

Fasciculations

Fasciculations are brief, flickering contractions of individual motor units in a denervated muscle, of which patients are usually not aware. They may be present in weak and wasted muscles but can also occur in muscles that appear unaffected. Fasciculations are particularly prevalent in motor neurone disease and motor neuropathies. Benign fasciculations are common in normal individuals. These are typically infrequent, localized to one muscle at a time, fast and may be noticed by the individual when associated with triggers such as stimulants, e.g., caffeine.

Pain and sensory disturbance

Sensory changes often occur in lesions of the spinal nerve roots, plexii and peripheral nerves. It should be noted that anterior horn cell disease, diseases of the neuromuscular junction and myopathies do not have objective sensory signs. Pain accompanies the sensory disturbance when the lesion is caused by infiltrating tumour, vasculitis or some toxins, e.g., alcohol.

Reduced tendon reflexes and flexor plantar responses

Tendon reflexes may be reduced or lost depending on the severity and distribution of the LMN lesion. Abdominal and

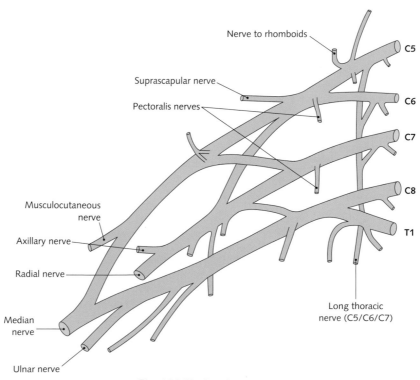

Fig. 14.3 The brachial plexus.

cremasteric reflexes are unaffected. Plantar responses are flexor unless there is severe loss of sensation or power to the big toe when the reflex may be completely absent.

1. **Anterior horn cells**, e.g., polio, motor neurone disease and syringomyelia
2. **Spinal nerves** or 'nerve roots', e.g., L5 radiculopathy
3. **Plexopathy**, e.g., brachial plexopathy (e.g., brachial neuritis)
4. **Peripheral neuropathy**, e.g., ulnar mononeuropathy or generalized polyneuropathy

Anterior horn cell disease

There are usually prominent fasciculations. Causes:

- motor neurone disease
- infective, e.g., poliomyelitis
- toxic, e.g., triorthocresyl phosphate
- local structural pathology, e.g., syringomyelia or intrinsic cord tumours

Radiculopathy and plexopathy

A knowledge of the myotomes is necessary to differentiate the site of a radiculopathy or plexopathy. A radiculopathy will cause muscle weakness and wasting in the myotome supplied by the affected single nerve root, with loss of the segmental tendon reflex, if there is one, and sensory loss in the corresponding dermatome (see Chapter 15). A polyradiculopathy is rare in isolation and indicates a lesion involving many roots but can be found in infiltrative processes such as a malignant radiculopathy. It may be differentiated from many peripheral neuropathies as it produces a more proximal weakness. It is often found in Guillain–Barré syndrome, which is also known as acute demyelinating polyradiculoneuropathy because it involves demyelination within multiple roots as well as nerves.

A plexus lesion will cause weakness and wasting in muscles innervated by several of the spinal nerves that form the plexus, as well as loss of corresponding reflexes. There may be accompanying sensory loss over several dermatomes (see Fig. 14.5). Only part of the plexus is usually involved, although characteristic patterns can often be seen.

Brachial plexopathy

The brachial plexus is illustrated in Fig. 14.3 and is discussed in detail in Chapter 26. The following are examples of brachial plexus syndromes:

- trauma and traction injuries
- neuralgic amyotrophy – usually associated with diabetes

- tumour infiltration
- radiotherapy-induced plexopathy
- idiopathic – can be preceded by viral infection
- Erb palsy (lateral cord: C5, C6) and Klumpke palsy (medial cord: C8, T1)

Lumbosacral plexopathy

In general, lesions of the lower plexus cause weakness and wasting of the hamstrings and foot muscles with loss of the ankle jerk and sensory loss on the posterior leg, whereas upper plexus lesions cause failure of hip flexion and adduction with anterior leg sensory loss (Fig. 14.4). Causes:

- trauma following abdominal or pelvic surgery, e.g., hysterectomy
- infiltration by neoplasia, e.g., cervical, ovarian and colorectal carcinoma, or granulomatous disease
- compression from an abdominal aortic aneurysm

Neuropathy

There are several types of peripheral neuropathy:

- **Mononeuropathy:** disease of a single peripheral nerve, e.g., lesion of the median nerve from compression in the carpal tunnel, lesion of the common peroneal nerve from trauma involving the fibular head.
- **Multiple mononeuropathy** or 'mononeuritis multiplex': this term is used when many single nerves are involved, such

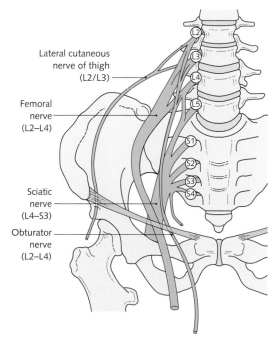

Lateral cutaneous nerve of thigh (L2/L3)

Femoral nerve (L2–L4)

Sciatic nerve (L4–S3)

Obturator nerve (L2–L4)

Fig. 14.4 The lumbosacral plexus.

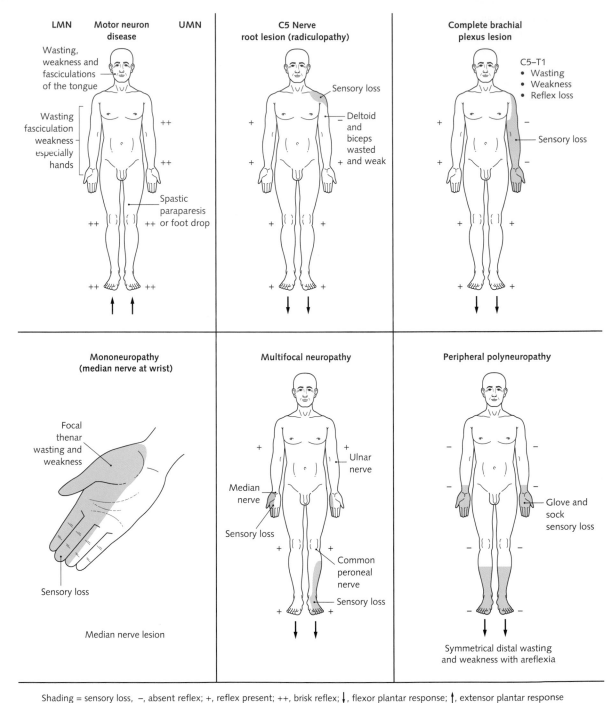

Shading = sensory loss, −, absent reflex; +, reflex present; ++, brisk reflex; ↓, flexor plantar response; ↑, extensor plantar response

Fig. 14.5 Patterns of weakness and sensory loss due to lower motor neurone lesions. The shaded areas indicate sensory loss. LMN, *Lower motor neurone;* UMN, *upper motor neurone.*

as in diabetes, sarcoid, leprosy and vasculitic disease, especially polyarteritis nodosa and neoplasia.

- **Polyneuropathy:** this is the more widespread involvement of the peripheral nerves and typically occurs in a symmetrical distal distribution, starting in the lower limbs, e.g., diabetic neuropathy, vitamin B_{12} deficiency, alcohol excess. Other polyneuropathies may exhibit some proximal signs as well as have a distal distribution, e.g., Guillain–Barré syndrome. Patterns of weakness caused by these disorders are shown in Fig. 14.5 (see also Chapter 27).

DISORDERS OF THE NEUROMUSCULAR JUNCTION

These include myasthenia gravis, Eaton–Lambert syndrome and iatrogenic syndromes.

HINTS AND TIPS

It can sometimes be difficult to identify the anatomical location of a lower motor neurone (LMN) lesion. The presence or absence of sensory loss can help: if there is LMN weakness without sensory loss, then anterior horn cell disease, myasthenia or myopathy are probable. Pure motor neuropathies are uncommon (e.g., porphyria, lead poisoning), but Guillain–Barré can mostly affect the motor system and other rare inflammatory neuropathies can be purely motor.

Myasthenia gravis is the most common disorder of the neuromuscular junction and the extraocular muscles are almost always affected at some point in the disease; they may be the only feature at presentation. There may also be weakness of the bulbar and respiratory muscles as well as proximal muscles, especially in the upper limbs.

The characteristic feature is fatigability of muscle strength, which can often be demonstrated clinically. Wasting is uncommon. Reflexes are usually normal and plantar responses are flexor. There is no sensory involvement or fasciculations (see also Chapter 28).

MYOPATHY

The limb weakness is usually bilateral and proximal in the shoulder and pelvic girdles and patients complain of an inability to stand from sitting, climb stairs, brush their hair or reach for objects above their head. Examples are Duchenne and Becker muscular dystrophy. Involvement of the face, neck and trunk occurs in many myopathic disorders. Dysphagia and respiratory muscle weakness might also occur (e.g., polymyositis). It is essential to also enquire about cardiac history as heart muscle involvement can often be life-threatening in these disorders. Muscle pain (myalgia) and cramps can occur, especially after exercise. Muscle wasting might be severe and tone is reduced. Reflexes are reduced in advanced myopathy but unaffected in the early stages. Plantar responses are flexor and there is no sensory disturbance.

Myopathies are discussed in more detail in Chapter 29.

Chapter Summary

- The motor pathway starts at the cerebral cortex and ends at the innervated muscle. It can be divided into upper motor neurones (UMNs) and lower motor neurones (LMNs).
- Clinically an UMN lesion can be differentiated from a LMN lesion (e.g., brisk reflexes associated with UMN and focal wasting associated with LMN).
- In spastic paraparesis or tetraparesis the lesion is likely to be in the spinal cord. The level at which the spinal cord is affected can be predicted by clinically assessing the extent of weakness.

UKMLA Conditions
Diabetic neuropathy
Motor neurone disease
Muscular dystrophies
Myasthenia gravis
Peripheral nerve injuries/palsies
Radiculopathies
Spinal cord compression
Spinal cord injury
Stroke

UKMLA Presentations
Back pain
Fasciculation
Limb weakness
Limp
Muscle pain/myalgia
Neuromuscular weakness

Limb sensory symptoms

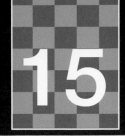

Sensory symptoms can arise from lesions at various levels within the central nervous system (cortex, subcortex, thalamus, brainstem, spinal cord) or from lesions of the peripheral sensory pathways (spinal nerve root, plexus, peripheral nerve). The anatomical distribution of sensory disturbance and the finding of other physical signs may help point towards a diagnosis.

Nerve endings in skin, joints, ligaments, tendons and muscle contain different receptors adapted to respond to a variety of sensory stimuli. The sensory information gathered by these receptors is carried back to the spinal cord by sensory nerves. There are two main pathways for the appreciation of different modalities of sensation:

1. Dorsal (posterior) column pathway (Fig. 15.1)
2. Spinothalamic pathway (see Fig. 15.1)

DORSAL (POSTERIOR) COLUMN PATHWAY

The dorsal column pathway carries information concerned with light touch, two-point discrimination, vibration and proprioception. Fibres carrying this information travel from the cutaneous nerves to the dorsal root ganglia, where their cell bodies lie and relay the information via the dorsal nerve roots to enter the spinal cord. These fibres ascend the spinal cord ipsilaterally in the dorsal columns and synapse in the gracile and cuneate nuclei of the lower medulla in the brainstem. They then decussate in the medulla and travel upwards as the medial lemniscus to synapse in the thalamus and then the parietal cortex. A somatotopic order is maintained throughout the pathway from the spinal cord to parietal cortex.

When pathology affects the dorsal column pathway, the patient may complain of numbness, pins and needles or lack of coordination of the hands or gait (a sensory ataxia) due to loss of proprioceptive information.

SPINOTHALAMIC PATHWAY

The spinothalamic pathway carries information about pain and temperature; it also carries itching and tickling sensations. The fibres travel within the peripheral nerves to the dorsal root ganglia and dorsal nerve roots (see Fig. 15.1). The fibres ascend or descend for one or two segments before synapsing in the dorsal horn. At this level, they decussate and ascend in the contralateral spinothalamic tract. In the brainstem, the tract becomes the lateral lemniscus and these fibres synapse in the thalamus and ultimately the parietal cortex. A somatotopic order is maintained throughout the central pathway, with the sacral fibres being outermost and the cervical fibres innermost.

Clinical manifestations of lesions of this pathway might include pins and needles, pain and impaired pain perception leading to painless burns and excessive wearing of the joints (which may become deformed and then called a Charcot joint).

TROPHIC SKIN CHANGES AND ULCERS

When patients lose the sensory supply to limbs, they are less able to prevent trauma and are less aware of the effect of prolonged pressure to their skin. This may result in ulcers, especially at pressure points, e.g., heels and sacrum. There is also loss of the autonomic supply to piloerector muscles, sweat glands and blood vessels. This can lead to a dry, pale, hairless skin that can become atrophic, swollen and shiny.

SENSORY SYNDROMES

Sensory symptoms may arise from a lesion involving the peripheral nerves, spinal nerves and dorsal roots ganglia or the central pathways. Lesions of the central pathways can be considered at the level of the spinal cord, brainstem, thalamus and parietal cortex. The distribution and pattern of sensory loss, together with associated physical signs, usually allows determination of the level of the sensory pathway affected and, possible differential diagnoses.

Lesions of peripheral nerves

Mononeuropathy

A lesion affecting sensory fibres in a peripheral nerve is accompanied by sensory impairment of all modalities in the corresponding anatomical distribution (Fig. 15.2). If a mixed motor and sensory nerve is involved, there will also be weakness of the muscles supplied by the nerve (see Chapter 27). The most common cause is entrapment neuropathy, e.g., median nerve at the wrist causing carpal tunnel syndrome.

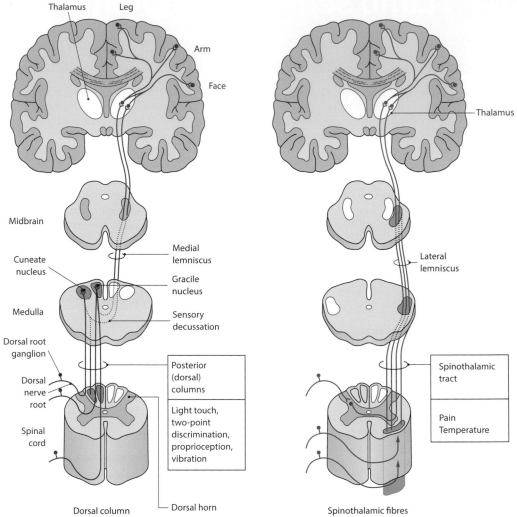

Fig. 15.1 Anatomy of the main sensory pathways in the spinal cord. Note that dorsal column fibres ascend on the ipsilateral side of the spinal cord and decussate in the medulla, whereas spinothalamic fibres cross the central grey matter of the spinal cord (after synapsing in the dorsal horn) and ascend on the opposite side of the cord.

Multiple mononeuropathy

Mononeuritis multiplex involves a number of individual nerves and occurs in diabetes, sarcoidosis, vasculitis, leprosy, amyloidosis and carcinomatous disease.

Polyneuropathy

Polyneuropathy most commonly results in a symmetrical impairment of all sensory modalities involving the feet and legs first, followed by hands and arms, due to length-related axonal loss; this is characteristically termed a glove and sock sensory loss. The reflexes are diminished or lost and, more rarely, there

may be accompanying muscle weakness. Causes of a polyneuropathy include diabetes, chronic alcohol abuse, vitamin B_{12} deficiency, paraproteinaemia and drugs (isoniazid, heavy metals, chemotherapeutic agents). Rarer causes may be inherited (e.g., Charcot–Marie–Tooth disease) or demyelinating (e.g., Guillain–Barré syndrome).

Lesions of the spinal nerve roots, dorsal roots and ganglia

Each dorsal nerve root carries sensory fibres of all modalities from an area on the skin called a dermatome (Fig. 15.2). The

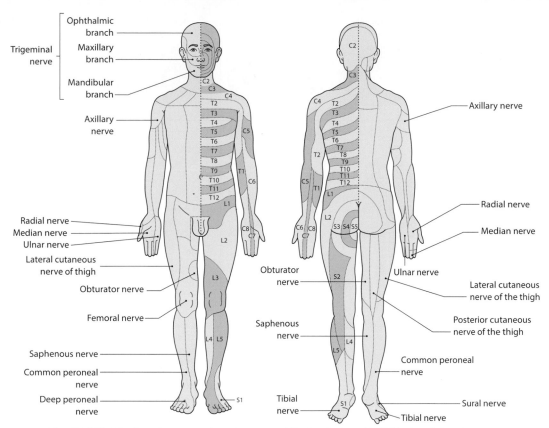

Fig. 15.2 Distribution of sensory dermatomes and the territories of individual peripheral nerves.

overlap of input from adjacent roots means that lesions of a single nerve root do not result in complete loss of sensation within the defined dermatome. The corresponding tendon reflexes may be diminished or lost. Lower motor neurone muscle weakness occurs if the anterior roots are also involved and is especially common in plexus lesions.

Reactivation of the herpes zoster virus (shingles) and prolapsed intervertebral discs can cause damage to the spinal nerves and dorsal roots.

Lesions of central nerves

Lesions of the spinal cord

Sensory disturbances arising from lesions of the spinal cord are illustrated in Fig. 15.3.

Transection of the cord

Transection of the cord causes bilateral impairment of all sensory modalities below the level of transection (as defined by the dermatomal pattern in Fig. 15.2). There is initially a flaccid and, eventually, a spastic paraplegia (thoracic and lumbar cord) or tetraplegia (cervical cord). Traumatic transection is the most common cause, e.g., road traffic accident.

Lesion of the posterior spinal cord

A lesion of the posterior spinal cord affects the dorsal columns, with sparing of the spinothalamic and corticospinal fibres. There is impaired light touch, two-point discrimination, vibration and proprioception below the level of the lesion. Motor function and perception of pain and temperature are spared unless the lesion progresses to involve the anterior part of the cord. Isolated loss of dorsal column function is rare but can occur in multiple sclerosis, spondylosis or prolapsed intervertebral discs and vitamin B_{12} deficiency.

Lesion of the anterior cord

A lesion of the anterior cord affects the spinothalamic and corticospinal tracts, with sparing of the dorsal columns. There is bilateral impairment of pain and temperature perception and a spastic paraplegia or tetraplegia below the level of the lesion. Anterior spinal artery occlusion is the most common cause of this syndrome.

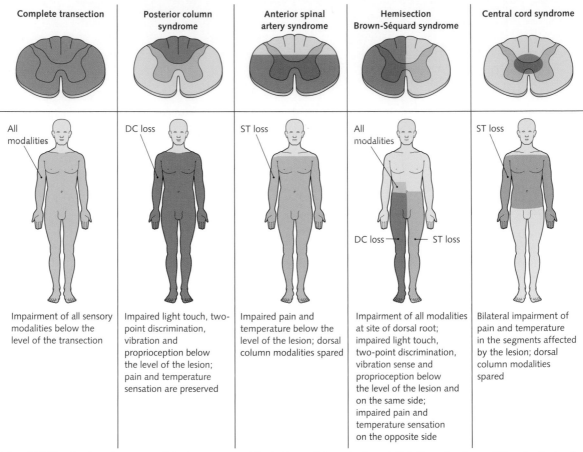

Fig. 15.3 Distribution of sensory disturbance caused by lesions of the spinal cord. *DC*, Dorsal column; *ST*, spinothalamic.

Hemisection of the cord (Brown–Séquard syndrome)

Hemisection of the cord causes impairment of light touch, two-point discrimination, vibration and proprioception below the level of the lesion on the same side (dorsal column) and impaired perception of pain and temperature on the opposite side (spinothalamic). Involvement of one or more nerve roots at the site of the lesion will result in impairment of all sensory modalities on that side within the distribution of the dermatomes affected. Upper motor neurone (UMN) weakness is present on the side of the lesion, due to the disruption of the corticospinal tracts prior to their decussation. Demyelination due to multiple sclerosis and asymmetrical central disc prolapse are the most common causes.

Central cord lesion

A central cord lesion affects the spinothalamic fibres and spares the dorsal columns. There is bilateral loss of pain and temperature perception in the segments affected by the lesion. Only the crossing fibres are involved so that a cape-like distribution of sensory loss occurs, e.g., a syrinx within the cervical cord. More commonly, a belt-like loss of sensation can occur and is often due to a multiple sclerosis plaque in the thoracic cord. The loss of spinothalamic sensation with preservation of dorsal column function is called a dissociated sensory loss. Wasting and weakness and loss of reflexes may occur from involvement of anterior horn cells and fibres subserving the reflex arc within the cord at the level of the lesion. If the lesion expands sufficiently, it might eventually involve the corticospinal tracts and cause UMN signs below the lesion.

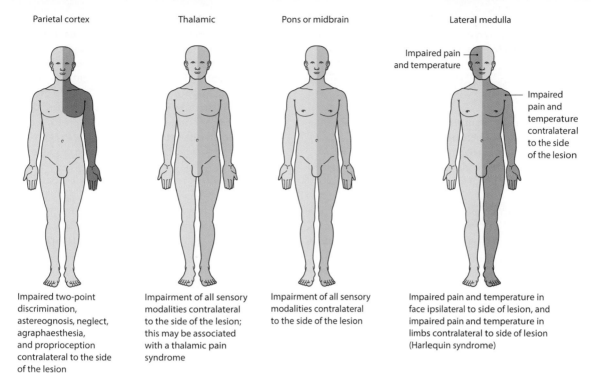

Parietal cortex   Thalamic   Pons or midbrain   Lateral medulla

Impaired pain and temperature

Impaired pain and temperature contralateral to the side of the lesion

Impaired two-point discrimination, astereognosis, neglect, agraphaesthesia, and proprioception contralateral to the side of the lesion

Impairment of all sensory modalities contralateral to the side of the lesion; this may be associated with a thalamic pain syndrome

Impairment of all sensory modalities contralateral to the side of the lesion

Impaired pain and temperature in face ipsilateral to side of lesion, and impaired pain and temperature in limbs contralateral to side of lesion (Harlequin syndrome)

Fig. 15.4 Distribution of sensory disturbance caused by cerebral and brainstem lesions.

HINTS AND TIPS

A dissociated pattern of sensory loss comprises loss of pain and temperature sensation (spinothalamic) with preservation of light touch, two-point discrimination, vibration and proprioception (dorsal columns). It can occur in:

- central cord lesions
- hemisection of the cord
- B_{12} deficiency
- anterior cord syndrome

Lesions of the brainstem

- Lower medulla: a unilateral lesion of the lower medulla (Fig. 15.4) causes impairment of pain and temperature perception of the face on the side of the lesion and on the opposite side of the body (Harlequin syndrome). Light touch, two-point discrimination, vibration and proprioception could be impaired on the side of the lesion, but this is usually spared in a lateral medullary infarction. This lesion involves the ipsilateral spinal trigeminal nucleus and tract and the spinothalamic tract subserving contralateral sensation.
- Pons and midbrain: a unilateral lesion of the pons or midbrain causes impairment of all sensory modalities on the opposite side of the body, including the face, because all the sensory tracts have already crossed, including the spinal nucleus and tract of the trigeminal nerve.

The brainstem syndromes discussed earlier can be accompanied by cranial nerve palsies and cerebellar signs ipsilateral to the lesion and by contralateral hemiparesis. In practice, brainstem lesions are often bilateral and, therefore, affect sensation in the face and all four limbs. In younger patients, multiple sclerosis is the most common cause of a brainstem pattern of sensory loss, while in older patients stroke and tumours are common causes.

Lesions of the thalamus

A thalamic lesion (see Fig. 15.4) causes impairment of all sensory modalities on the opposite side of the body, including the face. There may be spontaneous pain and dysaesthesia on the affected side: the thalamic pain syndrome. The most common causes of a thalamic pattern of sensory loss are stroke, tumours, multiple sclerosis and trauma.

Lesions of the parietal lobe

A parietal lobe lesion (see Fig. 15.4) causes:

- Loss of discriminative sensory function of the opposite side of the face and limbs. There is impaired two-point discrimination, lack of recognition of objects by touch (astereognosis) or figures drawn on the hand (agraphaesthesia) and loss of perception of limb position. However, the primary modalities of pain, temperature, touch and vibration are relatively preserved.
- Sensory inattention: this is usually caused by lesions of the nondominant parietal cortex. The patient fails to perceive stimuli on the opposite side of the body when the stimulus is applied bilaterally. However, when applied on the affected side only, the same stimulus is perceived normally. This inattentive defect or neglect might also apply when testing the visual fields, the phenomenon of visual inattention.

● **Chapter Summary**

- There are two main neuroanatomical pathways responsible for sensation: the dorsal column pathway subserving light touch, two-point discrimination, vibration and proprioception and the spinothalamic pathway subserving pain and temperature sensation.
- By assessing the anatomical sensory pattern, it is possible to differentiate clinically between diseases of the peripheral nerves (e.g., single nerve distribution), spinal cord (e.g., dermatomal distribution), brainstem and cerebral cortex (e.g., hemisensory involvement).
- Commonly affected dermatomes include C5/C6 (usually as a result of cervical spine pathology) and L5/S1 (usually as a result of lumbar spine pathology).

UKMLA Conditions
Diabetic neuropathy
Peripheral nerve injuries/palsies
Spinal cord compression
Spinal cord injury
Spinal fracture
Trauma

UKMLA Presentations
Altered sensation, numbness and tingling
Unsteadiness

Disorders of gait 16

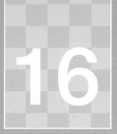

A patient's gait is a coordinated action requiring integration of motor, sensory, vestibular and visual functions. It therefore often provides clues to a patient's underlying diagnosis and is a critical part of any neurological examination. The most common gaits are:

- antalgic (painful)
- apraxic
- cerebellar/sensory ataxia
- functional (nonorganic)
- hemiparetic
- high stepping
- myopathic
- parkinsonian
- spastic paraparesis

PRACTICAL APPROACH TO THE ASSESSMENT OF GAIT

Always ensure the patient is safe to walk unaided prior to assessment. Watch the patient walk away from and back towards you along a stretch of corridor if possible. Analyse the gait in a systematic fashion, starting with an overall impression and then carefully assessing the gait from the feet upwards. Observe the upper and lower half of the patient's body from the front and back as they walk and watch how the patient turns:

- Does the patient walk with an aid: stick, crutches, rollator?
- How does the patient initiate movement? Patients who have apraxic gaits appear as if they have forgotten how to walk and may be rooted to the spot. Patients with an extrapyramidal syndrome may have difficulty in initiating walking.
- Look at the size of the paces the patient uses: small paces are typical of extrapyramidal syndromes or an apraxic gait.
- Look at the lateral distance between the feet. They may be widely separated in a broad-based gait, which is present in cerebellar or sensory ataxia or apraxic gaits. In a scissoring gait of a severe spastic paraparesis, the lateral distance is reduced and the legs may cross over with toes dragging.
- Does the patient walk in a straight line? Patients who have impairment of cerebellar or vestibular function or of postural sensation (sensory ataxia) are unsteady and may be unable to tandem walk, i.e., heel-to-toe walking.
- Look at the knees: in a high-stepping gait, they are lifted off the floor more than normal due to foot drop.

- Look at the pelvis and shoulders. In a waddling gait of proximal myopathies, there is marked rotation of both.
- Does the patient have normal arm swing? Arm swing may be reduced in patients who have an extrapyramidal syndrome. This is often more marked on one side than the other, especially in idiopathic Parkinson's disease.
- How well does the patient turn around? Patients who have an extrapyramidal syndrome or ataxia perform this with difficulty. Patients with idiopathic Parkinson's disease turn in a series of movements or *en bloc*.
- Ask the patient to walk on their toes (S1) and then heels (L5). Patients with a common peroneal nerve palsy and L5 or S1 radiculopathy will find this difficult.
- Perform Romberg test. Ask the patient to stand with feet together and eyes closed. The test is positive if the patient is more unsteady with eyes closed than with eyes open. This occurs in patients with a sensory ataxia who have impaired proprioception or, more rarely, vestibular dysfunction.

COMMON PITFALLS

Romberg test is a test for impaired proprioception and is not a test for cerebellar dysfunction. In addition, it cannot be tested reliably in patients with a cerebellar or vestibular disorder or moderate-to-severe weakness from any cause, because the patient will be unsteady irrespective of whether there is a sensory ataxia.

DIFFERENTIAL DIAGNOSIS OF GAIT DISORDERS

Gait of cerebellar ataxia

Patients with cerebellar ataxia stand and walk unsteadily, as if they are drunk. They soon begin to compensate for this by adopting a broad base with feet further apart. The gait is unsteady with irregularity of stride. Their trunk sways and the patient may veer towards one side. In mild cases, the only manifestation of gait disturbance may be difficulty in walking heel-toe in a straight line (i.e., tandem walking).

111

On neurological examination, there may also be nystagmus, dysarthria and cerebellar signs in the limbs. Ataxia may be absent in the limbs and apparent only in the gait when the lesion is in the midline (cerebellar vermis.), so-called truncal ataxia. See Chapter 12 for further information on cerebellar dysfunction.

Causes include:

- alcoholic cerebellar degeneration
- multiple sclerosis
- vascular disease, e.g., ischaemic, haemorrhagic, arteriovenous malformations
- anticonvulsant therapy, e.g., phenytoin, carbamazepine
- posterior fossa tumours
- cerebellar paraneoplastic syndrome
- hereditary cerebellar ataxias

Hemiparetic gait

Patients with a hemiparetic gait have a characteristic posture on one side of flexion and internal rotation of the upper limb and extension of the lower limb. The leg moves stiffly and is swung around in a semicircle to avoid scraping the foot across the floor. However, such scraping does occur to some extent and the toe and outer sole of the shoe become worn.

Causes include:

- cortical or internal capsular strokes
- cerebral hemispheric tumour
- traumatic lesions

Spastic gait

A spastic gait is seen in patients who have spastic paraparesis. The legs move slowly and stiffly and the thighs are strongly adducted such that in severe cases the legs may even cross as the patient walks (scissor gait). The feet may be plantar flexed and inverted and the toes may scuff the ground.

Causes include:

- spinal cord compression
- trauma/spinal surgery
- birth injuries or congenital deformities: cerebral palsy
- multiple sclerosis
- motor neurone disease
- parasagittal meningioma
- subacute combined degeneration of the cord

Parkinsonian gait

The patient often has a stooped and flexed posture with loss of arm swing, which is almost always more marked on one side in idiopathic Parkinson's disease. The steps are short and the patient shuffles. There may be difficulty starting and stopping. Turning may occur as multiple small steps or *en bloc* (i.e., not smoothly but in stiff, stuttering movements). Having started to walk, the patient leans forward and the pace quickens, as though the patient is attempting to catch up on himself (festinant gait).

Gait of sensory ataxia

Sensory ataxia arises from impaired proprioception caused by a lesion of the peripheral nerves, posterior roots, dorsal columns in the spinal cord or, rarely, the ascending afferent fibres to the parietal lobes. The gait is unsteady and wide-based and often stamping. Romberg test is positive and there is impaired perception of joint position on examination of the lower limbs.

Causes include:

1. Posterior spinal cord lesions:
   - multiple sclerosis
   - cervical spondylosis
   - tumours
   - vitamin B_{12} deficiency
   - tabes dorsalis (tertiary syphilis)
2. Sensory peripheral neuropathies:
   - hereditary: Charcot–Marie–Tooth disease
   - metabolic: diabetes
   - inflammatory: Guillain–Barré syndrome
   - malignancy: myeloma, paraneoplastic syndrome
   - toxic: alcohol, drugs (e.g., isoniazid)

Steppage gait

Steppage gait arises from weakness of the pretibial and peroneal muscles of lower motor neurone type. The patient has foot drop and is unable to dorsiflex and to evert the foot. The leg is lifted high on walking so that the toes clear the ground and there is, therefore, exaggerated hip flexion. On striking the floor again, there is a slapping noise. Shoe soles are worn on the anterior and lateral aspects.

Causes include:

1. Common peroneal nerve palsy, e.g., from
   - mechanical compression
   - fibular fracture (unilateral foot drop)
   - mononeuritis of the common peroneal nerve.
2. Anterior horn cell disease, e.g., polio, motor neurone disease (often asymmetrical foot drop).
3. Charcot–Marie–Tooth disease (bilateral foot drop).

Myopathic gait

The myopathic gait is often called a waddling gait and is caused by weakness of the proximal muscles of the lower limb girdle. The weight is alternately placed on each leg, with the opposite hip and side of the trunk tilting up towards the weight-bearing side. However, the weak gluteal muscles cannot stabilize the weight-bearing hip, which sways outward, with the opposite pelvis and trunk dropping. The patient will shift their weight over the weight-bearing leg so that the shoulders will drop on the side opposite to the hip drop.

Causes include:

- Muscular dystrophies: Duchenne, Becker, myotonic.
- Endocrine myopathies: Cushing disease, hypo- and hyperthyroidism.
- Inflammatory myopathies: polymyositis and dermatomyositis.

Apraxic gait

Disease of the frontal lobes gives rise to an apraxic gait. The patient walks with feet placed apart and with small, hesitant steps, which may be described as walking on ice or *marche au petit pas*. There is difficulty with initiation of walking and, in advanced cases, it might seem as though the patient's feet are stuck to the floor. There are no abnormalities of power, sensation or coordination. There may be other signs of frontal cortical dysfunction (e.g., a grasp or rooting reflex); the tendon reflexes may be brisk and the plantar responses extensor.

Causes include:

- subcortical ischaemic leucoencephalopathy 'small vessel disease'
- hydrocephalus including normal pressure hydrocephalus
- frontal lobe tumours, e.g., meningioma
- frontal subdural haematomas (bilateral)
- frontal contusions following head injury

Antalgic gait

The antalgic gait arises from pain (e.g., a painful hip or knee due to arthritis). The patient tends to bear weight mainly on the unaffected side, only briefly putting weight onto the affected side.

Functional gait

A functional or nonorganic gait might arise from psychological or behavioural disturbance. It does not conform to any of the descriptions given above. It can take a number of forms and is inconsistent in character. There are no objective abnormal neurological signs on formal examination. There are often other positive features of an underlying psychiatric disturbance.

> **HINTS AND TIPS**
>
> The character of a patient's gait will provide clues to the clinical signs that might be expected on further neurological examination. The abnormal types of gait are summarized below:
> - Ataxic: broad-based and unsteady
> - Hemiplegic: unilateral flexed posture of the upper limb and extended posture of the lower limb
> - Spastic paraparesis: stiff, slow movements of the legs; scissoring posture of the legs if severe
> - Parkinsonian: flexed posture, shuffling small-stepped gait with loss of arm swing
> - Sensory ataxia: high-stepped stamping gait
> - Steppage: foot drop
> - Myopathic: waddling gait
> - Apraxic: hesitant walking on ice gait
> - Nonorganic: bizarre and variable

● Chapter Summary

- Close examination of gait can often point towards the underlying neurological diagnosis. Assessment of stride length and stride width is of particular importance, because this can differentiate between different conditions such as ataxia (wide-based gait), Parkinson's disease (small shuffling steps) and spastic gait (stiff and slow).

UKMLA Conditions
Cerebral palsy and hypoxic–ischaemic encephalopathy
Muscular dystrophies
Parkinson's disease
Spinal cord compression
Spinal cord injury
Stroke

UKMLA Presentations
Abnormal development/developmental delay
Head injury
Limb weakness
Limp
Unsteadiness

The red, painful eye

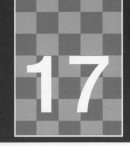

Red eye is among the commonest ophthalmic presentations to general practitioners, accident and emergency departments and high street opticians. It is usually accompanied by some degree of pain/discomfort, ranging from the mild (e.g., blepharitis and conjunctivitis) to the severe (e.g., scleritis, iritis and acute angle closure).

The red, painful eye usually suggests a disorder in the anterior segment – i.e., the front parts of the eye (conjunctiva, sclera/episclera, cornea, iris and lens).

It is important to be able to distinguish between mild, self-limiting causes of red eye, such as conjunctivitis, and sight-threatening causes, such as primary angle closure, iritis, scleritis and microbial keratitis.

DIFFERENTIAL DIAGNOSIS

Differential diagnoses are shown in Table 17.1.

RED FLAG

- Painful unilateral red eye
- Reduced visual acuity/vision loss
- Photophobia
- Unequal or misshapen pupils
- Headache

Table 17.1 Common differential diagnoses of a red, painful eye

Differential	Discharge	Vision	Conjunctiva	Pupil	Cornea	Anterior chamber	Eye pressure
Subconjunctival haemorrhage	No	Unaffected	Bright red	Normal	Clear	Quiet	Normal
Blepharitis	Occasional	Unaffected	Injected vessels	Normal	Clear	Quiet	Normal
Conjunctivitis	Yes	Unaffected	Injected vessels and formces	Normal	Clear	Quiet	Normal
Trauma – abrasion/FB	Watering	Depending on severity	Injected vessels	Normal	Abrasion/FB	Quiet	Normal
Keratitis	Watering	May be affected	Injected vessels	Normal	White lesions, hazy	Possible cells	Possibly elevated
Iritis	No	May be affected	Injected around cornea	Small, fixed, irregular	Keratic precipitates	Cells	Possibly elevated
Episcleritis	NO	Unaffected	Sectoral deep injection	Normal	Normal	Normal	Normal
Scleritis	No	Maybe affected	Sectoral deep 'brick red' injection	Normal	Normal	Possible cells	Normal
Primary angle closure	Watering	Reduced	Entre eye red	Fixed, mid-dilated	Hazy	Shallow cells	Elevated

FB, *Foreign body;* IOP, *intraocular pressure.*
(*From* Crash Course: ENT, Dermatology, and Ophthalmology. *3rd ed. Elsevier.*)

HISTORY

Description of pain:

- Grittiness and irritation – suggestive of conjunctivitis or blepharitis.
- Itching characteristic of allergic conjunctivitis.
- Sharp pain, if experienced after trauma, may suggest a corneal foreign body or corneal abrasion.
- Eye watering is usually an accompanying symptom.
- Pain exacerbated by bright lights – photophobia – is usually a feature of anterior uveitis/iritis.
- A dull, boring ache is characteristically described in anterior scleritis. Episcleritis can look similar, but the pain is usually milder, and patients will never volunteer that the pain is severe enough to keep them up at night, which they may do with scleritis.

DURATION OF SYMPTOMS

- Patients who have experienced trauma whether it be a corneal abrasion, corneal foreign body or a chemical injury will be symptomatic immediately and will present to emergency services accordingly.
- Viral (Fig. 17.1) and bacterial (Fig. 17.2) conjunctivitis may have a period of latency whereby the eye may be mildly irritated for up to 10 days before the redness and discharge develop.
- A red, discharging eye over a period of months is unlikely to be bacterial or viral conjunctivitis as these are self-limiting

conditions which resolve within 21 days. In these circumstances, one should consider the possibility of *Chlamydia* conjunctivitis, where there is a thick and rope-like mucopurulent discharge.

ASSOCIATED SYMPTOMS

Watering

Mild-to-moderate watering may be seen in blepharitis or conjunctivitis.

Excessive lacrimation may be seen in corneal abrasions, corneal foreign bodies, subtarsal foreign body (where a foreign body lodges under the top lid and scratches the corneal epithelium with each blink) and trichiasis (where a lash is misdirected onto the globe – this may be particularly uncomfortable if it rubs on the cornea).

Discharge

Clear discharge with stickiness of the eye lids in the morning is common in blepharitis. Discharge between viral and bacterial conjunctivitis may be indistinguishable, although in bacterial may be yellow/green compared to yellow/white in viral.

The discharge in *Chlamydia* conjunctivitis is thick and accumulates in rope-like strands. Gonococcal conjunctival discharge in babies (as ophthalmia neonatorum) is excessive, even 'explosive'.

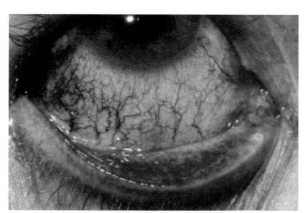

Fig. 17.1 Viral conjunctivitis, generalized conjunctival redness seen here. (From Boruchoff SA. *Anterior Segment Disease: A Diagnostic Color Atlas*. Boston: Butterworth-Heinemann. 2001; with permission.)

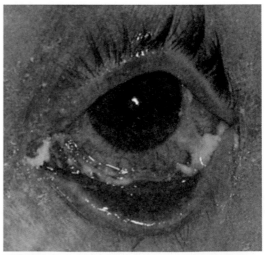

Fig. 17.2 Acute purulent conjunctivitis. (From Shiland B. *Medical Assistant: Integumentary, Sensory Systems, Patient Care and Communication—Module A*. Elsevier Inc. 2016.)

Photophobia

Photophobia is characteristic of anterior uveitis/iritis. However, it may also be a symptom of any condition which causes ciliary muscle spasms, including microbial keratitis, herpetic keratitis, corneal abrasion and recurrent erosion syndrome.

Visual loss

Conditions affecting the external lids (blepharitis), the conjunctiva (conjunctivitis) and the episclera (episcleritis) do not usually affect vision, except where the patient is viewing the world through a film of pus or tears (which can of course be wiped away).

Blurred vision in the context of a red, painful eye will usually suggest either corneal involvement (microbial keratitis, herpetic keratitis, corneal oedema in acute angle closure, large corneal abrasion) or a significant inflammatory component (scleritis or iritis).

Previous medical history

A number of underlying medical conditions may be associated with red, painful eyes. A recent history of upper respiratory tract viral illness such as a cough or sore throat may be associated with the onset of viral conjunctivitis.

Previous ophthalmic history

Ask about recent surgery. Acute iritis, and more seriously endophthalmitis, may occur following cataract surgery. In general, endophthalmitis occurs within 10 days of surgery, whereas iritis may occur weeks after the surgery.

Anterior uveitis/iritis and herpes simplex keratitis are recurrent conditions and patients may volunteer their diagnosis from the outset. Refractive error – acute angle closure is more likely to occur in elderly patients with short, hypermetropic (long-sighted) eyes with coexistent cataracts.

Always ask about history of contact lens use. Contact lenses predispose to microbial causes of keratitis, in particular soft lenses. Ask about whether patient sleeps in contact lenses or swims/showers in them (the latter may point to a diagnosis of acanthamoeba).

EXAMINATION

A systematic examination of the anterior segment structures should easily identify the cause of the red, painful eye.

External lids and adnexa

Before examining a patient's lids, look at their face. Do they have features of acne rosacea? Is there a vesicular rash over one side of the forehead (herpes zoster ophthalmicus – shingles)? Do they have features suggestive of thyroid eye disease, such as proptosis?

Inflammation, redness and swelling of the lids indicate cellulitis, either orbital or preseptal. As it is the more severe condition, one must exclude features of orbital cellulitis such as proptosis, double vision, loss of colour vision, reduced vision, and swollen optic disc.

If you suspect conjunctivitis, palpate the preauricular lymph nodes. Tender preauricular lymphadenopathy is a feature of viral conjunctivitis. Look for signs of herpetic lesions – cold sores or the vesicular lesions of herpes zoster (shingles).

Examine the lid margin looking for features of blepharitis which includes crusting of the lashes, telangiectatic vessels at the lid margin, irregular lid margin, meibomian gland orifice capping, and inflamed meibomian glands.

Internal lids

Always evert the lids; this way you will be able to identify and remove subtarsal foreign bodies.

Inspection of the inner aspect of the lids is a reliable way of diagnosing conjunctivitis (look for follicles and papillae).

Conjunctiva

If the conjunctiva is inflamed, injected with follicles +/– tender preauricular lymphadenopathy, viral conjunctivitis is likely. Subconjunctival haemorrhages and chemosis ('water-logged conjunctiva') may also occur in this condition (see Fig. 17.3).
If the conjunctiva is inflamed, injected with subtarsal and bulbar papillae and there is excessive purulent discharge, then bacterial conjunctivitis is likely (see Fig. 17.4).

Acute chemosis and papillae are a feature of allergic/atopic conjunctivitis, as well as chemical conjunctivitis which may be seen following a chemical injury.

Table 17.2 shows the features of bacterial and viral conjunctivitis.

Sclera/episclera

The redness seen in scleritis can be distinguished from episcleritis in a number of ways. In scleritis, the redness is sectoral but takes on a brick-like, violet colour with the distension of all the scleral and episcleral vessels which may appear tortuous. This redness is characteristic when viewed in room light. The patient may also report severe aching pain when the lid is pressed directly over the area of inflammation (see Fig. 17.5).

The injection in episcleritis is also sectoral, but much milder, with a less striking reddish hue. A single drop of phenylephrine 2.5% will allow the episcleral vessels to constrict in episcleritis,

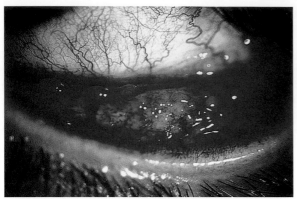

Fig. 17.3 Chronic follicular conjunctivitis. Follicles are small and resemble grains of rice, with a surrounding vascular bed. They are characteristic of viral and chlamydial conjunctivitis (where the follicles are much larger). (From Kanski JJ. *Clinical Ophthalmology: A Synopsis.* 5th ed. New York: Butterworth-Heinemann; 2004.)

Table 17.2 Features of bacterial and viral conjunctivitis

Type	Features
Bacterial conjunctivitis	• Inflamed conjunctiva • Purulent discharge • Eyes 'stuck together' in the morning • Papillae may be evident • Responds quickly to a broad-spectrum- topical antibiotic
Viral conjunctivitis	• Inflamed conjunctiva • Serous/watery discharge • Follicles are prominent • +/– tender preauricular lymphadenopathy • May have history of recent upper respiratory tract infection • Subconjunctival haemorrhage and chemosis ('waterlogged conjunctiva') may be present • No specific treatment in most cases

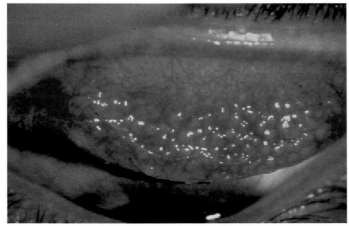

Fig. 17.4 Bacterial conjunctivitis with velvet-like appearance of papilla seen on upper eyelid. Papillae are larger polygonal 'bumps' with a central vascular core. They are nonspecific and may be seen in bacterial conjunctivitis, allergic conjunctivitis, foreign bodies (including chronic contact lens wear) and floppy eyelid syndrome. (From Adkinson NF, et al. *Middleton's Allergy 2-Volume Set.* 8th ed. Saunders; 2014.)

making the eye appear whiter (see Fig. 17.6). This does not happen in scleritis, which may be a useful feature in distinguishing between the two conditions.

An inflammatory 'nodule' may be present in both episcleritis and scleritis.

See Table 17.3 to differentiate episcleritis and scleritis.

Cornea

The appearance of whitish/cloudy lesions, called infiltrates, within the anterior corneal stroma is a feature of corneal inflammation – keratitis.

Where corneal infiltrates with overlying epithelial fluorescein staining occur in the context of contact lens wear, microbial keratitis is the most likely diagnosis. In this circumstance, one should treat as such, before microbiological confirmation from corneal scrapes (which takes 48 hours) is received.

Corneal oedema – waterlogging of the cornea – is usually apparent as a hazing and thickening of the cornea. It may be present in a localised form in any form of infective keratitis. A more diffuse, generalised form may occur in acute elevations of intraocular pressure, as may occur in acute angle closure.

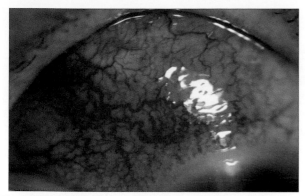

Fig. 17.5 Scleritis with a violaceous hue caused by deep inflammation. (From Yanoff M, Duker J. *Ophthalmology*. 6th ed. Elsevier; 2023.)

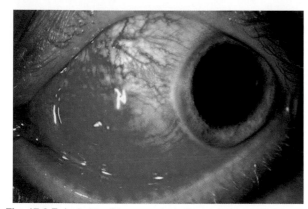

Fig. 17.6 Episcleritis. Close-up view of eye shows redness and visible blood vessels. (From Hegde V, et al. Episcleritis: an association with IgA nephropathy. *Cont Lens Anterior Eye*, 32(3):141–142, 2009.)

HINTS AND TIPS

The instillation of topical fluorescein and illumination with cobalt blue light is useful in detecting corneal epithelial pathology including:

• Corneal abrasions
• Dry eye – characterized by punctate ('spotty') fluorescein staining
• Microbial keratitis
• Viral keratitis (dendritic ulcers) – characteristic tree-like branching of herpes simplex

Anterior chamber

Full examination of the anterior chamber – the fluid space between the cornea and the iris – is difficult without the use of the slit lamp. There are some features which may be apparent using a pen torch or the direct ophthalmoscope:
See Table 17.4 and Figs 17.7–17.9 for features to look for when examining the anterior chamber.

Iris and pupil

Acute angle closure may present with a number of symptoms and iris/ pupil signs:

• Reduced vision.
• Nausea or vomiting.
• Fixed, mid-dilated pupil.
• Anterior iris bowing (iris bombé).
• Peripheral iridocorneal touch, as well as shallowing/ narrowing of the anterior chamber.

Table 17.3 Differentiating features between episcleritis and scleritis

Feature	Episcleritis	Scleritis
Incidence	Common	Rare
Red eye	Yes	Yes
Signs	Superficial, bright red	Black-blue hue
Pain	Nil to mild	Moderate to severe
Associated systemic disease	Rare	Common
Visual disturbances	Extremely rare	Not uncommon
Use of phenylephrine 2.5% drops	Blanches the conjunctival and episcleral vessels	Does not blanch scleral vessels
Management	Conservative – sometimes artificial drops may be used	Urgent referral to ophthalmologist – oral NSAIDs, glucocorticoids, or immunosuppressive drugs in severe cases

Table 17.4 Examination of anterior chamber using pen torch/direct ophthalmoscope and slit lamp

Examination of anterior chamber features	Description	Associated with	Seen by pen torch/ direct ophthalmoscope?	Seen by slit lamp?
Hypopyon	Settling of inflammatory cells	Endophthalmitis Infective keratitis Severe uveitis	Yes	Yes
Hyphaema	Settling of red blood cells	Recent trauma/surgery	Yes	Yes
Anterior chamber shallowing/flattening	Feature of acute angle glaucoma	Acute angle closure glaucoma	Difficult to assess	Yes, using angled slit beam
Cells and flare	Cells – circulating inflammatory cells Flare – protein exudate	Anterior uveitis	No	Yes

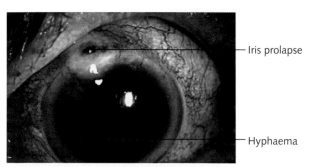

— Iris prolapse

— Hyphaema

Fig. 17.7 Blunt trauma. Hyphaema and globe rupture with iris prolapse. (From Feather A, et al. *Kumar and Clark's Clinical Medicine*. 10th ed. Elsevier; 2021.)

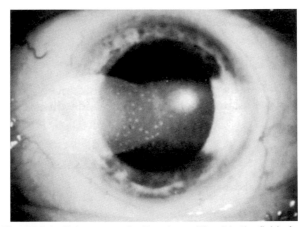

Fig. 17.9 A slit-lamp examination shows "flare" in the fluid of the anterior chamber (caused by increased protein content) and keratic precipitates on the posterior surface of the cornea, representing small collections of inflammatory cells). (Courtesy of Dr Henry J. Kaplan.)

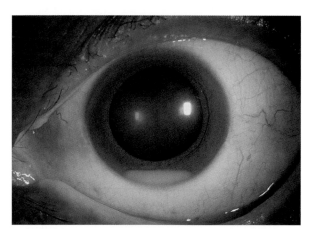

Fig. 17.8 Hypopyon. A creamy white exudate rich in white blood cells produced as a result of intense intraocular inflammation. The exudate settles in the dependent aspect of the anterior chamber due to gravity. (From Rich R, et al. *Clinical Immunology*. 6th ed. Elsevier; 2023.)

The cornea may be hazy secondary to oedema and the intra-ocular pressure is elevated. Cataract may also be a predisposing factor.

Iritis may be associated with:

- Posterior synechiae – these are inflammatory adhesions between the pupillary margin of the iris and the anterior lens capsule. When one attempts to dilate the pupil pharmacologically, the pupil may be so stuck down as to not dilate at all, or it may take on an irregular shape secondary to focal adhesions.
- Iris nodules (especially in sarcoid-related anterior uveitis).

Intraocular pressure

This may be elevated in a number of conditions but is seldom in itself a cause of pain, except when raised to high levels in a short time frame. Causes include:

- Acute angle closure.
- Rubeosis.
- Some forms of anterior uveitis – 'hypertensive uveitis'. Another, rarer form, Posner–Schlossman syndrome, is associated with high IOP, very mild anterior reaction and one or two keratic precipitates. Hypertensive uveitis is a common presenting feature of toxoplasma-associated uveitis, so always remember to look in the fundus for evidence of active toxoplasma retinitis. Herpes zoster uveitis is also frequently associated with raised pressure.

INVESTIGATIONS

In ophthalmology, most clinical diagnoses can be made on the basis of history and examination without recourse to specific tests. There are a few important investigations to be aware of when a patient presents with a red eye:

- Conjunctival swabs (viral, bacterial, chlamydial) if an infective conjunctivitis is suspected.
- Corneal scrapes – taken if a contact lens-related ulcer/infiltrate is seen. Specimens are plated onto a microscope slide (for rapid microscopy) and onto blood agar, chocolate agar, Sabouraud agar and brain–heart infusion broth (if fungi suspected), and *Escherichia coli* seeded nonnutrient agar (if acanthamoeba suspected).

Systemic investigations are rarely performed in first presentations of scleritis and iritis. Investigations are performed if the presentation is atypical or if recurrent:

- Iritis screen – chest X-ray (tuberculosis/sarcoid), serum ACE (sarcoid), VDRL (syphilis), HLA B27 (ankylosing spondylitis).
- Scleritis screen – cANCA (Wegener).

CT is useful in the diagnosis of orbital conditions. B-scan ultrasonography may be required if a view of the posterior segment is not possible, e.g., because of hyphema.

Chapter Summary

- Differentiation of the different causes of red eye is important in order to distinguish between ophthalmic emergencies that require a referral to ophthalmology and non sight-threatening causes that can be managed within a primary care setting.
- Identification of different types of conjunctivitis can be recognised through features of presentation. Bacterial conjunctivitis usually produces purulent discharge and presence of follicles, whereas viral conjunctivitis produces watery discharge and presence of papillae.
- Episcleritis and scleritis can be differentiated through the use of phenylephrine 2.5% drops which cause blanching of vessels in episcleritis and nonblanching in scleritis.
- When taking ophthalmic red eye history: description of pain, duration of symptoms, and associated symptoms including watering, discharge, photophobia and visual changes should be considered.
- Recognition of red flag symptoms such as acute painful red eye, photophobia and mid-dilated pupil should increase suspicion of acute angle closure glaucoma. This should be treated as an ophthalmic emergency.
- Anterior uveitis is the most common type of uveitis which involves the iris. Suspicion should indicate urgent referral to ophthalmologist.

UKMLA Conditions
Acute glaucoma
Conjunctivitis
Infective keratitis
Iritis
Scleritis
Uveitis

UKMLA Presentations
Acute change in or loss of vision
Eye pain/discomfort
Facial/periorbital swelling
Red eye

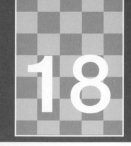
Patients with gradual change of vision usually present for the first time in an optometric practice, on the assumption that the problem will be remedied with the dispensing of glasses. Often the patient will have a refractive error and, as such, will usually improve with glasses.

DIFFERENTIAL DIAGNOSIS

The most common reason vision is affected in older age is usually secondary to cataract, where vision will also improve, up to a level, with refraction and updated glasses (See Fig. 18.1). Often presentation to hospital eye services is made when no improvement can be made on refraction (i.e., glasses do not help).

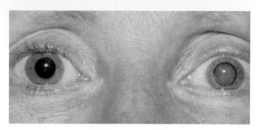

Fig. 18.1 Cataract. Notice the cloudiness of the left eye characteristic of advanced cataracts. The right eye is not cloudy. (From Patton K, et al. *The Human Body in Health & Disease.* 8th ed. Elsevier; 2024.)

- Toxic, drug-related.
- Tumours.

HINTS AND TIPS

COMMON REFRACTIVE ERRORS

- Myopia – short sightedness
- Hyperopia – long sightedness
- Astigmatism – 'rugby ball-shaped' cornea
- Presbyopia – middle age onset poor reading vision

Common causes of gradual visual loss

- Refractive error (see Fig. 18.3).
- Cataract
- Posterior capsular opacification (PCO) (post-cataract surgery)
- Age-related macular degeneration (ARMD)
- Primary open angle glaucoma (POAG)

Rarer causes of gradual visual loss

- Extremes of refractive error – keratoconus (see Fig. 18.2), myopic degeneration.
- Inherited eye disease.

HISTORY

Duration of symptoms

It can be difficult to get an accurate history of gradual visual loss in terms of time scale. Patients may attend an optometrist for a routine check-up and be found to have deteriorated since their visit the previous year; in this case, the patient will only become aware of the problem when it is pointed out by the optometrist. Detecting gradual monocular (in one eye) visual changes can be particularly difficult as the other (normal) eye will compensate.

Associated symptoms

- 'Negative' scotomata occur most commonly following optic nerve disease. The patient is not aware of their central field loss until they try to read.
- By contrast, patients are aware of 'positive' scotomata. Patients with macular degeneration are constantly aware of their central field deficit.
- Visual distortion (metamorphopsia), increase in image size (macropsia) and decrease in image size (micropsia) are reflections of changes in the relative positions of photoreceptors and are a feature of macular disease.

See Table 18.1 for common associated symptoms of gradual visual loss.

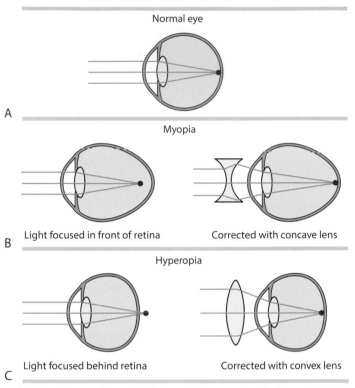

Fig. 18.3 Refraction in (A) normal vision; (B) myopia and (C) hyperopia/hypermetropia. (From Shiland B. *Medical Assistant: Integumentary, Sensory Systems, Patient Care and Communication—Module A.* Elsevier Inc.; 2016.)

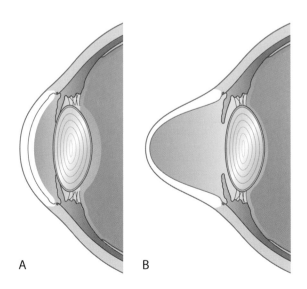

Fig. 18.2 (A) Normal eye. (B) Keratoconus. Note thinning of the cornea as well as the forward protrusion. (From Stein HA, et al. *The Ophthalmic Assistant: A Text for Allied and Associated Ophthalmic Personnel.* 11th ed. Elsevier; 2023.)

HINTS AND TIPS

Remember to ask about conditions that could increase the risk of developing gradual loss of vision including, diabetes mellitus (cataract, ARMD, POAG), hypertension (ARMD and POAG), and dyslipidaemia.

Table 18.1 Common associated symptoms of gradual visual loss with relevant pathologies

Symptom	Pathology
Glare	Cataract
Floaters	Vitritis, retinal detachment
Night blindness (nyctalopia)	Retinitis pigmentosa (RP)
Peripheral visual loss ('bumping into things')	Late-stage glaucoma, RP
Positive central (dark) scotoma	Age-related macular degeneration (ARMD)
Visual distortion (metamorphopsia)	Wet age-related macular degeneration ARMD

Family history

Family history is important as it may point to an inherited condition such as retinitis pigmentosa or Stargardt disease. If a hereditary disorder is suspected, you should always map out a family tree.

Drug history

Do not forget to take a detailed drug history as some chronic medications may cause poor vision, vigabatrin, tamoxifen, chloroquine, and ethambutol being well-known examples. Long-term corticosteroid use can cause cataract and secondary raised eye pressure (glaucoma).

Alcohol and tobacco intake may be useful in identifying patients at risk of vitamin B_{12} and folate deficiency that can cause an optic neuropathy. Smoking tobacco also increases the likelihood of developing cataracts and ARMD.

EXAMINATION

Visual acuity

An accurate assessment of visual acuity (VA) (by Snellen or Log-MAR chart) is essential, if possible, with the patient wearing their current spectacles (if any) as this is how they 'see the world'.

Rechecking VA using a pinhole is essential; an improvement in vision usually points to a condition that may be improved with up-to-date glasses (e.g. cataract or refractive error).

Colour vision

- Usually assessed using Ishihara colour plates.
- Loss of colour vision is an early sign of optic neuropathy.

Visual field

- May be examined by confrontation, or more formally by static automated perimetry.
- Central scotoma is a feature of macular disease. An Amsler grid is useful for examining the central field in macular disease and the presence of metamorphopsia.
- An enlarged blind spot is a feature of chronic optic nerve swelling (e.g., idiopathic intracranial hypertension – IIH).

Pupils

A relative afferent pupillary defect is ocular examination finding that suggests asymmetric disease of the optic nerve or retina (see Fig. 18.4). Causes include optic neuropathies, retinal artery or vein occlusions and retinal detachment.

Red reflex

Opacities within the red reflex may be observed in cataract. 'Hazy' visual media may be seen in cataract, PCO or corneal pathology. Loss of the red reflex is apparent in vitreous haemorrhage, retinal detachment and ocular tumours.

Fundoscopy

Systemic examination of:

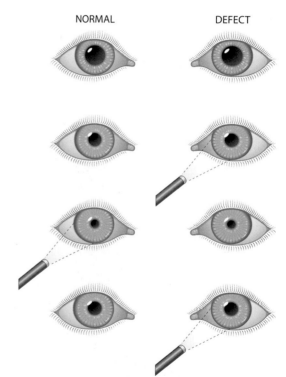

NORMAL   DEFECT

Fig. 18.4 Relative afferent pupillary defect (Marcus Gunn pupil). This patient has an abnormal left optic nerve. In ambient light (*top row*), the pupils are equal. As the abnormal eye is illuminated (*second row*), only modest constriction is noted. As the light is swung to the normal eye (*third row*), the pupils constrict briskly. When the light is swung back to the abnormal eye (*bottom row*), paradoxical dilation is noted. (From Friedman JN, Kaiser PK, Pineda A. *Massachusetts Ear & Eye Infirmary Illustrated Manual of Ophthalmology*. 3rd ed. Philadelphia, Saunders; 2009.)

Optic nerve

- Optic disc pallor suggests chronic optic neuropathy (see Fig. 18.5).
- Optic disc 'cupping' (enlarged optic disc cup with thinning of the neuroretinal rim) is a characteristic feature of glaucomatous optic neuropathy.

Macula

Drusen (deep yellow flecks) at the macula are a characteristic feature of macular degeneration. As 'dry' macular degeneration progresses, dark pigmentary changes as well as atrophy may be observed at the macula (see Fig. 18.6).

Retinal periphery and vasculature

Peripheral patchy 'bone spicule' pigmentation is a feature of retinitis pigmentosa. The retinal vessels may also be attenuated (the optic disc may also display 'waxy pallor') (see Fig. 18.7).

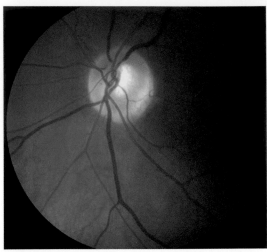

Fig. 18.5 Optic atrophy. Note disc pallor and lack of visible nerve fiber layer striations. (From Aminoff MJ, Josephson SA. *Aminoff's Neurology and General Medicine.* 6th ed. Elsevier; 2021.)

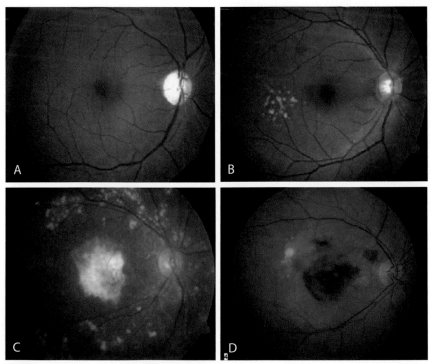

Fig. 18.6 Example of AMD's symptoms: (A) image fundus image of healthy eye; (B) image fundus with drusens; (C) dry (atrophic) AMD; (D) wet (neovascular or exudative) AMD. *AMD*, Age-related macular degeneration. (El-Baz AS, Suri J. *State of the Art in Neural Networks and their Applications.* Academic Press; 2021.)

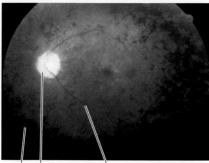

Bone spicules   Waxy pallor   Attenuated vessels

Fig. 18.7 Retinitis pigmentosa demonstrating dense retinal pigment epithelium changes, optic disc pallor and attenuated retinal vessels. (From Friedman NJ, Kaiser PK, Pineda II R. *The Massachusetts Eye and Ear Infirmary Illustrated Manual of Ophthalmology.* 5th ed. Elsevier; 2021.)

INVESTIGATIONS

These are often not necessary as the diagnosis should normally be apparent from history and examination:

B-scan ultrasound – may be necessary if fundal examination is precluded by a dense cataract. This is needed to exclude the possibility of a 'sudden' cause for visual loss, given that the cataract is of chronic onset.

Blood tests – in particular B_{12} and folate; may be useful to rule out nutritional optic neuropathy.

Electrodiagnostic testing (visual evoked potential, electro-oculogram, electro-retinogram) has two important roles in gradual visual loss:

- Can identify the location (i.e., rod, cone, macular, optic nerve) of the visual dysfunction.
- Can be used to identify nonorganic (i.e., 'functional') visual loss. By the same token, it can be used to estimate what the VA should be given the observed integrity of the visual pathway.

● Chapter Summary

- The most common cause of gradual change in vision in older age is cataract and age-related macular degeneration. Recognizing risk factors for these conditions is essential, e.g., smoking, diabetes mellitus.
- Most patients present when refractive correction is unable to solve their vision.
- Examination with fundoscopy is essential for identification of conditions such as age-related macular degeneration and primary open angle glaucoma.
- Investigations are not essential for majority of diagnoses of gradual loss of vision and should be apparent from history and examination alone.

UKMLA Conditions
Cataracts
Chronic glaucoma
Macular degeneration
Optic neuritis
Visual field defect

UKMLA Presentations
Gradual change in vision
Loss of red reflex

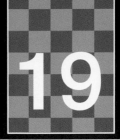
DIFFERENTIAL DIAGNOSIS

The causes of sudden change in vision may be classified as either painful or painless. See Tables 19.2 and 19.3 for common causes of painful/painless, suddden change in vision.

See Table 19.1 for list of differentials for sudden change in vision.

HINTS AND TIPS

When confronted with a patient complaining of a sudden change in vision, it is important to remember that common things are common. Certain disorders get more common according to the demographics of the patient. Bear this in mind, so you can narrow down your differential even before you take the history.

Patient demographics

Age

Some conditions are unlikely under the age of 60, particularly ischaemic optic neuropathy; the arteritic form (i.e., giant cell arteritis) is vanishingly rare in this group. Retino-vascular occlusive conditions (venous and arterial occlusions) are also relatively unusual in a younger age group; if encountered one should suspect an underlying thrombophilic tendency.

Sex

Benign intracranial hypertension is almost exclusively a condition affecting young (usually overweight) females. Demyelinating optic neuritis is also far more common in young females.

Race

Afro-Caribbean descent – always consider the possibility of sickle cell (SC) retinopathy (SC trait); this may present with a vitreous haemorrhage.

Indian subcontinent diabetics – more prone to severe retinopathy (both proliferative complications and maculopathy).

Some forms of uveitis are more common in certain groups:

- Turks/Greeks – Behcet's
- South Americans – toxoplasmosis
- Africans – sarcoidosis

History

Duration of symptoms:

- Immediate loss of vision – suggests a vascular 'event' (venous or arterial occlusion).
- Progressive loss of field over hours, days – retinal detachment.
- Progressive dimming of vision – optic nerve pathology.
- Transient visual loss, lasting seconds, hours – migraine, giant cell arteritis, benign intracranial hypertension.

Associated symptoms

- Painful eye – iritis, scleritis, keratitis and primary angle closure (all may have photophobia too!).
- Headache – headache on waking may be a feature of benign intracranial hypertension (as is buzzing in the ear). The headache in temporal arteritis is characteristically centred on the patient's temple; there may be associated pain in the jaw on chewing ('jaw claudication'). Headache preceded by scintillating lights or 'fortification spectra' is a feature of migraine.
- Photopsia (flashing lights) – this may precede a retinal detachment (or retinal tear). In migraine they are more commonly bilateral; there may be scintillating lights or zig-zag lines.
- Floaters – a sudden increase in floaters may precede retinal detachment. Vitreous haemorrhage and vitritis are also present with floaters.
- Loss of colour appreciation – a characteristic feature of demyelinating optic neuritis.
- Distortion of vision ('metamorphopsia') – exudative (wet) macular degeneration.

Previous ophthalmic history

Certain ophthalmic conditions predispose to particular causes of sudden visual loss:

- Myopia (short-sightedness) – the risk of retinal detachment increases with high myopia.
- Hypermetropia (long-sightedness) – these patients are more prone to primary angle closure, particularly in combination with dense cataract. Also, hypermetropic patients are more likely to have small, crowded optic discs which are more prone to ischaemic optic neuropathy, particularly if the patient is hypertensive.
- Ocular hypertension/glaucoma – predisposes to central retinal vein occlusion.

Table 19.1 Differentials of sudden change in vision

	Retinal detachment (RD)	Posterior vitreous detachment (PVD)	Central retinal artery occlusion (CRAO)	Central retinal vein occlusion (CRVO)	Vitreous haemorrhage	Optic neuritis	Anterior ischemic optic neuropathy
Visual acuity	Sudden loss	Normal	Sudden loss	Sudden loss	Variable – Depending on extent of bleed	Variable Mild – no perception of light	Sudden loss of vision
Other visual symptoms	Flashes (Photopsia) Floaters	Shower of floaters	None	None	Dark floaters	Loss of colour vision (dyschromatopsia) Central scotoma	Nonarteritic – Altitudinal visual field defect; Arteritic - No visual field defect
Pain?	No	No	No	No	No	Yes, especially on eye movement	Yes
Other symptoms	None	None	None	None	None	Multiple sclerosis symptoms: – Uhthoff's phenomenon – Internuclear ophthalmoplegia	Exclude GCA – Jaw claudication – Headache – Tender, palpable temporal artery
Signs	– Visible retinal detachment (looking like a hill) – Retinal breaks – Macula on/off – on requires urgent treatment – RAPD	Weiss ring May be retinal detachment present	– Pale retina – Cherry red spots – There may be RAPD	– Flame haemorrhages – Optic disc oedema There may be RAPD	RBC in anterior vitreous humour	– RAPD – Loss of colour vision – Swollen optic disc – Later progress to pallor of optic disc – Optic atrophy	– RAPD – Swollen optic disc
Investigations	Not required usually clinical diagnosis ?USS/OCT if unsure	None	?USS or fluorescein angiography – retinal blood supply	?USS or fluorescein angiography	None – clinical diagnosis	MRI brain – White matter abnormalities	– ESR – CRP – Platelets – Raised platelets = Temporal artery biopsy
Management	Surgical options Vitrectomy with gas or oil tamponade Scleral buccal Retinal pneumopexy	– None If no associated RD or tears – Retinal breaks = laser to prevent RD	Ocular massage – dislodge the thrombus Lower IOP – acetazolamide ?Ant. chamber paracentesis ?Intra-arterial thrombolysis	? –Pan retinal photocoagulation – Anti-VEGF – If risk of neovascularization	Reassure patient to consider different ways of lying down If it doesn't clear/ associated retinal detachment consider vitrectomy	High-dose steroids	– Arteritic = steroids (high-dose prednisolone/IV methylprednisolone) to be given prior to biopsy results – Nonarteritic = aspirin

RAPD, Relative afferent pupillary defect; GCA, Giant cell arteritis; RBC, Red blood cells; USS, Ultrasound; OCT, Ocular computerised tomography; ESR, Ethrythocye sedimentation rate; CRP, C-reactive protein; RD, Retinal detachment

Table 19.2 Common causes of painful, sudden change in vision

Anatomical location	Examples
Anterior segment	Iritis, scleritis, keratitis, primary angle closure glaucoma
Optic nerve	Optic neuritis (demyelinating), arteritic ischemic optic neuropathy
Intercranial	Migraine, idiopathic intracranial hypertension

Table 19.3 Common causes of painless, sudden change in vision

Anatomical location	Examples
Vitreous	Vitritis, vitreous haemorrhage
Retinal – vascular	Branch retinal vein occlusion Central retinal vein occlusion Branch retinal artery occlusion Central retinal artery occlusion
Retinal – macula	Exudative (wet) age-related macular degeneration, diabetic maculopathy
Retinal	Retinal detachment, retinitis, retinochoroiditis
Optic nerve	Nonarteritic ischaemic optic neuropathy, compressive optic neuropathy
Intracerebral	Stroke

Previous medical history

Hypertension

High blood pressure predisposes patients to venous and arterial occlusions, as well as nonarteritic ischaemic optic neuropathy and stroke.

Diabetes

The commonest presentation of sudden visual loss in a diabetic is vitreous haemorrhage in proliferative diabetic retinopathy, although retinal vein occlusions may also present in this way.

Thyroid/Graves disease

Visual loss in thyroid eye disease may be caused by three mechanisms:

1. Corneal scarring.
2. Raised intraocular pressure.
3. Compressive optic neuropathy.

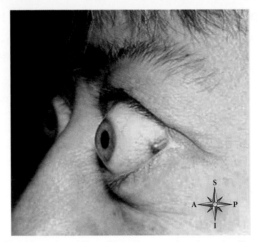

Fig. 19.1 Hyperthyroidism. Note the prominent, protruding eyes (exophthalmos) of this person with Graves' disease. (From Patton K, et al. *The Human Body in Health and Disease*. 8th ed. Elsevier; 2024.)

The last presents acutely. It is important that colour vision and visual field are checked in any patient with thyroid eye disease complaining of reduced vision (Fig. 19.1).

EXAMINATION

Visual acuity

A Snellen chart can be used to examine the visual acuity. (See Chapter 2.)

Colour vision

Ishihara plates can be used to assess colour vision. It is usually reduced in optic nerve parthologies. (See Chapter 2.)

Visual fields

Either to confrontation or by formal perimetry (static or kinetic). Following is a list of visual field defects:

- Homonymous field defects (quadrantinopias, hemianopias) are a feature of stroke.
- Altitudinal defects are a feature of nonarteritic ischaemic optic neuropathy.
- Central scotomata – optic neuritis, macular degeneration.
- Peripheral field loss – retinal detachment.
- Enlarged blind spots – idiopathic intracranial hypertension.

Amsler grid examination is useful for examining the macular central field and to illicit metamorphopsia.

Pupils

An RAPD (relative afferent pupillary defect) is a feature of optic nerve, not macular pathology. It may also be a feature of retinal detachment.

A fixed mid-dilated pupil is a feature of primary angle closure, whereas a small irregular pupil is a feature of anterior uveitis/iritis.

Anterior segment examination

As in Chapter 2, slit lamp examination of the anterior chamber will be helpful in identifying iritis, scleritis and primary angle closure.

Fundoscopy

Vitreous

A dense vitreous haemorrhage may preclude a view of the fundus. Inflammatory cells and debris within the vitreous cavity are a feature of vitritis. Pigment cells in the vitreous are strongly suggestive of a retinal break (tear/hole) or detachment.

Macular pathology

Look for haemorrhages, exudates and oedema which are features of vein occlusion and diabetic maculopathy. Haemorrhages in exudative macular degeneration may present in the preretinal zone, within the retina and in the subretinal space. Drusen may also be present.

Optic nerve pathology

Disc swelling is a feature of most acute optic neuropathies (except retrobulbar neuritis). Disc swelling may also be present in central retinal vein occlusion, posterior scleritis and bilaterally in idiopathic intracranial hypertension.

Retinal vasculature

Dot, blot haemorrhages and exudates in one sector in the distribution of a vein (which may be seen to be occluded – pale) are features of branch vein occlusion (see Fig. 19.3). Central retinal vein occlusions, in contrast, have haemorrhages present in all four quadrants of the retina. In a retinal arterial occlusion, the affected area of retina appears pale yellow owing to retinal oedema; the fovea appears as a cherry red spot (see Fig. 19.2).

Retinal periphery

Retinal detachments appear as mobile retinal 'curtains', billowing with eye movement. They arise from the retinal periphery, where a retinal hole or tear may be observed, and progress towards the posterior pole as fluid collects behind the detaching retina.

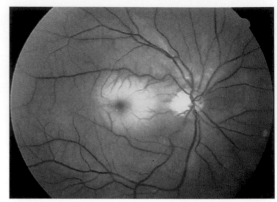

Fig. 19.2 Central retinal artery occlusion. Note the cherry red spot in the centre of the macula, with surrounding whitening of the retina. (From Jankovic J, et al. *Bradley and Daroff's neurology in clinical practice*. 8th ed. Philadelphia, Elsevier; 2022.)

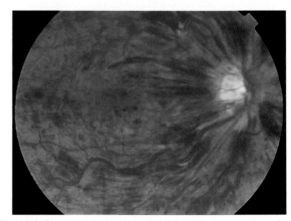

Fig. 19.3 Central retinal vein occlusion with venous tortuosity and dilation, and extensive flame-shaped haemorrhages. (From Kanski J, Bowling B. *Clinical Ophthalmology—a Systematic Approach*. 7th ed. Edinburgh: Saunders; 2011.)

INVESTIGATIONS

Blood tests

ESR and CRP are usually elevated in giant cell arteritis. It is important to check both in patients over 60 who have any features of temporal arteritis, disc swelling or retinal artery occlusion. They should also be checked in patients over 60 with episodes of transient visual loss or unexplained visual loss.

In cases of retinal vein occlusion, full blood count, renal function, lipid screen and glucose should be checked in all cases (as well as blood pressure). In atypical cases (e.g., younger subjects, multiple or recurrent), a thrombophilia screen should be carried out.

B-scan ultrasonography

Useful in cases of vitreous haemorrhage as it can help exclude a retinal detachment, which would require urgent surgical intervention.

Fluorescein angiography

This is a particularly useful photographic test that enables the perfusion of the retinal vasculature to be assessed. It is possible to identify areas of vascular leakage and vascular nonperfusion. It is therefore particularly useful in the diagnosis and in the guiding of the management of exudative vascular conditions (macular degeneration, diabetic retinopathy, vein occlusions, inflammatory vasculopathies) and ischaemic retinopathies (diabetes, vein occlusions).

Imaging

CT of the orbits is useful for excluding any compressive orbital or 'intraconal' cause of reduced vision.

MRI of the brain is required to confirm demyelination as a cause of optic neuritis. An MRI of the brain and orbits should be considered in any cases of unexplained reduced vision or field loss.

Electrodiagnostic testing

In patients with unexplained visual loss, electrodiagnostics may be required to identify a nonorganic cause (i.e., malingering).

● Chapter Summary

- Sudden change in vision can be classified into painful and painless causes where you can then differentiate between different causes.
- Important to consider the history of the duration of symptoms and extent of change in vision as it can help you classify the anatomical location of the pathology (e.g., immediate loss of vision suggests a vascular event (CRAO, CRVO)).
- Past medical history such as hypertension, diabetes and thyroid disease can increase the likelihood of certain pathologies – be sure to ask about them when taking a history.
- Examination with fundoscopy is important to assess the vitreous, macula, optic nerve and retinal vasculature that may reveal features of the cause of the sudden change in vision.
- Suspicion of giant cell arteritis is an ophthalmic sight-threatening emergency and high-dose steroid/IV methylprednisolone should be given prior to confirmation of diagnosis via temporal artery biopsy.

UKMLA Conditions
Central retinal arterial occlusion
Diabetic eye disease
Retinal detachment
Thyroid eye disease
Visual field defects

UKMLA Presentations
Acute change in or loss of vision
Flashes and floaters in visual fields
Eye pain/discomfort

EYELID MALPOSITION

The commonest eyelid malposition's are:

- Ptosis – droopy upper lid.
- Entropion – turned in lid margin (see Fig. 20.1).
- Ectropion – turned out lid margin (see Fig. 20.2).

PTOSIS

Differential diagnosis

See Table 20.1 to see the differentials for ptosis.

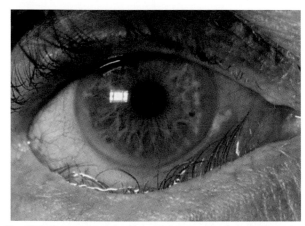

Fig. 20.1 Entropion of the lower lid. (From Kanski JJ, Nischal KK. *Ophthalmology: Clinical Signs and Differential Diagnosis.* St. Louis: Mosby; 2000.)

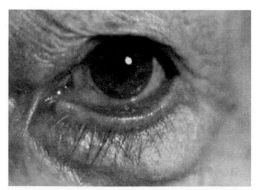

Fig. 20.2 Ectropion of the lower lid. (From Shiland BJ. *Mastering Healthcare Terminology.* 7th ed. Elsevier; 2023.)

History

Ask about symptoms of:

- Headache – important for third nerve palsies.
- Diplopia – third nerve palsy, myasthenia.
- Fatiguability – myasthenia.
- History of contact lens use – commonly can cause aponeurotic dehiscence.

Examination

Observation

Things to look for can include:

- Anisocoria (difference in pupil size – important for Horner and third nerve palsy).
- Heterochromia (congenital Horner).

Table 20.1 Common causes of ptosis

Cause	Features
Congenital ptosis	Presence since birth, if untreated affected eye may be amblyopic, frontalis overaction (raise eyebrow to lift lid), low skin crease, reduced levator function.
Aponeurotic dehiscence	Usually older patients, also contact lens wearers with high skin crease.
Cranial nerve III palsy	Full ptosis, affected eye deviated down and out ± pupil dilation.
Horner syndrome	Partial ptosis, pupil miosis, hemifacial anhidrosis. If congenital, iris colour may be different in one eye compared to the other (heterochromia).
Myasthenia	Ptosis increases with fatigue; variable or bilateral ptosis improves with application of ice pack to closed lids.
Pseudo-ptosis	Ptosis lid retraction in fellow eye (i.e., in thyroid eye disease). Empty socket syndrome in patients with prosthetic eye.

- Symmetry – look at whole face, eyebrow height and compare.

Ask yourself: does the patient have an obvious squint, prosthetic eye or features of thyroid eye disease?

Ptosis assessment

Using a ruler, you can measure:

- The palpebral aperture (the distance between the upper and lower lids – normally approximately 10 12 mm).
- The height of the skin crease (low in congenital, high in aponeurotic dehiscence, normally approximately 4–5 mm).
- Levator function (normally approximately >12 mm, reduced in congenital ptosis and in myogenic causes such as myasthenia and myotonic dystrophy).

Levator function needs to be checked in isolation; therefore, fix the brow in place and then measure the upper lid margin excursion from down gaze to full up gaze.

Look to see if there is fatiguability by measuring the palpebral aperture before and after 1 min of up gaze; the palpebral aperture will reduce in myasthenia as the levator becomes fatigued.

Ocular motility

Check ocular motility to confirm third nerve palsy. Motility will also be disordered in myasthenia.

Investigations

Magnetic resonance imaging (MRI) should be performed if an intracranial cause is suspected. ACh receptor antibodies are useful to confirm a diagnosis of myasthenia; the 'tensilon' test is very rarely performed these days in the ophthalmology setting.

Ectropion and entropion

Both of these conditions are extremely common among the elderly, where loss of tissue elasticity results in the lid either slipping over the tarsal plate, causing the lashes to point in the direction of the globe (entropion), or to slip downwards, withdrawing the lid margin away from the globe (ectropion). Lid margin malposition may also be a consequence of trauma, scarring (cicatricial), inflammatory conditions or tumours (e.g. basal cell carcinoma). Patients may present with epiphora and/or a red eye.

EYELID LUMPS AND BUMPS

Common eyelid bumps are:

- chalazion – or meibomian cyst
- hordeolum – stye
- inclusion cyst

- sebaceous cyst
- papilloma

One must always beware of potentially malignant lesions. The commonest are:

- basal cell carcinoma
- squamous cell carcinoma
- melanoma

HINTS AND TIPS

Most lumps and bumps can be excised as a minor operative procedure. Usually this is done on cosmetic grounds at the patient's request. If there is any suspicion of malignancy, the excised material should be sent for histology. In older patients, presenting with a suspicious lid lesion, a biopsy should be performed first, to ensure that a complete excision can be planned.

EYELID SWELLING

There are many causes of a swollen eyelid:

- allergy
- inflamed cyst – e.g., chalazion
- conjunctivitis
- bruising/black eye

The most important condition to be aware of is orbital cellulitis. Red, inflamed lids may be 'preseptal' only – i.e., involving the most anterior lid tissues. It is important to recognize features suggestive of orbital cellulitis, as this is sight and potentially life-threatening.

HINTS AND TIPS

The following signs must be absent for a diagnosis of preseptal cellulitis, their presence would indicate orbital cellulitis:

- pain on movement of the eye
- restriction of eye movements
- proptosis
- visual disturbance
- chemosis
- RAPD

The above must be absent for a diagnosis of preseptal cellulitis, their presence would indicate orbital cellulitis.

History

The episode may be preceded by trauma such as a bite. The condition is rapidly progressive. Children may be profoundly unwell – parents may describe the child as being febrile and listless. Ask about double vision or reduced vision.

Examination

Crucial signs of orbital cellulitis that should not be missed are:

- Proptosis.
- Reduced ocular motility – in some cases the globe may be 'frozen'.
- Reduced colour vision.
- Reduced vision.
- Swollen optic nerve.

Any children with preseptal cellulitis should be observed for development of these signs.

Investigations

Orbital cellulitis is an emergency and requires systemic antibiotics as soon as suspected. It is therefore likely that treatment will commence before investigations can be performed. Computed tomography (CT) of the orbits is useful for identifying whether there is a subperiosteal or intracranial abscess requiring drainage. Blood cultures should also be performed if the patient is febrile.

PROPTOSIS

By far the commonest cause of proptosis, whether bilateral or unilateral, is thyroid eye disease. Other causes include:

- Orbital myositis.
- Orbital cellulitis.
- Orbital apex tumours (e.g., lymphoma).

- Orbital inflammatory disorders (e.g., Wegener, sarcoidosis).
- Vascular anomalies (e.g., orbital varices, caroticocavernous sinus fistula).

The eye may look proptosed if it is very big, as in high myopia.

Thyroid eye disease

Features include:

- Adnexal soft tissue swelling – periorbital oedema.
- Lid retraction.
- Proptosis.
- Restriction of eye movement.
- Injection over the horizontal recti insertions, chemosis.
- Raised intraocular pressure, particularly on up gaze.
- Corneal exposure with punctate fluorescein staining.

Patients are at risk of visual loss from:

- Corneal scarring secondary to exposure.
- Glaucoma secondary to raised intraocular pressure.
- Optic neuropathy secondary to compression from engorged orbital contents.

Examination

1. Exophthalmometry.
2. Ocular motility +/– orthoptic assessment.
3. Visual acuity.
4. Colour vision.
5. Visual fields.
6. Pupils – check for RAPD.
7. Intraocular pressure (both straight ahead and in up gaze).
8. Fundoscopy – look for swollen discs and choroidal folds.

If acute compressive thyroid ophthalmopathy is suspected, high-dose oral steroids (or even pulsed intravenous) should be commenced as soon as possible. The patient may require referral on to an orbital specialist for consideration of surgical decompression.

Chapter Summary

- Common eyelid malpositions include ptosis, entropion and ectropion. This may be a consequence of trauma, scarring, inflammatory conditions or tumours such as basal cell carcinoma, squamous cell carcinoma or melanoma.
- Common causes of ptosis have characteristic features, e.g. Horner syndrome – partial ptosis, pupil miosis, anhidrosis of half the face.
- CN III produces ptosis and a 'down and out' eye deviation.
- Common eyelid bumps include chalazion, hordeolum, sebaceous cyst and papilloma.
- Orbital cellulitis is an ophthalmic emergency – key symptoms if present should increase suspicion: pain on movement of eye, RAPD, proptosis, and restriction of eye movements.

UKMLA Conditions
Benign eyelid disorders
Periorbital and orbital cellulitis
Thyroid eye disease

UKMLA Presentations
Diplopia
Eye pain/discomfort
Facial/periorbital swelling
Ptosis

Diseases and Disorders

Dementia

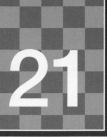

DEFINITION

Dementia is a syndrome and not a single disease entity. It refers to progressive impairment of higher cortical functions, including memory, orientation, comprehension, calculation, learning capacity, language and judgement. The dominant symptoms depend on the brain region most affected by disease. It is often accompanied or preceded by deterioration in emotional control, social behaviour or motivation. In the initial stages, there are often focal cortical deficits, and as it progresses it is eventually associated with diffuse involvement of both cerebral hemispheres. The patient is often alert in the early and middle stages of the disease. This is in contrast to delirium (acute confusional state), in which alteration of level of consciousness is a defining feature. There are many causes of dementia, but the most common are degenerative.

DIFFERENTIAL DIAGNOSES

- Primary neurodegenerative diseases, e.g., Alzheimer's disease, dementia with Lewy bodies, Parkinson's disease, frontotemporal lobar degeneration (including Pick disease), Huntington's disease.
- Vascular, e.g., small vessel disease, multiple cortical infarcts.
- Metabolic, e.g., hypothyroidism, vitamin B_{12} and folate deficiency.
- Infections, e.g., HIV, prion disease, syphilis, progressive multifocal leucoencephalopathy, subacute sclerosing panencephalitis.
- Inflammatory disorders, e.g., central nervous system (CNS) vasculitis, neurosarcoidosis, multiple sclerosis.

- Neoplastic/paraneoplastic, e.g., tumour (primary or secondary), limbic encephalitis.
- Normal pressure hydrocephalus.
- Head injury, e.g., chronic subdural haematoma.
- Repeated exposure to toxins, e.g., alcohol, heavy metal poisoning, organic solvents.
- Depression: pseudodementia (patients who are depressed may appear demented).

EPIDEMIOLOGY

The most common causes of dementia are Alzheimer's disease and vascular dementia and these are predominantly diseases of the elderly. The prevalence of dementia in persons aged between 50 and 70 years is about 1%, and in those approaching 90 years of age it reaches 50%. The annual incidence rate is 190/100,000 and, with an increasingly ageing population, it is expected to rise even further.

GENERAL CLINICAL FEATURES

In the assessment of a patient with dementia, several key factors should be addressed to aid diagnosis. First, dementia must be distinguished from acute confusional states (delirium) and psychiatric disorders (Table 21.1). The earliest symptoms and length of the history, along with the tempo of the disease (fluctuant, gradually or rapidly progressive or a stepwise deterioration), should be elicited. Finally, the impact on the social and occupational functioning should be explored. In the examination, one should try to distinguish the pattern of cognitive impairment and look for any other abnormalities apart from dementia.

Table 21.1 Differentiating dementia from delirium and depression as causes of cognitive impairment

	Dementia	Delirium	Depression
Conscious state	Alert	Impaired	Alert
Onset	Insidious/gradual	Abrupt	Variable
Course tempo	Gradually progressive	Fluctuant – may be circadian disruption	Fluctuant
Orientation	Initially preserved	Early prominent disorientation	Variable
Hallucinations	Late feature	Prominent	Rare (auditory typically)
Behaviour	Depends on cause	Restless	Withdrawn

141

History

It is essential to obtain a history from a relative or friend, as well as from the patient, to assess the features associated with dementia such as rate of intellectual decline, how functional status and activities of daily living have been affected, changes in behaviour and relevant past history (e.g., previous stroke or head injury) and family history of young-onset dementia. The rate of progression of dementia depends on the underlying cause:

- Alzheimer's disease: slowly progressive over years.
- Vascular dementia: repeated large vessel occlusion causes stepwise deterioration, whereas small vessel disease causes a progressive decline without steps. They often coexist.
- Prion disease or CNS vasculitis: progressive over months.
- Encephalitis: over days to weeks.

The earliest symptoms described tend to correlate with the area of the brain first affected. As disease spreads through the brain, other symptoms develop. Therefore, in Alzheimer's disease, recent memory impairment is the most common initial complaint and reflects early degeneration of the hippocampal areas. In frontotemporal dementia, changes in personality can often be reported, reflecting early involvement of frontal structures.

> **COMMUNICATION**
>
> It is vital to take a history from a relative or friend who knows the patient well. Patients with dementia, especially with frontal lobe disease, are often completely unaware of any problem. The relative should ideally be interviewed separately from the patient or given a questionnaire to fill in, as personality change, especially when related to disinhibition, can be difficult for the relative to talk about in front of the patient.

EXAMINATION

A careful physical and cognitive examination may reveal clues as to the aetiology. In the physical examination, you should specifically look for evidence of:

- focal signs
- involuntary movements
- pseudobulbar signs
- primitive reflexes, e.g., pout, grasp and rooting reflexes
- apraxia
- gait disorder

There are a number of tests that can be used to assess the pattern of cognitive impairment including a mini-mental test (quick to perform but superficial), Montreal Cognitive Assessment or the Addenbrooke's Cognitive Examination, which is lengthy to perform but comprehensive. These tests are designed to test memory, abstract thought, judgement and specific higher cortical functions (see Chapter 2).

> **HINTS AND TIPS**
>
> It is vital to take a good social and psychiatric history in patients with dementia. The social circumstances surrounding a patient with dementia are critical for optimal management, e.g., familiar environments and routine. Remember that the carers also need social support.

INVESTIGATIONS

It is important to carry out a number of investigations to exclude potentially treatable causes of dementia.

Blood tests

Routine blood tests may be necessary to exclude:

- hypothyroidism
- vitamin B_{12} and folate deficiency
- syphilis

  Specific blood tests for rare causes of dementia include:

- metabolic disorders, e.g., Wilson disease, leucodystrophies
- HIV (AIDS dementia)
- vasculitis and inflammatory diseases
- limbic encephalitis

Imaging of the brain

Imaging of the brain is obligatory in a patient with dementia and can be performed using computed tomography (CT) and preferably magnetic resonance imaging (MRI). The primary goal is to exclude:

- Space-occupying lesions: especially chronic subdural haematoma in the elderly following a fall.
- Normal-pressure hydrocephalus: dilated ventricles without cortical atrophy. This presents with cognitive decline, urinary incontinence and gait apraxia. The diagnosis may be supported by a lumbar puncture,

removing up to 50 mL of CSF, which should result in improvement in the clinical features. It can be treated by ventriculoperitoneal shunting.

Typically, variable degrees of cerebral atrophy with enlarged ventricles are seen with most forms of dementia. However, MRI can also be used to allow assessment of signal change and patterns of atrophy consistent with specific forms of dementia. For example, increased T2 signal in the thalami is characteristic of variant Creutzfeldt–Jakob disease (CJD). Bilateral hippocampal and temporal lobe atrophy is seen in Alzheimer's disease and asymmetrical anterior hippocampal, amygdala and temporal lobe atrophy is seen in frontotemporal lobar degeneration (FTLD). In cerebrovascular disease, imaging can demonstrate multiple infarcts or significant small vessel disease.

Lumbar puncture

The National Institute for Health and Care Excellence (NICE) guidelines recommend the use of cerebrospinal fluid (CSF) examination in those patients under 65 years to exclude potentially treatable causes of dementia. For example, a lymphocytic CSF may point to an infective or inflammatory disorder. The presence of oligoclonal bands might suggest an immune process (e.g., limbic encephalitis). The CSF levels of tau (increased) and beta-42 (decreased) can sometimes help with the diagnosis of Alzheimer's disease but tend to be measured only in specialist centres. Similarly, elevated S100 and protein 14-3-3 and a positive real-time quaking-induced conversion (RT-QuIC) assay are supportive of a diagnosis of CJD.

Neuropsychometry

Neuropsychologists test the different domains of cognitive function in considerable detail. This helps with diagnosis, with the pattern of deficits indicating which regions of the brain are involved in the disease process. Formal neuropsychometry is especially useful when performed at intervals. This enables comparison of intellectual function within a patient over time. It can be a reliable indicator of either progression in disease (suggesting an organic dementia) compared with improvement or plateau in decline of intellectual function, which can be seen in patients with treated depression or functional memory loss.

Electroencephalography

Periodic complexes on the electroencephalogram tracing may indicate prion disease such as CJD. This group of disorders is associated with a rapidly progressive course, which is usually an important diagnostic feature.

Genetic testing

The following genetic mutations can be associated with dementia:

- Huntington mutation: Huntington's disease.
- Young-onset Alzheimer's disease: amyloid precursor protein (*APP*), presenilin 1 and 2 and apolipoprotein E4 mutations.
- Familial CJD: prion protein gene mutation.
- FTLD: tau, progranulin and *C9orf72* mutations.

Brain biopsy

Brain biopsy is rarely performed but might be indicated if a disease is rapidly progressive or a treatable cause of dementia is suspected and other investigations fail to reach a diagnosis (e.g., cerebral vasculitis).

MANAGEMENT

Treatable causes of dementia should be addressed. Some of these are potentially reversible or their clinical course can be stabilized (e.g., vasculitis, hydrocephalus and depressive pseudodementia).

Management of most cases of dementia requires careful advice and counselling of the patient and family and shared care involving the family, carers, hospital specialists, general practitioner and community psychiatric services. Long-term residential care is often required.

In other cases such as Alzheimer's disease, depression and any underlying systemic disorders should be treated to maximize cognitive function. The use of centrally acting cholinergic drugs for primary neurodegenerative dementias is discussed in the following section. Neuroleptic medication may be required for behavioural disturbance but can exacerbate extrapyramidal features, such as slowing of movements.

PRIMARY NEURODEGENERATIVE DEMENTIAS

Alzheimer's disease

Alzheimer's disease is the most common cause of dementia in the developed world. There are approximately 500,000 cases in the United Kingdom at any one time. It is rarely seen in persons under the age of 45 years, except in familial cases, and the incidence increases dramatically with age, especially in patients aged over 70 years.

Familial Alzheimer's disease is rare. Mutations in the amyloid precursor protein (*APP*) gene on chromosome 21, presenilin 1 and 2 genes are associated with young-onset AD. There is also an association of late-onset disease with the apolipoprotein E4 genotype. Individuals with Down syndrome develop the full neuropathological and clinical changes of Alzheimer's disease by the age of 30 to 40 years, probably contributed to by the excessive *APP* produced by a 50% increase in gene dosage due to the extra chromosome 21.

Pathology

Alzheimer's disease is identified by the presence of extracellular amyloid plaques and intracellular neurofibrillary tangles in the brain. The plaques consist of dystrophic neurites clustered around a core of β-amyloid protein, which is derived from the larger precursor protein, APP. Amyloid can also be deposited in cerebral blood vessels, leading to amyloid angiopathy.

Neurofibrillary tangles are derived from the microtubule-associated protein tau, which is in an abnormally hyperphosphorylated state and causes protein aggregation. The majority of the pathology affects the hippocampus, temporal and parietal lobes. Typically, the primary motor and sensory cortex are spared.

Clinical features

Alzheimer's disease presents with features of progressive episodic (knowledge of events) memory loss and evolves over many years. Patients might become repetitive in their questioning, forget to pass on messages and misplace items around the house. Dysphasia, apraxia, visuospatial deficits and topographical disorientation are also common early features reflecting involvement of the parietal lobes. Patients may fail to recognize previously familiar environments and faces. They may have difficulty with naming and using common household objects or dressing. There might be problems in executive function such as planning, decision-making and sequencing. Seizures and myoclonus are relatively common in late disease. Agitation and delusions (often paranoid in ideation) can also occur late in disease. Pyramidal and extrapyramidal features rarely occur.

There are several rare, atypical presentations of Alzheimer's disease. These include posterior cortical atrophy, where visuospatial problems predominate; language-dominant presentations; and frontal variants, where behavioural problems are seen early.

Diagnosis

A definite diagnosis of Alzheimer's disease can be made only from pathological findings. In practice, a typical history with progressive episodic memory loss and negative routine tests will allow a diagnosis of probable Alzheimer's disease. If cognitive impairment is demonstrated that does not yet affect the patient's functional status, this is termed mild cognitive impairment (MCI). Amnestic MCI is frequently a prodrome to Alzheimer's disease.

CT scans show nonspecific generalized cerebral atrophy with a compensatory enlargement of ventricles due to loss of brain tissue rather than hydrocephalus. The temporal lobes may be more severely atrophic. Serial volumetric analysis of the temporal lobes and hippocampi using MRI may show atrophy of these areas and may enable a more specific diagnosis.

Drug treatment

The acetylcholinesterase inhibitor tacrine is licensed in the United States and France, and donepezil, galantamine and rivastigmine are licensed in the United Kingdom. In general, these drugs arrest symptoms by approximately 6 months of having diseases but do not alter the course of the neurodegenerative process. NICE recommend their use in patients with mild-to-moderate disease and patients need to be monitored carefully for cholinergic side effects (e.g., bowel disturbance).

Memantine has also been demonstrated to improve symptoms in advanced disease and might have an additional benefit in combination with anticholinesterase inhibitors. NICE recommends its use in patients with moderate disease who are intolerant of acetylcholinesterase inhibitors or in patients with severe disease.

Prognosis

In spite of recent advances in our understanding and treatment, the prognosis of Alzheimer's disease is very poor, with relentless progression to death, which is often due to bronchopneumonia. The mean survival is 8 years from the onset of the disease.

Dementia with Lewy bodies

Dementia with Lewy bodies (DLB) has only been recognized as a separate clinical entity relatively recently. It is associated with prominent early visual hallucinations, memory disturbance and fluctuations in the clinical course even from day to day. The visual hallucinations often do not upset patients (compared with drug-induced visual hallucinations in idiopathic Parkinson's disease) and patients need to be directly asked about them because information is often not volunteered. The extrapyramidal features in DLB are similar to those in idiopathic Parkinson's disease, except the characteristic resting tremor may be absent, there is a poor response to L-DOPA therapy and the clinical signs are often symmetrical. In contrast to dementia seen in the later stages of idiopathic Parkinson's disease, the dementia often predates the onset of parkinsonism in DLB. DLB and Parkinson's disease dementia together make up the third most common cause of dementia in later life. The neuropathology is a mixture of that seen in Parkinson's disease with Lewy bodies (eosinophilic intraneuronal inclusions containing α-synuclein, aggregated with abnormally phosphorylated neurofilaments and ubiquitin) in the substantia nigra, but also in the cerebral cortex, as well as Alzheimer's disease type pathology such as amyloid plaques and neurofibrillary tangles.

Management

The patients often develop prominent psychiatric side effects with dopamine agonists, such as confusion and hallucinations. Patients are also very sensitive to neuroleptics, developing profound rigidity and akinesia. Clinical trials have shown that acetylcholinesterase inhibitors can produce significant improvement in the symptoms of DLB, including noncognitive symptoms for which NICE recommends their use.

Frontotemporal lobar dementia

Frontotemporal lobar dementia (FTLD) is a relatively rare cause of dementia, accounting for 20% of young-onset dementia and 5% to 10% dementia overall. It is more common in women: up to 50% of cases are genetic (see earlier). It tends to occur between the ages of 50 and 65 years, which is younger than sporadic Alzheimer's disease.

It is accompanied by marked cerebral atrophy in the frontal and anterior temporal lobes with relative sparing of the parietal lobes in contrast to Alzheimer's disease. The neuropathology of FTLD is heterogeneous. Some cases demonstrate argyrophilic inclusions (i.e., pieces of protein that stain with silver), which are called Pick bodies. They are found within the neuronal cytoplasm and contain the protein tau. Some cases have inclusions that contain tau but are not Pick bodies and other cases contain inclusions that are ubiquitin positive and tau negative.

Clinical features

FTLD can manifest as one of three syndromes. The behavioural variant FTLD presents with prominent frontal features, with behavioural and psychiatric features at presentation, and is frequently misdiagnosed. The remaining two presentations (semantic dementia and progressive nonfluent aphasia) of FTLD are language-dominant disorders and together are known as primary progressive aphasia. A subgroup of patients develop additional signs of weakness and wasting in bulbar and/or limb muscles in a pattern similar to that of amyotrophic lateral sclerosis (ALS). These cases have ubiquitin-positive pathology and are termed FTD-MND (frontotemporal dementia associated with MND). CT or MRI scans show prominent frontotemporal atrophy.

No specific treatment has been found and the disease progresses to death over 6 to 12 years.

Vascular dementia

Cerebrovascular disease is a major cause of cognitive impairment in isolation or in combination with Alzheimer's disease. It is the second most common cause of dementia. Histopathologically, a spectrum of changes can be apparent, from large vessel atheromatous change to prominent small vessel disease and ischaemic changes including lacunar and microinfarcts, leukoaraiosis, gliosis and demyelination.

Patients present in a variety of ways. The classic description is of multiinfarct dementia, which describes a stepwise deterioration due to recurrent strokes. A frontosubcortical pattern of presentation is common, reflecting the vulnerability of these structures to vascular damage. Patients present with executive and attentional impairment, behavioural change and cognitive slowing, with relative sparing of memory. Strategically localized single brain lesions may also profoundly affect specific cognitive functions (e.g., language or memory) without causing global dementia. Finally, vascular dementia can also present with gradual cognitive decline and no history of vascular episodes. This results from diffuse small vessel disease causing widespread white matter change. Patients present with marked slowness of thinking and memory retrieval and frontal deficits. Examination might reveal focal signs, brisk reflexes, pseudobulbar palsy or gait apraxia. This is called subcortical ischaemic leucoencephalopathy.

Diagnosis

The diagnosis of multiinfarct dementia is based on the history and the presence of multiple areas of large vessel infarction and/or prominent small vessel disease on CT or MRI. Patients often also have evidence of other vascular disease (e.g., ischaemic heart disease, peripheral vascular disease) or vascular risk factors.

Treatment

Secondary prevention of atherosclerosis in established cases can be achieved with good control of hypertension, hyperlipidaemia and antiplatelet agents such as aspirin if strokes have occurred. Current NICE guidelines do not recommend the use of cholinesterase inhibitors in vascular dementia.

Vasculitis

Vasculitis is an uncommon cause of dementia but should be recognized as most cases respond to treatment. They include:

- polyarteritis nodosa
- primary granulomatous angiitis: isolated vasculitis of the central nervous system
- systemic lupus erythematosus
- giant cell arteritis
- thrombotic microangiopathies

Dementia as part of other degenerative diseases

In the following conditions, dementia may be a prominent finding with other neurological features:

- Parkinson's disease (frontotemporal)
- Huntington's disease (frontal/subcortical)
- Progressive supranuclear palsy (frontal)
- Corticobasal degeneration (hemispheric cortex)
- Motor neuron disease (frontotemporal)

Pseudodementia

Depression in the elderly can mimic the initial phases of dementia and is termed pseudodementia. Pseudodementia can be successfully treated with antidepressant medications and counselling if necessary.

Chapter Summary

- Dementia is the progressive decline in higher cortical function. Delirium is an acute confusional disorder that is usually reversible.
- In assessing higher cortical function in a patient, obtaining a collateral history from the main carer is crucial as the patient may forget or trivialize important parts of the history.
- There are a number of potentially treatable causes of dementia (e.g., hypothyroidism, B_{12} deficiency) that need to be excluded before specific neurodegenerative disorders such as Alzheimer's disease are considered.
- Alzheimer's disease is the most common form of dementia worldwide and presents predominantly with features of progressive episodic (knowledge of events) memory loss.

UKMLA Conditions
Dementias
Parkinson's disease

UKMLA Presentations
Behaviour/personality change
Confusion
Memory loss

DEFINITIONS

- Epileptic seizure: a paroxysmal, synchronous and excessive discharge of neurons in the cerebral cortex manifesting as a stereotyped disturbance of consciousness, behaviour, emotion, motor function or sensation. An epileptic seizure typically has sudden onset, lasts seconds to minutes and usually ceases spontaneously. They often recur.
- Epilepsy: the condition in which there is a propensity to have recurrent and unprovoked seizures. A single seizure is therefore not usually sufficient to make a diagnosis of epilepsy and seizures occurring solely in association with precipitants (e.g., fever in young children, metabolic disturbance, alcohol or drug abuse, acute head injury) are termed acute symptomatic and are not considered as epilepsy.
- Status epilepticus: a state of continuous seizure activity for 5 min or more or recurrent seizures, with failure to regain consciousness between seizures. This is a medical emergency and mortality is 10% to 15%.
- Prodrome: premonitory changes in mood or behaviour, which might precede the attack by some hours.
- Aura: the subjective sensation or phenomenon that might precede and mark the onset of the epileptic seizure. It might localize the seizure origin within the brain.
- Ictus: the attack or seizure itself.
- Postictal period: the time after the ictus during which the patient may be drowsy, confused and disorientated. The patient may also have residual focal neurological signs, e.g., Todd paralysis.

EPIDEMIOLOGY

Between 3% and 5% of the population suffer one or two seizures during their lives. Recurrent seizures occur in 0.5% to 1% of the population; 70% of these cases are well controlled with drugs and have prolonged remissions.

Epilepsy more commonly presents during childhood or adolescence but can occur at any age. Incidence rates vary with age, between 20 and 70 cases per 100,000 persons a year. There are two peaks in the incidence of grand mal seizures. The first occurs in children and adolescents, in whom no cause can usually be found. The second occurs in patients aged between 50 and 70 years, in whom the disease is probably caused by subcortical ischaemic changes secondary to hypertension.

AETIOLOGY

Epilepsy is a symptom of numerous disorders, but in over 50% of patients with epilepsy, no apparent cause is found, in spite of full investigation.

Of the symptomatic causes in adults, vascular disease (especially stroke), alcohol abuse, cerebral tumours and head injury are the most common. With modern neuroimaging, structural causes of focal epilepsies such as hippocampal sclerosis and neuronal migrational defects have grown in importance.

Family history

There is an increased susceptibility to seizures in relatives of patients with epilepsy. This is especially true in the case of absence seizures, where up to 40% of cases have a family history. No single genetic trait can account for the vast heterogeneity of all epileptic syndromes. The mechanism probably involves factors that alter membrane structure or function or channel dysfunction, which might then lead to a lowered seizure threshold.

Antenatal and perinatal factors

Intrauterine infections such as rubella and toxoplasmosis, as well as maternal drug abuse and irradiation in early gestation, can produce brain damage and neonatal seizures. Perinatal trauma and anoxia, when sufficiently severe to cause brain injury, might also result in epilepsy.

Trauma and surgery

Severe closed or open head trauma is often followed by seizures. These can be within the first week (early) or might be delayed up to several months or years (late), when the likelihood of chronic epilepsy is greater. Surgery to the cerebral hemispheres is followed by seizures in about 10% of patients.

Metabolic causes

Many electrolyte disturbances can cause neuronal irritability and seizures such as hyponatraemia and hypernatraemia, hypocalcaemia, hypomagnesaemia and hypoglycaemia. Other metabolic causes include uraemia and hepatic failure.

Toxic causes

Drugs such as phenothiazines, monoamine oxidase inhibitors, tricyclic antidepressants, amphetamines, lidocaine (lignocaine) and nalidixic acid might provoke fits, either in overdose or at therapeutic levels in patients with a lowered seizure threshold. Withdrawal of antiepileptic medication and benzodiazepines might also cause seizures, especially when done rapidly.

Chronic alcohol abuse is a very common cause of seizures. These might occur while drinking, during a withdrawal phase or secondary to hypoglycaemia or trauma. Other toxic agents capable of causing seizures include carbon monoxide, lead and mercury.

Infectious and inflammatory causes

Seizures might be the presenting feature or part of the course of encephalitis, meningitis, cerebral abscess or neurosyphilis and usually indicate a poorer prognosis in these conditions. High fevers secondary to noncerebral infections in children aged over 6 months and under 6 years of age are a common cause of generalized seizures (febrile convulsion). These are usually self-limiting and seizures do not tend to recur in adult life.

Vascular causes

Up to 15% of patients with cerebrovascular disease experience seizures, especially with large areas of infarction or haemorrhage. Less common vascular causes of seizures include cortical venous thrombosis and vasculitis (e.g., polyarteritis nodosa) as well as vascular malformations.

Intracranial tumours

Sudden onset of seizures in adult life, especially if partial, should always raise the possibility of an intracranial tumour.

Hypoxia

Seizures can develop during or following respiratory or cardiac arrest secondary to anoxic encephalopathy. This can sometimes be confused with generalized myoclonus (see Chapter 5).

Degenerative diseases

All patients with degenerative cortical neuronal diseases of the brain have an increased risk of seizures (e.g., Alzheimer's disease).

Seizure precipitants

Flashing lights, flickering television or computer screens precipitate some seizure types; this is called photosensitivity. Sleep deprivation and increased stress often precipitate seizures in susceptible patients.

HINTS AND TIPS

Failure to comply with medication is a very common cause of seizures, including status epilepticus. Usually, the patient fails to comply because of side effects of the anticonvulsants or difficulty coming to terms with their condition psychologically. It is therefore important to ask about troublesome side effects and discuss alternatives with the patient and the general practitioner.

CLINICAL FEATURES

The diagnosis of epilepsy is primarily clinical. A detailed history is therefore essential and usually requires eyewitness reports, particularly when consciousness is lost during the event.

If an aura preceded the attack, the patient might be able to describe this, which might help localize the focus. The patient might not remember the aura, especially if there is secondary generalization.

Focal seizures

Focal seizures arise from a localized area of cerebral cortex. The clinical manifestations of the seizure depend on where in the cortex the seizure arises (see Table 22.1) and how fast and far it spreads. Sixty percent of partial seizures originate in the temporal lobes and the remainder mostly originate from the frontal lobes. Seizures originating from the parietal or occipital regions are rare. Focal seizures can be subdivided into focal aware, focal impaired awareness and focal to bilateral.

Focal aware seizures

Focal aware seizures are seizures in which consciousness is not impaired and in which the discharge remains localized. They are typically brief and involve focal symptoms. A structural brain lesion must be excluded (e.g., stroke, tumour or abscess).

Focal impaired awareness

Focal impaired awareness seizures might have similar features to focal aware seizures, but by definition impairment of consciousness is always involved. They usually originate in the temporal or frontal lobe and cause a disturbance of consciousness usually without loss of postural control, i.e., the patient remains standing. The actual attack varies between and within individuals.

Table 22.1 Common clinical features of seizures

Seizure	Clinical features
Temporal lobe seizures	• Aura: epigastric sensation, olfactory or gustatory hallucinations, autonomic symptoms (e.g., change in pulse or blood pressure, facial flushing), affective symptoms (e.g., fear, depersonalization), déjà vu • Seizure: motor arrest and absence prominent, automatisms (e.g., lip smacking, chewing, fidgeting, walking), automatic speech (if nondominant hemisphere onset), contralateral dystonia • Duration: slow evolution over 1–2 minutes • Postictal: confusion common, postictal dysphasia (if dominant hemisphere onset)
Frontal lobe seizures	• Aura: typically abrupt onset with variable aura, often indescribable, forced thinking, ideational or emotional manifestations • Seizure: vocalization/shrill cry, violent and bizarre automatisms, cycling movements of legs, ictal posturing and tonic spasms, version of head and eyes contralateral to side of seizure focus, fencing posture (extension and abduction of one arm with rotation of head to same side and flexion of the other arm), sexual automatisms with pelvic thrusting, obscene gestures and genital manipulation • Duration: typically very brief (~30 s) • Postictal: confusion brief with rapid recovery
Parietal lobe seizures	• Somatosensory symptoms common, e.g., tingling, pain, numbness, prickling, vertigo, distortions of space • Automatisms and secondary generalization may occur
Occipital lobe seizures	• Visual hallucinations common, e.g., seeing flashing lights or geometrical figures, sometimes complex hallucinations of objects/people if seizures arise from visual association cortex • Eyelids might flutter, occasional eye turning or rapid blinking • Automatisms and secondary generalization might occur

They can start as a focal aware seizure and then progress or they can involve alteration of consciousness from the outset. Focal impaired awareness seizures typically last 2 to 3 minutes but can continue for several hours as a part of nonconvulsive status epilepticus. Patients are typically amnesic of the event.

Focal to bilateral

These are focal seizures in which the epileptic discharge spreads to both cerebral hemispheres, resulting in a generalized (usually tonic–clonic) seizure. The spread of the seizure may be so rapid that no features of the localized onset are apparent.

Generalized seizures

Generalized seizures are characterized by the bilateral involvement of the cortex at the onset of the seizure. Patients lose consciousness at seizure onset, so there is usually no warning.

Generalized tonic–clonic seizures

These seizures typically have no warning, although in some cases of epilepsy they might be preceded by increasing frequency of myoclonic jerks or absences. Tonic–clonic seizures start with a sudden loss of consciousness and the subject falls to the ground. This is followed by the tonic phase, which lasts for about 10 s, when the body is stiff, the elbows are flexed and the legs extended. Breathing stops and the patient may turn cyanotic.

The tonic phase is followed by the clonic phase, which usually lasts for 1 to 2 minutes, during which time there is violent generalized rhythmical shaking. The eyes are open and roll back, the tongue may be bitten and there is tachycardia. Bladder and bowel control may be lost. The frequency of the clonic movements gradually decreases and, eventually, ceases, marking the end of the seizure. Following a tonic–clonic seizure, the patient often cannot be roused for several minutes and awakes with confusion (postictal confusion), headache, myalgia and some retrograde amnesia. It is not unusual for patients to fall asleep after a convulsion and this can sometimes be mistaken for unconsciousness.

Clonic seizures are similar to tonic–clonic seizures, but without an initial tonic phase.

Absence seizures

Typical absence seizures have onset between 4 and 12 years of age. The attacks may occur several times a day, lasting 5 to 15 s. The patient suddenly stares vacantly. There may be eye blinking and myoclonic jerks. They are often diagnosed following complaints about an inattentive child with poor academic performance. Typical absence seizures are associated with a characteristic electroencephalogram (EEG) pattern of three-per-second generalized spike-and-wave discharges. Atypical absence seizures are associated with more severe epilepsy syndromes such as Lennox–Gastaut syndrome and the EEG usually shows less specific changes. The seizures themselves have a less abrupt onset/cessation, with more marked eyelid fluttering and myoclonic jerking.

Myoclonic seizures

Myoclonic seizures are abrupt, brief involuntary movements that can involve the whole body or parts of it such as the arms or head. Not all myoclonus is the result of epilepsy; it is epileptic if it occurs in the context of a seizure disorder and is cortical (rather than brainstem or spinal cord) in origin.

Atonic and tonic seizures

These are rare, generalized seizures and are often termed drop attacks. They typically occur in severe epilepsy syndromes. Atonic seizures involve a sudden loss of tone in the postural muscles, causing a patient to fall. Tonic seizures involve a sudden increase in muscle tone, causing a patient to become rigid and fall.

HISTORY AND INVESTIGATIONS TO AID DIAGNOSIS

The diagnosis of a seizure is based on the clinical history. Additional information can be provided by brain imaging, the EEG or blood tests. The use of neuroimaging is more important in cases with late onset (over the age of 25 years), that are focal, are refractory to treatment, and are associated with persisting abnormal clinical signs or when the presentation is with status epilepticus.

Clinical features during an attack that support the diagnosis of a seizure include pupil dilatation, raised blood pressure and heart rate, extensor plantar responses and central and peripheral cyanosis.

In generalized seizures, the PO_2 and pH can be lowered and the creatine kinase (CK) and lactate might be elevated.

An EEG is extremely useful if recorded during an attack and may show spike-and-wave activity. Interictal EEGs might show focal spikes or slow waves suggesting subclinical seizure activity, but they can be normal in 50% of adults with epilepsy. In some cases, abnormal activity can be provoked by hyperventilation or photic stimulation (flashing light). This is especially true for absence seizures. Prolonged EEG in the form of video telemetry or ambulatory EEG may increase the probability of recording ictal EEG.

COMMON PITFALLS

A normal electroencephalogram (EEG) does not exclude epilepsy. Not all cortical spikes are recorded by scalp EEG, especially in the case of focal seizures. Conversely, an EEG with suggestive or definite epileptic features is very helpful in making a diagnosis of epilepsy. Ultimately, however, epilepsy is a clinical diagnosis.

Computed tomography or magnetic resonance imaging might reveal structural lesions that have caused the seizures, especially if there is focal onset.

DIFFERENTIAL DIAGNOSES

It is important to distinguish epilepsy from other causes of transient focal dysfunction or loss of consciousness, as there are social and economic implications when a diagnosis of epilepsy is made, e.g., the patient is unable to drive or operate certain machinery.

The most common differentials of a convulsive seizure include:

1. Syncope (see Chapter 5).
2. Nonepileptic or functional seizures, which are surprisingly common, especially in patients with known epilepsy. The following features help to differentiate a pseudoseizure from an epileptic seizure: more common in young women with a past psychiatric history; seizures tend to be refractory to all drugs; pupils, blood pressure, heart rate, PO_2 and pH might remain unchanged during seizure; plantar responses are flexor; the EEG shows no seizure activity during the episode and no postictal slowing.
3. Transient ischaemic attacks: these can include transient loss of consciousness when the posterior circulation is involved, but this is very uncommon and often overdiagnosed.
4. Migraine: syncope can occur during migraine, causing confusion with epileptic seizures. In addition, migraine preceded by visual or sensory disturbances can be mistaken for focal epilepsies, as seizures are commonly followed by headache. However, the progression of visual and sensory symptoms is usually much more rapid in epilepsy than migraine.
5. Hypoglycaemia: this can cause behavioural disturbance and seizures.

DRUG TREATMENT

When to start drug treatment

Research shows that after one seizure only 30% to 60% of patients have recurrence within 2 years. Moreover, if there is an identifiable provoking factor (e.g., alcohol), recurrence rates are higher. Recurrence rates rise to 80% to 90% following two or more seizures within 1 year. For this reason, antiepileptic treatment should typically be considered when two or more unprovoked seizures have occurred within a short period. However, in certain circumstances it may be prudent to start treatment after a single unprovoked seizure. This includes a seizure associated with a clearly abnormal EEG, seizures associated with a neurological deficit present since birth and seizures associated with a progressive neurological disorder.

What drugs to choose

Whenever possible, treatment should involve only one drug to avoid interaction between the anticonvulsants and additive side effects. Treatment is aimed at making the patient seizure-free while minimizing drug side effects. Seizure freedom can be achieved with monotherapy in about 80% of patients with epilepsy.

The most common anticonvulsants in current clinical use are carbamazepine, sodium valproate, lamotrigine, levetiracetam and phenytoin. Second-line drugs include clobazam, clonazepam, gabapentin, topiramate, pregabalin, zonisamide, lacosamide, rufinamide, oxcarbazepine and phenobarbital. NICE guidelines state that the first-line drugs for primary generalized epilepsy in adults are sodium valproate lamotrigine or levetiracetam; for absence epilepsy in children ethosuximide or sodium valproate; and for focal seizures carbamazepine or lamotrigine. Many patients still take phenobarbital and phenytoin for generalized seizures but these are less commonly prescribed because of their side effects. Some patients might still be taking vigabatrin, but this is rarely used because it can cause progressive and irreversible visual field defects.

If one anticonvulsant fails at the maximum tolerated dose, it is substituted by another first-line drug. The first-line drugs are then tried in combination and finally second-line anticonvulsants are added.

Whichever drug is used, the dose should be built up slowly. Measurement of blood drug concentrations is important for phenytoin, as it displays zero-order kinetics and small increases in dose can cause it to reach toxic levels. For other drugs, therapeutic drug monitoring, if available, can be used to check compliance or to confirm clinically diagnosed toxicity.

Pharmacokinetics of antiepileptic drugs

Phenytoin, phenobarbital, topiramate and carbamazepine are known to induce enzymes within the liver that metabolize other drugs. This effect is particularly important when the patient is on the combined oral contraceptive pill, which can be rendered ineffective unless higher doses are used. Many of the antiepileptic drugs also block pathways within the liver for metabolism of drugs, e.g., sodium valproate prolongs the half-life of lamotrigine. Care must be taken when prescribing these drugs, especially in combination, to avoid toxic levels and other adverse reactions.

Adverse effects of antiepileptic drugs

All antiepileptic drugs can produce acute, dose-related, idiosyncratic or chronic toxicity and variable degrees of teratogenicity (damage to the developing foetus).

Acute toxicity

Allergic skin reactions occur in up to 10% of patients on phenytoin and in up to 15% on carbamazepine. Lamotrigine can be associated with a particularly severe skin rash (Stevens–Johnson syndrome). These can be reduced by introducing these drugs slowly at low doses and building up to therapeutic levels. Patients being started on lamotrigine must be warned about a rash and asked to stop the medication and seek urgent medical help should they develop a rash. Bone marrow aplasia is a rare idiosyncratic complication of carbamazepine.

Chronic toxicity

Chronic toxicity is especially associated with phenytoin and includes the development of coarsened facies, acne, hirsutism, gum hypertrophy and possibly peripheral neuropathy. All anticonvulsants appear to have some effect on cognitive function and can cause drowsiness. This is especially a problem with phenytoin. Carbamazepine and phenytoin can cause a cerebellar ataxia in a dose-related manner. Generally, carbamazepine and sodium valproate have fewer chronic effects than phenytoin. Lamotrigine is increasingly used for many types of epilepsy because of its low side effect profile. Levetiracetam is also being used more frequently because of a relatively lower incidence of side effects and absence of effect on hepatic metabolism.

Teratogenicity and pregnancy

The background risk of major foetal malformations in the general population is 1% to 2%. This increases to 3% in patients who have epilepsy but do not take anticonvulsants and to 4% to 9% in those patients who do take anticonvulsants. This risk increases in those with high plasma anticonvulsant concentrations and is higher in those on polytherapy. Sodium valproate (particularly doses >800 mg) appears to have the highest individual risk of the anticonvulsants and is associated with an increase in learning difficulties. The aim of drug treatment during pregnancy is to minimize drug exposure while maintaining seizure control and safety of mother and foetus. In addition, NICE recommends that a 5 mg dose of folic acid should be taken prior to conception by women with epilepsy and for the first trimester of pregnancy. Valproate must not be used in any woman or girl able to have children unless there is a Pregnancy Prevention Programme (PPP) in place. The use of sodium valproate and topiramate in particular in pregnancy is associated with neural tube defects. Women on these drugs need early screening using ultrasound +/− amniocentesis (to test for alpha-fetoprotein) for early detection of neural tube defects.

Patients with epilepsy and on treatment who wish to become pregnant should seek specialist advice before conception and require regular follow-up by a neurologist during the pregnancy. The pharmacokinetics might markedly change during pregnancy, necessitating regular monitoring of seizures and serum drug concentrations. Breastfeeding is not contraindicated, except for women taking phenobarbital or ethosuximide, which can be excreted in significant quantities in breast milk.

STATUS EPILEPTICUS

Status epilepticus is now defined as a seizure lasting longer than 5 minutes, necessitating emergency treatment, or a series of seizures without recovery lasting 30 minutes and usually indicating neuronal death. Convulsive status epilepticus is particularly important, as it is associated with mortality of up to 20%.

Patients with status epilepticus require immediate resuscitation. This involves establishing an airway and venous access and administering oxygen. Circulation should be assessed and an infusion set up with normal saline.

Blood tests comprise blood gases, glucose, electrolytes, renal and liver function and anticonvulsant levels if the patient has known epilepsy.

COMMON PITFALLS

If hypoglycaemia is suspected in a patient with a possible history of alcohol abuse or malnutrition, thiamine must be given with intravenous glucose, as glucose alone can precipitate Wernicke encephalopathy.

Drug treatment

It is helpful to plan therapy in a series of progressive phases:

- Premonitory stage (0–10 minutes): rapid treatment might prevent the evolution to status. Lorazepam, diazepam or midazolam can be used at this stage.
- First-line therapies: a dose of fast-acting intravenous benzodiazepines such as lorazepam. This can be repeated once if seizures continue. Repeated doses of benzodiazepines might lead to an accumulation and an increased risk of respiratory depression, especially with diazepam.
- Second-line therapies: phenytoin or fosphenytoin is usually given at this stage with intravenous loading doses. Alternatives include the use of intravenous sodium valproate or levetiracetam.

- Third-line therapies: by this stage, anaesthesia is required, with ventilation and intensive care treatment. The most common agents used are intravenous thiopental or propofol. EEG monitoring is very helpful to confirm when status has been aborted. In all cases, neuromuscular blockade should be avoided if possible, because if the seizures return, the patient's muscles will be paralysed, and therefore the return of seizure activity might not be noticed.

Once the patient is stable, further investigations might be necessary to elucidate the cause of the status epilepticus.

NEUROSURGICAL TREATMENT OF EPILEPSY

The indication for surgical treatment requires the accurate identification of a localized site of onset of seizures or the ability to disconnect epileptogenic zones and prevent spread as a palliative procedure. Patients should also have been shown to have epilepsy that is intractable (adequate trials of therapy with at least two first-line drugs) to medical therapy.

The majority of the procedures undertaken in centres worldwide involve some form of temporal lobe surgery. Less commonly, extratemporal cortical excisions, hemispherectomies and corpus callosotomy are carried out. Temporal lobe and extratemporal surgery can result in up to 80% and 40%, respectively, of patients becoming seizure-free in the first year after surgery.

MORTALITY OF EPILEPSY

Deaths directly related to epilepsy fall into several categories: status epilepticus, accidents as a consequence of a seizure and sudden unexpected death in epilepsy (SUDEP). SUDEP is defined as a nontraumatic, unwitnessed death occurring in a patient with epilepsy who had previously been healthy, for which no cause is found even after a thorough postmortem examination. There are many postulated mechanisms of death, including respiratory or cardiovascular arrest, but the underlying pathophysiology is still unknown. Annual mortality is 1 per 1000 epilepsy patients in the community, but this increases to 1 per 200 per year for those with refractory epilepsy.

DRIVING AND EPILEPSY

The Driver and Vehicle Licensing Agency (DVLA) can revoke a British driving licence in any individual felt to be unsafe to himself/herself and/or the public. Patients who have had one or more seizures need to contact the DVLA regarding the length of period they are not allowed to drive. As a guide, the following conditions need to apply before the patient can return to driving with or without treatment, although it should be noted that those drivers with group 2 licences have more severe restrictions:

- Patients who have a diagnosis of epilepsy cannot drive for 1 year after a single seizure.
- Patients who have only nocturnal seizures may drive if they are seizure-free during the daytime for 3 years or 1 year if they have only ever had nocturnal seizures.

- For single seizures with a specific provocative cause (acute symptomatic seizure) that is unlikely to recur, the DVLA will deal with drivers on an individual basis.
- Following a single unprovoked epileptic seizure or isolated seizure, patients are barred from driving for 6 months, provided there is no history of epilepsy, previous solitary seizures or a high risk of recurrence, in which case they are prevented from driving for 12 months.
- Patients who are driving and taking antiepileptic drugs but who wish to stop epileptic medication are recommended to stop driving during cessation and for 6 months following the last dose of their drug.

● Chapter Summary

- A seizure is defined as a synchronous and excessive discharge of neurons in the cerebral cortex. They can be characterized clinically into focal (with or without impairment of consciousness), focal to bilateral and generalized.
- Epilepsy is initially treated with antiepileptic medication (AEDs), with an 80% chance of seizure freedom. However, AEDs are associated with potential acute reactions (e.g., skin rash with lamotrigine), side effects with chronic use (e.g., tremor with valproate) and drug interactions (e.g., phenytoin). In addition, there is increased risk of birth defects with some AEDs taken during pregnancy.
- Status epilepticus is now defined as a seizure that lasts longer than 5 minutes or when seizures occur close together without recovery in between. Urgent acute resuscitation and administration of antiepileptic medication is required in these patients to improve outcome.

UKMLA Conditions
Cerebral palsy and hypoxic–ischaemic
  encephalopathy
Epilepsy

UKMLA Presentations
Abnormal development/developmental delay
Blackouts and faints
Decreased/loss of consciousness
Driving advice
Fits/seizures

Parkinson's disease and other extrapyramidal disorders

AKINETIC–RIGID SYNDROMES

Akinetic–rigid syndromes are defined by akinesia, which encompasses three main features: a poverty of movement (hypokinesia), a slowness of movement (bradykinesia) and fatiguing of repetitive movement. The definition also includes muscle stiffness with and a resistance to passive movement referred to as rigidity. These conditions are caused by neurodegeneration of, or lesions in, the basal ganglia and their connections and are also referred to as extrapyramidal syndromes. The basal ganglia consist of the caudate nucleus, globus pallidus, putamen, substantia nigra and subthalamic nucleus (Fig. 13.1). The akinetic rigid syndromes can be divided into the most common, namely Parkinson's disease, and the atypical parkinsonian disorders of multiple system atrophy (MSA), progressive supranuclear palsy (PSP) and corticobasal degeneration (CBD).

Parkinson's disease

Parkinson's disease was first described by James Parkinson in 1817, who named it the shaking palsy. It is the most common of all the akinetic–rigid syndromes, with a prevalence of 170 per 100,000 of population in the United Kingdom. It is more common in men than in women and the average age at disease onset is 60 years. It is a slowly progressive, degenerative disease involving the basal ganglia as well as other brain areas. It causes an akinetic–rigid syndrome, commonly associated with a rest tremor, which is later accompanied by a flexed posture, shuffling gait and impaired balance. The disease also manifests with a variety of nonmotor symptoms, cognitive and psychiatric complications.

Pathology

There is progressive degeneration of cells within the pars compacta of the substantia nigra in the midbrain. These neurons are dopaminergic. Eosinophilic intraneuronal inclusions called Lewy bodies can be found in the surviving neurons of the substantia nigra. These contain the protein α-synuclein, aggregated with abnormally phosphorylated neurofilaments and ubiquitin. The nigral cells projecting to the striatum are mostly affected (the nigrostriatal pathway). This causes a loss of dopamine in the striatum. Pathological changes may also be seen in other nondopaminergic brainstem nuclei such as locus ceruleus. The involvement of the nondopaminergic system might account for the lack of response of some features of Parkinson's disease to dopamine replacement therapy and the development of nonmotor complications.

Aetiology

The cause of Parkinson's disease is unknown. Twin studies have provided conflicting information about the possible genetic component of Parkinson's disease. Recently, several family pedigrees have been described with familial Parkinson's disease. These include rare autosomal dominant gene mutations in α-synuclein and LRKK2 and autosomal recessive gene mutations in Parkin, *PINK1* or *DJ1* genes.

A consistent environmental factor has not been elucidated. Increased interest in exogenous toxins as a cause arose with the finding that drug addicts taking heroin contaminated with 1-methyl-4-phenyl-1,2,3,6-tetrahydropyridine developed a similar condition, with selective destruction of the nigral cells and their striatal connections. There is also some evidence that pesticides and herbicides increase the risk of developing Parkinson's disease.

Clinical features

Clinical features of Parkinson's disease comprise the classical triad of rest tremor, limb rigidity and not only bradykinesia but also akinesia, with progressive fatiguing of movements, in association with changes in posture and gait and a host of nonmotor symptoms and cognitive decline.

An important and characteristic feature of Parkinson's disease is the striking asymmetry of the clinical signs. If a patient presents with symmetrical parkinsonian clinical signs, they are unlikely to have idiopathic Parkinson's disease.

Tremor

Tremor is the initial presenting symptoms in about 60% of patients with Parkinson's disease. This is a characteristic coarse resting tremor (4–7 Hz) of the hands and can affect any part of the body, including the chin, tongue and legs. It can be exacerbated by emotion and distraction, e.g., walking or using the contralateral limbs. The rest tremor disappears in sleep. It is often pill-rolling in nature on account of the thumb moving rhythmically backwards and forwards on the palmar surface of the fingers. The rest tremor might lessen or disappear during voluntary movement (e.g., when raising arms in front of body), but then reappears after a delay, in the new position (reemergent tremor).

Rigidity

There is stiffness of the limbs, which can be felt as resistance throughout the full range of passive movement in the arms.

This is termed lead-pipe rigidity. When combined with the tremor, which can be subclinical, there is a jerky element (cog-wheel rigidity). The increase in tone can be felt most easily when the wrist is rotated in both clockwise and anticlockwise directions and can be made more apparent when the patient is asked to move voluntarily the opposite limb (synkinesis). The rigidity is usually asymmetrical in the limbs.

COMMON PITFALLS

Both rigidity and spasticity produce an increase in tone, but there are important differences (Table 23.1).

Bradykinesia, hypokinesia and akinesia

Akinesia is often the most disabling feature of Parkinson's disease. It is a grouping of symptoms that includes bradykinesia (slowness of movement with decrement of repetitive alternating movements) and hypokinesia (reduced amplitude of movements). Bradykinesia and hypokinesia affect not only the limbs but also the muscles of facial expression to give mask-like facies known as hypomimia and reduced blinking. The muscles of mastication, speech and voluntary swallowing and some of the axial muscles can also be involved. There is particular difficulty in initiating and terminating movements.

Speech is altered, producing a monotonous, hypophonic dysarthria, due to a combination of bradykinesia, rigidity and tremor. Power is usually preserved, although in advanced disease the slowness (bradykinesia) and rigidity make testing power difficult. Sensory examination is also normal, although patients can often describe discomfort and sensory abnormalities in the legs. Handwriting reduces in size and becomes spidery (micrographia).

Postural changes

The posture is characteristically stooped (Fig. 23.1), with a shuffling, flexed, festinant (steps that become increasingly fast) gait with poor asymmetrical arm swing. Falls are common later in the disease process, as the normal righting reflexes are affected. There may be difficulty in initiating gait (start hesitation) and when the patient tries to turn either when walking or lying (e.g., in bed), there are great difficulties (freezing) and the patient is said to move *en bloc*.

Nonmotor, cognitive and psychiatric features

Constipation is usual and urinary difficulties are common, especially in men. Depression is also common. Cognitive function is preserved in the early stages, but dementia is a common complication later in the disease. Anosmia can precede the onset of Parkinson's disease by several years.

HINTS AND TIPS

Patients with Parkinson's disease often have additional nonmotor symptoms that are equally important to manage. These may result directly from the disease or drug therapy. They include cognitive decline, depression, impulsivity, gastrointestinal complaints (e.g., weight loss and constipation), erectile dysfunction in men, postural hypotension and intrusive REM sleep behavioural disorder.

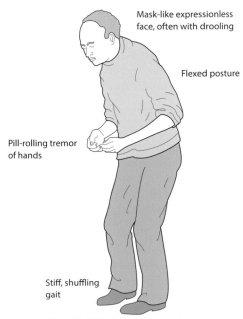

Mask-like expressionless face, often with drooling

Flexed posture

Pill-rolling tremor of hands

Stiff, shuffling gait

Fig. 23.1 Parkinsonian posture.

Table 23.1 The differences between spasticity and rigidity	
Spasticity	Rigidity
Lesion in upper motor neuron	Lesion in basal ganglia and connections
Increased tone more marked in flexors in arms and extensors in legs	Increased tone equal in flexors and extensors
Increased tone most apparent early during movement (clasp-knife effect)	Increased tone apparent throughout range of movement (lead-pipe rigidity)
Reflexes brisk with extensor plantars	Normal reflexes with flexor plantars

Natural history

Parkinson's disease progresses usually over 10 to 15 years with worsening mobility, falls and cognitive decline. The cumulative incidence of dementia approximates to 80%. If falls occur early within the disease, other akinetic–rigid syndromes, e.g., MSA, should be considered as the diagnosis. Death is usually from bronchopneumonia.

Investigations

Parkinson's disease is a clinical diagnosis and a magnetic resonance image (MRI) of the brain in uncomplicated disease is typically normal. A dopamine transporter (DaT) single-photon emission computed tomography scan typically shows decreased DaT binding in the basal ganglia. DaT scans should not be routinely used to confirm a diagnosis of Parkinson's disease, nor can they distinguish between Parkinson's disease, MSA and PSP. NICE recommends its use where it is difficult to differentiate essential tremor from parkinsonism.

Treatment

The main aim of treatment is to restore the dopamine levels within the striatum. A patient's clinical and lifestyle characteristics, together with their preference once fully informed about medication options, should be taken into consideration. The medications for Parkinson's disease and their mechanisms are shown in Fig. 23.2.

Levodopa (L-DOPA)

L-DOPA forms the mainstay of treatment for most patients with Parkinson's disease. It is given in a combined form with a peripheral decarboxylase inhibitor (benserazide, as Madopar; carbidopa, as Sinemet) to prevent the peripheral conversion of the inactive L-DOPA to the active form, dopamine, reducing the peripheral side effects of nausea, vomiting and hypotension. The conversion to dopamine still occurs within the central nervous system (CNS) because benserazide and carbidopa cannot cross the blood–brain barrier, but L-DOPA can.

L-DOPA improves bradykinesia and rigidity but has a variable effect on tremor. However, the majority of patients with Parkinson's disease respond well to treatment and this is often used as additional support for the diagnosis. As the disease progresses, the duration of action of the medication decreases and marked fluctuations in motor symptoms occur with L-DOPA–responsive phases called the on period, followed by off periods where medication overtly wears off or does not take effect. The on periods can become associated with dyskinesias, which are excessive choreiform movements caused by the use of L-DOPA, which can be troubling, and the off periods can become associated with sudden and unpredictable periods of immobility or freezing. Other side effects of L-DOPA include drowsiness, postural hypotension and psychiatric complications such as vivid dreams, nightmares, illusions, hallucinations and impulse control disorders.

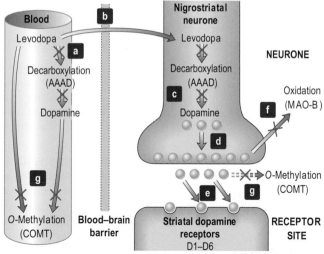

Fig. 23.2 Medications in Parkinson's disease. Levodopa crosses the blood–brain barrier and is converted to dopamine. (a) Carbidopa and benserazide reduce the peripheral conversion of levodopa to dopamine. This leads to a reduction in the side effects of circulating dopamine. (b) Dietary amino acids from high-protein meals can inhibit active transport across the blood–brain barrier by competing with levodopa. (c) Levodopa is converted (aromatic amino acid decarboxylase, AAAD) to dopamine. (d) Amantadine enhances dopamine release. (e) Dopamine agonists activate dopamine receptors. (f) Monoamine oxidase (MAO)-B inhibitors prevent the breakdown of dopamine. (g) Catechol-*O*-methyl transferase (COMT) inhibitors increase the activity of dopamine by blocking its breakdown. (From Feather A, Randall D, Waterhouse M. *Kumar & Clark's Clinical Medicine.* 9th ed. Elsevier; 2017.)

Dopamine agonists

Dopamine agonists are analogues of dopamine and directly stimulate the dopamine receptors. The most effective anti-parkinsonian dopamine agonists stimulate D_2 receptors predominantly, but other types of dopamine receptor stimulation are probably important.

Dopamine agonists have varying selectivity and include bromocriptine, cabergoline, pergolide, ropinirole, pramipexole and apomorphine. Apomorphine is administered as individual subcutaneous injections or as a subcutaneous infusion and is usually reserved for patients at the end stages of the disease, particularly those with severe motor fluctuations or dyskinesias. The dopamine agonists are sometimes prescribed alone as the first-line treatment of Parkinson's disease in younger patients, to delay the use of L-DOPA and therefore early and troublesome dyskinesias. They rarely produce the same dramatic motor response as L-DOPA. Dopamine agonists share a similar side effect profile to L-DOPA but might cause more marked nausea and vomiting and in the elderly can have such particularly severe psychiatric side effects that they are often avoided. Older agonists (pergolide, cabergoline, bromocriptine) are associated with a long-term risk of pleuro-pulmonary-retroperitoneal and cardiac valve fibrosis and for this reason they are avoided.

Anticholinergic drugs

Anticholinergic drugs include benzhexol (trihexyphenidyl), benztropine and procyclidine, which are antimuscarinic agents that penetrate the CNS. They can be effective in reducing tremor, although not so effective in reducing rigidity and bradykinesia. Side effects such as dry mouth, constipation, urinary retention, visual blurring, hallucinations, confusion and memory impairment often prevent their use, especially in the elderly. Amantadine is an antiviral agent, which has some dopamine reuptake blocking and anticholinergic activity and releases stored dopamine. It can be useful in the early stages of the disease and for L-DOPA-induced dyskinesias. Side effects include ankle swelling, skin changes and confusion.

Monoamine oxidase B inhibitors

Selegiline and rasagiline are irreversible inhibitors of monoamine oxidase B (MAO-B), which act to block the degradation of dopamine in the CNS. Its use can prolong the duration of action of L-DOPA.

Catechol-*O*-methyltransferase inhibitors

Dopamine is broken down peripherally by both dopa decarboxylase and catechol-*O*-methyltransferase (COMT). The rationale of these drugs is, therefore, to prevent the additional COMT-mediated breakdown and increase dopamine availability centrally. They are used in conjunction with L-DOPA to reduce the L-DOPA dose and to increase its duration of action. Entacapone is the most widely used drug in this group, while tolcapone is a second-line agent due to a risk of liver failure and rhabdomyolysis.

Surgery

Functional stereotactic neurosurgery for Parkinson's disease is also included in the management of patients with complex disease. Deep brain stimulation of the subthalamic nucleus or globus pallidus can have a significant effect on underlying parkinsonism, including tremor and dyskinesias.

Differential diagnosis of Parkinson's disease

Parkinsonism refers to a syndrome where the clinical features resemble Parkinson's disease but have a different pathological basis. Hypothyroidism and depression may superficially mimic Parkinson's disease but will have no physical signs of parkinsonism.

Causes of parkinsonism include:

- Medications: dopamine antagonists (e.g., phenothiazines, reserpine, haloperidol), lithium.
- Trauma: subdural haematomas, repetitive head injury, e.g., boxing.
- Cerebrovascular disease: lacunar infarcts of the basal ganglia and small vessel disease of the cerebral white matter.
- Hydrocephalus or tumour.
- Infections such as encephalitis lethargica and Japanese B encephalitis.
- Atypical parkinsonian disorders: multisystem atrophy, PSP and CBA (see next section).

The atypical parkinsonian disorders

The atypical or Parkinson plus syndromes refer to other forms of parkinsonism that have clinical features not typical of Parkinson's disease. These include symmetrical parkinsonism, little or no tremor and a poor or an absent response to L-DOPA therapy. There are also additional neurological symptoms and signs.

Progressive supranuclear palsy

PSP is a rare condition with a mean age of onset of 63 years and an average survival of 7 years. It is characterized by falls early on, symmetrical parkinsonism and a prominence of axial features with cognitive decline, dysarthria, dysphagia and a striking supranuclear gaze palsy that initially affects vertical gaze but subsequently might affect all eye movements. The speed and range of voluntary eye movements are limited and can be overcome with the doll's head or oculocephalic manoeuvre, which demonstrates a full range of eye movements. There might be an astonished facial expression with overreaction and increased wrinkling of the frontalis muscle. There is usually a history of falling backwards early in the disease and PSP should be strongly considered in any patient with parkinsonian signs who suffers frequent falls within the first few years of onset. A pseudobulbar palsy develops insidiously with dysarthria, dysphagia and prominent emotional lability. Cognitive decline is common, particularly with frontal release signs and dysexecutive features. Pathological findings include neuronal loss, gliosis and aggregates of tau protein and neurofibrillary tangles in the brainstem, basal ganglia and cerebral cortex. The diagnosis is based on the clinical features and the MRI might identify atrophy of the midbrain (the hummingbird sign) and superior cerebellar peduncles. There is usually little response to treatment with L-DOPA, but amantadine might be useful.

Multisystem atrophy

MSA is a neurodegenerative disorder characterized by parkinsonism and cerebellar signs or autonomic failure. It is rare, with a mean age of onset of 57 years and an average survival of 7 years. Two forms are recognized: MSA-P and MSA-C. MSA-P is associated with asymmetrical parkinsonism that is poorly responsive to L-DOPA and autonomic failure. The latter includes a postural drop in blood pressure, loss of sweating, urinary incontinence or retention and early erectile dysfunction.

In MSA-C, a cerebellar ataxia predominates with autonomic failure. Other features that occur in MSA and might help to differentiate it from other parkinsonian conditions include postural instability, orofacial dystonia and anterocollis, myoclonus that manifests as an irregular and jerky tremor of the upper limbs, pyramidal signs, abnormal respiratory patterns (e.g., stridor, gasps and sleep apnoea) and prominent emotional lability referred to as emotional incontinence. Cognitive decline is not a feature of MSA. The pathological hallmark of the disease is glial cytoplasmic inclusions that contain α-synuclein in the basal ganglia, cerebellum, pons/medulla and motor cortex. Cell loss and gliosis are also seen in Onuf nucleus in the spinal cord, which underly the intrusive dysfunction of bladder and bowel. The diagnosis is a clinical one that can be supported by an MRI, which might show degeneration of the middle cerebellar peduncles and pons (hot cross bun sign). Abnormal autonomic function tests might also aid in diagnosis. Treatment is essentially symptomatic, although amantadine and L-DOPA should be trialled.

Corticobasal degeneration

CBD is a rare disorder that is characterized by strikingly unilateral involvement with rigidity and dystonia in an arm. There is no tremor, but other parkinsonian symptoms and signs are often prominent in addition to cognitive and visuospatial neglect, limb apraxia (inability to make purposeful movements) and myoclonus of the affected arm. Dysphasia and dysphagia might also occur. Patients also report alien limb phenomenon where the arm appears to have a mind of its own and also appears alien. The arm might eventually become functionally useless. Initial symptoms typically begin at the age of 60 years. As the disease progresses, both sides are affected. Patients usually become bed-bound through immobility and die within 6 to 8 years. Treatment is mainly supportive and L-DOPA has little or no effect. Postmortem examination of the brain demonstrates tau inclusions.

Other parkinsonian syndromes

Medication-induced parkinsonism

Medications that have dopamine antagonist effects can cause a parkinsonian syndrome with bradykinesia and rigidity and tremor. The neuroleptics, which include the phenothiazines (e.g., chlorpromazine), butyrophenones (e.g., haloperidol), thioxanthenes (e.g., flupentixol) and substituted benzamides (e.g., sulpiride), can commonly cause parkinsonian or extrapyramidal side effects. These typically resolve after drug withdrawal, although some of the effects might be irreversible despite discontinuing the offending drug. Other commonly used dopamine receptor–blocking drugs include prochlorperazine, metoclopramide and flunarizine, which are commonly used to treat vertigo, nausea and vomiting and migraine.

Cerebrovascular disease

The pathological basis of cerebrovascular disease causing parkinsonism is usually multifocal small vessel disease, particularly subcortical ischaemia and lacunar infarcts. Patients often have a degree of cognitive impairment and pyramidal signs in the limbs with symmetrical bradykinesia and rigidity and little resting tremor. It typically affects the lower limbs and is sometimes called lower limb parkinsonism. Patients typically have a small-stepped gait called *marche à petit pas* with an upright stance (as compared with the stooped posture of Parkinson's disease) and an unsteady wide-based gait. Treatment is aimed at secondary prevention by treating underlying cardiovascular risk factors, especially hypertension.

Wilson disease

Wilson disease is an inherited autosomal recessive disorder of copper metabolism, resulting in low levels of the copper-binding protein caeruloplasmin. This causes elevated levels of free copper in the blood, which results in copper deposition in the brain, particularly in the basal ganglia, in the Descemet membrane in the cornea (Kayser–Fleischer rings only seen on slit lamp examination of the eyes) and in the liver, which causes cirrhosis. Patients typically present in their teens or early adult life with atypical parkinsonism, tremor, dystonia, cerebellar signs and cognitive decline. Patients can also present with prominent psychiatric symptoms, including a personality change, emotional lability and psychosis. It is uncommon for neurological manifestations to occur after the age of 40 years. The diagnosis is made by identifying low levels of caeruloplasmin with high free copper in the urine and serum after a penicillamine challenge. An MRI of the brain might show cortical atrophy or signal change in the putamen and a liver biopsy can provide a tissue diagnosis. Genetic testing is not practical due to the large number of mutations that have been found. The disease is treated with copper-binding agents such as penicillamine, zinc acetate or trientine and the neurological damage may be partly reversible.

HINTS AND TIPS

Idiopathic Parkinson's disease can be differentiated from other parkinsonian syndromes by:

- An excellent response to L-DOPA.
- Asymmetrical onset of the bradykinesia, rigidity and usually tremor.
- Absence of other neurological system involvement, e.g., pyramidal system.

NEUROLEPTIC-INDUCED MOVEMENT DISORDERS

Dopamine-blocking drugs used to treat psychiatric illness or as antiemetics or vestibular sedatives can cause a variety of movement disorders.

Acute dystonic reactions

Dystonia develops in 2% to 5% of patients on neuroleptics or antiemetics (metoclopramide and prochlorperazine). This reaction is unpredictable and can occur even after single dose of the medication. The range of dystonias includes torticollis, oculogyric crisis and trismus. They respond rapidly to intravenous injection of an anticholinergic drug (e.g., procyclidine or benztropine). Some patients on neuroleptics who develop these reactions are also treated or cotreated with an oral anticholinergic.

Medication-induced parkinsonism

See earlier.

Akathisia

Akathisia is a restless, repetitive and irresistible need to move, usually caused by neuroleptics. It may cease with drug withdrawal or be treated with a benzodiazepine or propranolol.

Tardive dyskinesia

Tardive dyskinesia is a movement disorder that develops after chronic exposure to neuroleptics. It can be irreversible and might worsen when the offending medication is stopped. Involuntary movements affect the face, mouth and tongue (orobuccolingual movements), causing lip smacking, grimacing and dystonic grimacing. It can be avoided by using newer atypical neuroleptics. It is thought to be due to drug-induced supersensitivity of the dopamine receptors.

Neuroleptic malignant syndrome

Occasionally, dopamine receptor–blocking drugs can cause this syndrome, which manifests with extreme rigidity, fluctuating conscious level, fever, autonomic disturbance and elevated serum creatine kinase. The drug in question should be withdrawn and the patient treated with a dopamine agonist/levodopa and dantrolene.

RESTLESS LEG SYNDROME

This is a common syndrome that can be familial or sporadic. It can be associated with iron deficiency, anaemia, pregnancy, peripheral neuropathy or uraemia. Patients complain of an unpleasant sensation in their legs and an irresistible urge to move their legs, which is worse at night when they are resting or inactive. Symptoms are relieved by movement and can be treated with iron replacement if serum ferritin levels are below the recommended range and dopaminergic medication.

Chapter Summary

- The akinetic–rigid syndromes are defined by hypokinesia (reduced movement), bradykinesia (slow movement) and limb rigidity. The most notable example is Parkinson's disease.
- The hallmark characteristics of Parkinson's disease include an asymmetrical resting tremor, lead-pipe limb rigidity and akinesia, especially in relation to gait. Postural instability and psychiatric/cognitive decline are other important features.
- Atypical parkinsonian diseases have shared features with Parkinson's disease but additional exclusive characteristics such as supranuclear gaze palsy (progressive supranuclear palsy), cerebellar disease (multiple system atrophy) and prominent apraxia (corticobasal degeneration).

UKMLA Conditions
Dementias
Parkinson's disease

UKMLA Presentations
Abnormal involuntary movements
Anosmia
Behaviour/personality change
Memory loss
Speech and language problems
Tremor
Unsteadiness
Urinary symptoms

Diseases affecting the spinal cord (myelopathy) 24

ANATOMY

The spinal cord extends from the top of the C1 vertebra to the bottom of the body of the L1 or L2 vertebra in adults. There is an expansion in the diameter of the cord in the cervical and lumbar regions due to increased numbers of anterior horn motor cells in the arms and legs. The lower end of the spinal cord is known as the conus medullaris (Fig. 24.1). The spinal cord is continuous superiorly with the medulla oblongata and inferiorly with the cauda equina and filum terminale. This is a thin connective tissue filament that descends from the conus medullaris with the spinal nerve roots. Thus, pathology at T12 and L1 affects the lumbar cord, pathology at L2 affects the conus medullaris and lesions below L2 involve the cauda equina and represent injuries to the spinal roots, rather than the spinal cord.

The spinal cord, cauda equina and filum terminale, down to the S2 level, are surrounded by a thick covering of dura mater, which is separated from the fine arachnoid mater by the potential subdural space. The arachnoid mater is separated from the pia mater, which invests the spinal cord and nerve roots, by the subarachnoid space.

A representative part of the spinal cord in cross-section is shown in Fig. 24.2. It contains the central grey matter, consisting of neuronal cell bodies and the peripheral white matter, which contains the ascending and descending axonal pathways. The ascending pathways relay sensory information from the periphery to the brain, brainstem and cerebellum and the descending pathways relay motor instructions from the brain. There are three main white matter tracts. The two main ascending tracts are the spinothalamic tract and dorsal columns and the main descending pathway is the lateral corticospinal tract (see Fig. 24.2 and Chapters 14 and 15).

Most of the main sensory and motor pathways cross to the contralateral side during their course in the central nervous system (CNS). It is important to know these sites of decussation because clinically different syndromes result from interruption of the pathways at various levels.

THE CLINICAL SYNDROMES OF SPINAL CORD DISEASE

There are three main motor syndromes associated with spinal cord disease:

- Paraparesis: upper motor neurone (UMN) involvement of legs only.
- Tetraparesis: UMN involvement of all four limbs.
- Brown–Séquard syndrome: unilateral lesion causing UMN involvement of one side.

These three patterns of weakness are often associated with sensory signs. They might develop rapidly or slowly over days, months or years, depending on the cause. Any lesion involving the spinal cord results in a syndrome called myelopathy. If the lesion damages the anterior horn cells as well as the corticospinal tracts, the patient will have UMN signs below the level of the lesion and lower motor neurone (LMN) signs at about the level of the lesion. If myelopathy occurs with radiculopathy (i.e., root involvement), the condition is called myeloradiculopathy. For example, the most common cause of compression of the cervical spinal cord is due to wear and tear osteoarthritis and degenerative changes within the cervical vertebrae or cervical spondylosis. This leads to damage to the corticospinal tracts in the cervical cord, resulting in UMN signs in the legs (paraparesis) and sensory loss below the level of the lesion (sensory level) (i.e., myelopathy), as well as LMN signs in the arms due to damage of spinal roots at the level of the spondylotic lesion, i.e., radiculopathy.

Paraparesis (spastic paraparesis or paraplegia)

Paraparesis indicates bilateral UMN damage involving the axons that innervate the legs from both corticospinal tracts. The clinical signs include increased tone with spasticity, pyramidal distribution of weakness, increased reflexes with clonus and extensor plantar responses. The abdominal and cremasteric reflexes or cutaneous reflexes might be absent (Fig. 24.3). There is often involvement of the two sensory pathways from the level below the lesion. This is called a sensory level. Sphincter dysfunction is also typical of spinal cord disease and occurs early with intrinsic spinal cord lesions and later in the course of extrinsic spinal cord lesions.

Tetraparesis (spastic tetraparesis, tetraplegia, quadriparesis and quadriplegia)

Spastic tetraparesis produces the same clinical picture as paraparesis but involves both arms and legs. It is usually caused by a lesion in the high cervical cord but is occasionally due to brainstem or bilateral cortical damage.

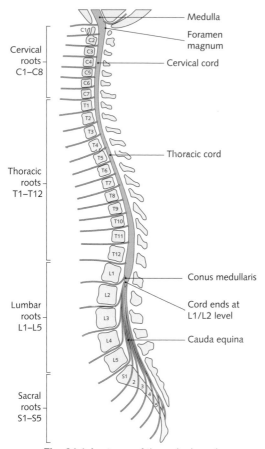

Fig. 24.1 Anatomy of the spinal cord.

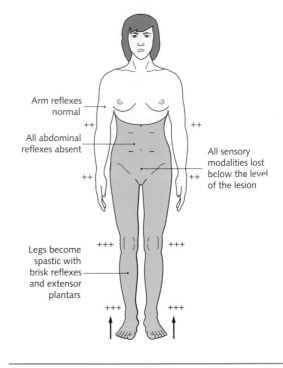

−, Absent reflex; +, Reduced reflex; ++, Normal
+++, Pathologically brisk reflex; ↑, Extensor plantar

Fig. 24.3 Clinical signs of cord compression caused by a lesion of the thoracic cord at the T7 level.

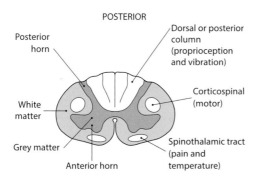

Fig. 24.2 A cross-section of the spinal cord, showing the positions of the major pathways.

Brown–Séquard syndrome (unilateral cord lesion)

Brown–Séquard syndrome is rare in its pure form but partial forms are more common.

The pure Brown–Séquard clinical picture (Fig. 24.4) consists of:

- Ipsilateral spastic leg and sometimes arm if the lesion is above C5, with brisk reflexes and an extensor plantar response.
- Ipsilateral loss of joint-position sense and vibration (dorsal columns).
- Contralateral loss of pain and temperature (spinothalamic tracts cross at their level of entry).

The sensory level is often a few segments lower than the level of the lesion because pain fibres ascend a few spinal segments before entering the dorsal horn to synapse then cross (see Chapter 15).

CAUSES OF SPINAL CORD DISEASE

Transection of the cord

Spinal cord transection is usually the result of trauma following anterior dislocation of one vertebra on another. It causes loss of all motor, sensory and autonomic function, including the sphincters, below the level of the lesion either immediately, if the transection is complete, or within hours if the damage is

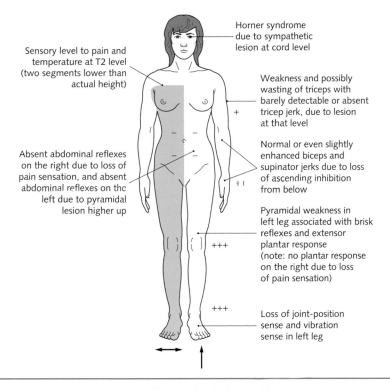

Horner syndrome due to sympathetic lesion at cord level

Sensory level to pain and temperature at T2 level (two segments lower than actual height)

Weakness and possibly wasting of triceps with barely detectable or absent tricep jerk, due to lesion at that level

Absent abdominal reflexes on the right due to loss of pain sensation, and absent abdominal reflexes on the left due to pyramidal lesion higher up

Normal or even slightly enhanced biceps and supinator jerks due to loss of ascending inhibition from below

Pyramidal weakness in left leg associated with brisk reflexes and extensor plantar response (note: no plantar response on the right due to loss of pain sensation)

Loss of joint-position sense and vibration sense in left leg

−, Absent reflex; +, Reduced reflex; ++, Normal
+++, Pathologically brisk reflex; ↑, Extensor plantar

Fig. 24.4 Clinical signs of a Brown–Séquard lesion at level C7 on the left.

partial, but later results in secondary oedema causing involvement of the whole spinal cord at the level of the partial lesion.

With any severe, acute spinal cord lesion, there are usually two clinical stages:

- Spinal shock: initially, there is loss of all reflex activity below the level of the lesion, with flaccid limbs, atonic bladder with overflow incontinence, atonic bowel, gastric dilatation and loss of genital reflexes and vasomotor control.
- Heightened reflex activity: this occurs after about 1 to 2 weeks and is associated with spasticity of the limbs, brisk reflexes and extensor plantar responses. Patients develop a spastic bladder (small capacity with urgency, frequency and automatic emptying) and hyperactive autonomic function (sweating and vasomotor changes).

HINTS AND TIPS

The supply to the diaphragm is via the phrenic nerve (C3, C4 and C5) and therefore any cord lesion above C3 can cause neuromuscular respiratory failure.

COMMON PITFALLS

Bilateral upper motor neurone signs in the legs (with or without arm involvement) with no cranial nerve signs usually indicate spinal cord pathology. The lesion must be above the body of L1, because the spinal cord ends at this level and lesions below this level involve the cauda equina and therefore cause lower motor neurone signs.

Differential diagnosis

In the absence of trauma, similar symptoms and signs of a very severe cord lesion might indicate the following:

- Ischaemic infarction of the cord: occlusion of a major segmental artery, dissecting aortic aneurysm or anterior spinal artery thrombosis.
- Haemorrhage into the spinal cord from an arteriovenous malformation (AVM), epidural or subdural haemorrhage.
- Acute or subacute necrotizing or demyelinating myelopathy.

- Epidural abscess.
- Acute vertebral collapse: usually associated with neoplastic disease of the vertebrae.

Treatment

Complete transection of the spinal cord has a very poor neurological outcome. It is more usual for incomplete cord transection to occur. In this scenario, it is vital to treat any spinal fracture and instability with orthopaedic or neurosurgical input, as this might prevent secondary damage to the intact cord from the spinal injury. The reduction of spinal cord oedema with immediate administration of high-dose corticosteroids might help.

Spinal cord compression

The site of compression or inflammation will determine the clinical picture. Pain is the most commonly presenting symptom, followed by limb weakness, sensory loss and sphincter disturbance. Lesions affecting the cord below T1 will not involve the arms, whereas lesions between C5 and T1 cause LMN and sometimes UMN signs in the arms and UMN signs in the legs. Lesions above C5 cause UMN signs in the arms and legs. Compressive lesions might spare sphincter function until the patient has severe disease. Therefore, any patient with sphincter involvement needs urgent investigation.

Causes

- Trauma (see above).
- Degenerative disease: spondylotic/disc disease and spinal canal stenosis.
- Tumours: metastatic or myeloma.
- Infective lesions: epidural abscess, tuberculoma, HIV, human T-cell lymphocytic virus type 1 (HTLV-1), granuloma.
- Epidural haemorrhage.

Degenerative disease: spondylotic/ disc disease and spinal canal stenosis

Spondylosis means degenerative changes within the spine that occur during ageing or secondary to trauma or rheumatological disease. The degenerative process starts with dehydration and disintegration of the disc. This then causes loading and hypertrophy of the facet joints, bulging of the discs and ligamentum flavum hypertrophy, all of which contribute to narrowing of the spinal canal. Clinically, the degenerative processes manifest in two ways: disc protrusion and spinal canal stenosis.

Damaged discs usually protrude laterally and cause compression of the nerve roots, resulting in an LMN lesion. However, discs can protrude centrally and posteriorly (see Chapter 26).

In the cervical/thoracic spine, canal stenosis will cause compression of the spinal cord causing a cervical spondylotic myelopathy.

This might present clinically with a stepwise neurological deterioration. Initially, symptoms might begin in the legs with unsteadiness and difficulty walking and there might be only mild signs in the arms. In the lumbar spine, canal stenosis might lead to compression of the cauda equina and cause neurogenic claudication. This manifests as neurological symptoms of calf pain, weakness and sensory disturbance that worsen with walking, standing or maintaining certain postures, but ease with bending forwards, sitting or lying, which enlarges the diameter of the spinal canal. Localized areas of narrowing might cause compression of an individual nerve root, manifesting as a painful radiculopathy. This is typically shooting in nature and referred into the dermatome of the affected root. Treatment for degenerative spinal disease might be conservative (analgesia, antiinflammatory medication, exercise and physiotherapy) or surgical when there is neurological compromise.

> **COMMON PITFALLS**
>
> It is important to remember that cervical cord compression can lead to a neurological deficit being confined to the legs, with only mild and subtle signs in the arms. Therefore, when requesting imaging studies for someone with symptoms and signs in the legs, the cervical spine should be assessed as well as the thoracic and lumbar spine.

Spinal cord tumours

Spinal cord tumours can be:

- Intramedullary (within the substance of the spinal cord): these are usually malignant, e.g., glioma, ependymoma or astrocytoma, causing an intrinsic cord lesion.
- Intradural but extramedullary, i.e., on the surface of the cord arising from the meninges (meningioma) or spinal root (schwannoma or neurofibroma), but within the dural sac. These are usually benign and present with spinal cord compression and back pain.
- Extradural (in the epidural space or within/between vertebrae): these are usually manifestations of multifocal systemic neoplasia, e.g., metastatic carcinoma, lymphoma, myeloma, or can be other mass lesions, e.g., abscess, lipoma. Extradural tumours typically present with vertebral collapse or spinal cord compression.

Infective lesions

Epidural abscess

Infections in the spinal column occur in the facet joints (septic arthritis), the intervertebral disc (discitis) or within the vertebral bodies (osteomyelitis). Infections in the epidural space give rise to epidural abscesses and are most often caused by *Staphylococcus aureus*. The organism usually reaches the cord via the bloodstream but may spread directly from skin/soft tissue infections or from sites of invasive procedures or spinal surgery. Damage occurs through direct compression of nerve tissue or blood supply, thrombosis of veins, focal vasculitis or inflammation. The classic clinical triad consists of fever, spinal pain and neurological deficits. Diagnosis is made with magnetic resonance imaging (MRI) and lumbar puncture. Treatment is with appropriate antibiotics and surgical drainage. The treatment of the underlying source of infection is also important.

Tuberculoma

Tuberculomas are a frequent cause of cord compression in areas where tuberculosis (TB) is common (e.g., India, Pakistan, Africa and in any areas populated from these countries of origin). It often occurs in the absence of pulmonary disease. Infection typically starts in a disc space, before spreading to form an epidural or paravertebral abscess. There may be destruction of vertebral bodies and spread of infection along the extradural space. This results in cord compression and paraparesis or Pott paraplegia. The clinical signs of TB meningitis might coexist. Diagnosis requires a high index of suspicion. The tuberculoma can be seen on MRI and *Mycobacterium tuberculosis* can be seen or grown from samples of cerebrospinal fluid. Treatment is with antituberculous therapy, as guided by the local microbiology sensitivities, but triple and quadruple therapy is often needed. This is continued for at least 9 months and can be used in conjunction with the judicious use of corticosteroids for coexisting oedema.

HIV

Immunocompromised HIV patients carry an increased risk of pyogenic spinal infections, including *Staphylococcus aureus* and tuberculosis. In addition, they have a risk of opportunistic infections and, therefore, there should be a low threshold for investigating patients with HIV presenting with back pain, particularly those with a low CD4 count or high viral load. Patients with HIV are also at risk of developing spinal cord disease as a result of demyelination or vacuolar myelopathy.

HTLV-1: tropical spastic paraparesis

HTLV-1 causes a progressive myelopathy, primarily of the thoracic cord. Patients from tropical regions develop a progressive spastic paraparesis and urinary disturbance with sparing of the posterior columns.

Epidural haemorrhage and haematoma

Epidural or extradural haemorrhage and haematoma are rare sequelae of anticoagulant therapy, bleeding diatheses and trauma, including lumbar puncture. They often result in a rapidly progressive cord or cauda equina lesion, associated with severe pain. Treatment is surgical decompression and management of any underlying disorder.

Vascular cord lesions

Anterior spinal artery occlusion

Infarction of the spinal cord is rare in comparison with that of the brain. The blood supply of the spinal cord is predominantly from a single anterior and two posterior spinal arteries. The anterior artery supplies the anterior two-thirds of the spinal cord. It arises from the vertebral arteries in the neck and is supported by radicular branches from the aorta. Anterior spinal artery occlusion is caused by thrombus or embolism and the risk factors for these are identical to those for cerebral infarcts. Spinal cord infarction can also occur in the context of severe systemic hypotension or vasospasm, e.g., cocaine use. In an anterior spinal infarct, onset of symptoms is sudden and not usually associated with back pain. Symptoms include paralysis, loss of bladder function and loss of pain and temperature below the level of the lesion. Position and vibration sense are spared. In the acute stage, the weakness might be flaccid due to spinal shock, but this can progress to spasticity over time. The mid to lower thoracic region is the most vulnerable to ischaemia as it is a watershed area for blood supply.

Dural arteriovenous fistulas

These are rare acquired lesions most typically seen in men over the age of 50 years. They exist on the dural surface and often affect the lower part of the spinal cord, including the conus medullaris. The most common presentation is of a progressive, stepwise myeloradiculopathy (or conus syndrome), probably related to venous hypertension. There is gradual loss of lower limb function with combined UMN and LMN signs and mixed cord and root sensory loss with saddle anaesthesia and bowel and bladder sphincter dysfunction. The diagnosis is typically established with MRI, magnetic resonance angiography (MRA) and spinal angiography and treatment involves endovascular embolization or surgical occlusion.

Intramedullary spinal arteriovenous malformations

Similar to dural AVMs, intramedullary spinal AVMs are congenital abnormalities consisting of arterial feeding vessels that drain into dilated, tortuous veins, which are under high pressure. They can either remain asymptomatic or present in young adults. Presentation can be with sudden loss of neurological function below the level of the lesion as a result of haemorrhage or infarction. Patients can also present with stepwise neurological symptoms due to the mass effect of the lesion or due to spinal cord ischaemia resulting from vascular steal or venous hypertension. MRI/MRA can be used to diagnose these lesions and they can be treated with endovascular occlusion or surgical resection.

Cavernous haemangiomas

These are capillary malformations that can occur within the spinal cord and in approximately one-third of cases are familial and might be multiple. The whole spine and brain should, therefore, be imaged to exclude multiple lesions. Bleeding can occur from them, causing gradual loss of cord function distal to the lesion. The diagnosis is based on MRI alone, as angiography is unhelpful, and treatment is surgical.

Inflammatory lesions and transverse myelitis

Transverse myelitis is a broad term used to describe segmental inflammation of the cord with resultant paraparesis (or tetraparesis), arising from a wide range of diseases. Most cases are idiopathic but probably arise from an autoimmune process triggered by a preceding infection. The inflammation of transverse myelitis is typically restricted to one or two segments and symptoms usually develop over several hours. Typically, the inflammation is bilateral with variable loss of distal motor, sensory and sphincter function, although unilateral syndromes have also been described. Pain and tingling are common and back and radicular pain may occur. The diagnosis is based on the clinical picture, MRI spine and CSF results. Treatment depends on the underlying cause but can include steroids.

Multiple sclerosis and neuromyelitis optica

Multiple sclerosis is a chronic inflammatory disease of the CNS (see Chapter 33). It can cause lesions in the brain and spinal cord, with spinal cord lesions more likely to produce clinical symptoms. Lesions appear as white matter hyperintensities on MRI. Neuromyelitis optica is a chronic CNS inflammatory disease similar to multiple sclerosis but is exclusively immune-mediated. It presents with optic neuritis and/or transverse myelitis. Typical MRI findings are that of longitudinally extensive lesions spanning three or more vertebral segments. Patients usually show positive aquaporin-4 antibodies in serum and treatment is immunosuppressive with steroids and later steroid-sparing agents.

Viral transverse myelitis

A number of viruses can cause transverse myelitis, either as a direct result of infection or postviral demyelination. Examples include Epstein–Barr virus, varicella zoster, cytomegalovirus, herpes simplex virus and HIV. It should be noted that some viruses (e.g., enteroviruses such as poliovirus) selectively invade the anterior horn cells to produce asymmetrical flaccid weakness with absent reflexes and no sensory signs.

Granulomatous and connective tissue disease

Connective tissue diseases can also cause transverse myelitis, e.g., systemic lupus erythematosus, Sjögren syndrome, scleroderma, antiphospholipid syndrome and rheumatoid arthritis.

Metabolic and toxic cord disease

Subacute combined degeneration of the cord

Subacute combined degeneration of the cord (SCDC) is the most notable example of metabolic disease affecting the spinal cord and is caused by deficiency of functional vitamin B_{12}. The deficiency might result from nutritional deficiency (especially in vegans), pernicious anaemia, gastrectomy or disease of the terminal ileum (e.g., Crohn disease). The deficiency causes a dorsal spinal cord syndrome; there is demyelination of the dorsal and lateral white matter of the spinal cord, producing a slowly progressive paraparesis, sensory ataxia and paraesthesia. Vitamin B_{12} deficiency can also cause damage to the peripheral nerves, i.e., a peripheral neuropathy that can exacerbate the sensory ataxia. Patients can also develop optic atrophy and a mild dementia. It is also important to ask about recreational use of nitrous oxide, which can cause a similar syndrome. Nitrous oxide causes a functional inactivation of vitamin B_{12}, and vitamin B_{12} serum levels may be normal, with elevated homocysteine and/or methylmalonic acid levels, and these should both also be measured if vitamin B_{12} deficiency is suspected. Not all patients will have subacute combined degeneration, with some nitrous oxide users developing a sensorimotor neuropathy with demyelinating features.

A similar syndrome to subacute combined degeneration (SCDC) as a result of vitamin B_{12} deficiency can occur with acquired copper deficiency.

A megaloblastic anaemia might be present on routine blood screen with associated low B_{12} levels; however, neither are a requisite for diagnosis. Treatment is with parenteral vitamin B_{12} therapy.

HINTS AND TIPS

There are only a few common causes of absent ankle jerks (i.e., lower motor neurone) and extensor plantar responses (i.e., upper motor neurone). These include:

- combined pathology, e.g., cervical spondylosis and peripheral neuropathy
- motor neurone disease (see Chapter 25)
- conus medullaris lesions (see anatomy)
- subacute combined degeneration of the cord (vitamin B_{12} myelopathy)
- Friedreich ataxia (see Chapter 36)
- tabes dorsalis/tertiary neurosyphilis (see Chapter 32)

Intrinsic cord lesions

The signs of an intrinsic cord lesion are usually caused by MS. Much rarer causes include an intrinsic tumour or a syrinx (syringomyelia).

Syringomyelia and syringobulbia

Syringomyelia (relatively common) and syringobulbia (very rare) are caused by a fluid-filled cavity (syrinx) within the spinal cord and brainstem, respectively.

The cavitation of the cervical cord is associated, in the majority of cases, with a congenital abnormality of the foramen magnum, which is usually an Arnold–Chiari malformation. This causes the cerebellar tonsils to lie in the posterior foramen magnum and potentially they can compress the brainstem. A syrinx can also arise due to an intrinsic tumour or following trauma, infection or inflammatory pathology. Most lesions are between C2 and T9, although they can extend upwards or downwards.

Clinically, the picture evolves because the expanding cavity damages the various neurones and pathways (Fig. 24.5). The signs can be unilateral, especially at presentation, but are ultimately bilateral, although there may be asymmetry:

- Pain in the upper limbs is often an early feature, which may be exacerbated by coughing or straining if associated with an Arnold–Chiari malformation.
- Dissociated spinothalamic sensory loss (i.e., loss of crossing pain and temperature fibres, but preservation of vibration and joint position pathways) in a cape-like or suspended distribution (i.e., the dermatomes above and below the level of the syrinx are spared). In advanced cases, the impairment of pain sensation can lead to the development of neuropathic or Charcot joints in the hand, elbow or shoulder.
- There is unilateral or bilateral Horner syndrome (meiosis, ptosis and anhydrosis) due to damage to sympathetic fibres within the spinal cord down to T1.
- There is wasting and weakness of the small muscles of the hand due to damage of the anterior horn cells at the T1 level (a common site for a syrinx).

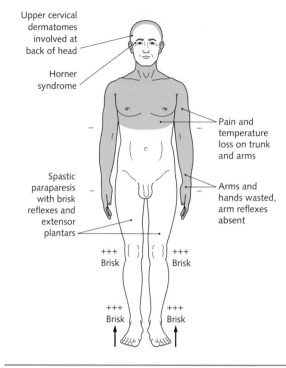

−, Absent reflex; ++, Normal; +++ Brisk; ↑, Extensor plantar

Fig. 24.5 The evolving pattern of an intrinsic cord lesion at T1. This pattern may be seen with syringomyelia and intrinsic cord tumours, e.g., glioma, ependymoma and astrocytoma.

- Spastic paraparesis develops only after the cavity is markedly distended and compresses on the corticospinal tracts.

With syringobulbia, there is also:

- bilateral wasting and weakness of the tongue
- hearing loss
- vestibular involvement with nystagmus
- facial sensory loss

Treatment of a syrinx associated with a Chiari malformation is surgical decompression of the foramen magnum.

Diseases affecting the spinal cord (myelopathy)

● **Chapter Summary**

- The spinal cord extends from the top of the C1 vertebra to the bottom of the body of the L1 or L2 vertebrae. Below L2 is the cauda equina.
- There are three main white matter tracts in the spinal cord: the two main ascending tracts are the spinothalamic tract and dorsal columns and the main descending pathway is the lateral corticospinal tract.
- The three main clinical presentations associated with cord disease are paraparesis (legs affected), quadriparesis (arms and legs affected) and Brown–Séquard (dissociated signs).
- Spinal cord disease can have a number of aetiologies: vascular (spinal cord infarct), infective (transverse myelitis), inflammatory (multiple sclerosis), metabolic (B_{12} deficiency) and malignancy.

UKMLA Conditions
Multiple sclerosis
Peripheral nerve injuries/palsies
Radiculopathies
Spinal cord compression
Spinal cord injury
Spinal fracture

UKMLA Presentations
Altered sensation, numbness and tingling
Back pain
Limb weakness
Neck pain/stiffness
Trauma

170

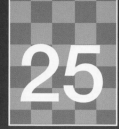
TYPES AND CLINICAL FEATURES OF MOTOR NEURONE DISEASE

Motor neurone disease (MND) is a disease in which there is progressive degeneration of motor neurones in the motor cortex and in the anterior horns of the spinal cord. There is also degeneration of the cells within the somatic motor nuclei of the cranial nerves within the brainstem.

MND encompasses a number of conditions that affect motor neurones. These include amyotrophic lateral sclerosis (ALS), progressive bulbar palsy, primary lateral sclerosis and progressive muscular atrophy (PMA). These categories do not represent distinct aetiological or pathological mechanisms and often merge as the disease progresses. Although MND predominantly affects motor neurones, it is increasingly recognized that other systems, including cognitive centres, cerebellar and extrapyramidal pathways, can be affected.

Amyotrophic lateral sclerosis

ALS is often used synonymously with MND in the United States and in Europe. It has an incidence of 2 per 100,000 per year, affects males more than females (M:F = 2:1), a mean age of onset of 60 years and a mean duration of survival of 3 years. In the United Kingdom, it is used to represent a particular form of MND with a mixture of upper motor neurone (UMN) and lower motor neurone (LMN) signs in the limbs, head, neck and bulbar region (Fig. 25.1). Degeneration of the UMNs gives rise to increased tone, pyramidal distribution weakness and brisk reflexes with extensor plantars. LMN involvement might give rise to muscle cramps, fasciculations, including of the tongue, wasting and weakness. All these features might occur in combination within a body region (Table 25.1).

Onset of disease tends to be focal, distal and asymmetrical and progresses in a segmental fashion from one limb to another. A small proportion of patients might present with symmetrical, proximal flaccid weakness of the arms, with sparing elsewhere, although as the disease progresses, UMN signs will develop. This is known as the flail arm variant of MND.

In addition to motor features, it is now also increasingly recognized that up to 50% of patients with MND may also have cognitive impairment, with up to 10% fulfilling the diagnostic criteria for frontotemporal dementia (FTD). Thus, MND and FTD represent two ends of a disease continuum, and these diseases are on a clinical, genetic and pathological spectrum.

Progressive muscular atrophy

Progressive muscular atrophy (PMA) is associated with LMN signs (wasting, weakness and fasciculations, although tendon reflexes are usually preserved), which often begin asymmetrically in the small muscles of the hands or feet and spread. This form often progresses to include UMN signs with time.

Progressive bulbar and pseudobulbar palsy

Bulbar refers to the lower brainstem motor nuclei. Bulbar palsy usually refers to involvement of the LMN with prominent fasciculations in the tongue, often with wasting, in addition to a

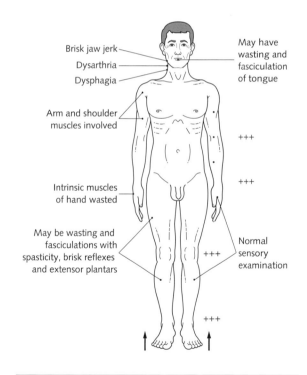

++, Normal; +++, Pathologically brisk reflex; ↑, Extensor plantar

Fig. 25.1 Clinical findings in a patient with classic amyotrophic lateral sclerosis with a mixture of upper and lower motor neurone signs. There is often a mixed bulbar and pseudobulbar picture, e.g., wasted, fasciculating tongue with a spastic palate, which may remain isolated or be the presenting feature of amyotrophic lateral sclerosis.

Table 25.1 Features of upper and lower motor neurone lesions

Upper motor neurone	Lower motor neurone
Spastic paralysis	Flaccid paralysis
No wasting	Muscle wasting
No fasciculations	Fasciculations present
Brisk reflexes	Reduced or absent reflexes
Clonus	No clonus
Extensor plantar response (Babinski)	Plantar response flexor or absent

weak palate with nasal regurgitation and a nasal voice. Pseudobulbar palsy involves the UMN bilaterally and leads to a spastic dysarthria (Donald Duck voice), dysphagia, hypersalivation, laryngospasm and emotional lability (pseudobulbar affect). Approximately 25% of MND patients might present with bulbar onset, with symptoms and signs restricted to the tongue and muscles innervated by the lower cranial nerves. Most of these patients will develop classic ALS/MND. Those in whom the disease remains restricted to the bulbar region tend to have a worse prognosis, due to an increased risk of aspiration. These patients often lose the ability to speak, due to lack of movement of the tongue, palate and mouth.

Primary lateral sclerosis

A small number of patients (typically 1%–5%) might present solely with UMN signs, typically initially in the legs before progressing to involve the arms and bulbar muscles. This variant is known as primary lateral sclerosis and the diagnosis can only be made once other conditions are excluded and the signs have remained solely UMN for at least 3 years. Unlike the other variants, these patients tend to have a slower progression and better prognosis.

Eye movements and sphincter involvement are never affected in MND and their abnormality virtually excludes the diagnosis. Patients might complain of sensory symptoms, including pain in the limbs, but have no sensory signs. They might also experience troublesome cramps, especially at night.

COMMON PITFALLS

Some groups of motor neurones are not affected by motor neurone disease. These include motor nerves from the oculomotor nuclei responsible for eye movements and those from the Onuf nucleus in the sacral spinal cord, which are important for bladder and bowel control.

PATHOGENESIS

The majority of cases of MND are sporadic with no family history. Familial cases account for between 5% and 10% of patients. The most common familial form is due to a hexanucleotide repeat expansion in the first intron of the *C9orf72* gene on chromosome 9. Another common genetic cause is abnormal expression of the superoxide dismutase-1 gene (*SOD-1*) found on chromosome 21, which typically causes autosomal dominant ALS. Understanding of the genetic basis of this condition has recently improved, with the discovery that in both familial and sporadic ALS, ubiquitin-positive neuronal cytoplasmic inclusions within the motor neurones are present and these contain the nuclear RNA- and DNA-binding protein TDP-43. This protein is also found in ubiquitin-positive frontotemporal lobe dementia. The pathological overlap between these two conditions mirrors the clinical overlap described earlier and a number of genetic mutations are now being identified that are thought to play a role in this overlap, the most recent and important being the *C9orf72* repeat expansion described earlier.

DIFFERENTIAL DIAGNOSIS

The differential diagnosis depends on the mode of presentation.

Amyotrophic lateral sclerosis

Differential diagnoses for ALS include conditions that present with a mixture of UMN and LMN signs:

- Cervical spondylotic radiculomyelopathy: a combination of spinal cord compression (UMN), spinal root compression and anterior horn cell loss (LMN).
- Spinal tumours: these can cause LMN signs at the level of the pathology and also UMN signs below the level of the lesion.
- Spinal conus medullaris lesions: these can present with a mixture of UMN and LMN features.
- Hyperthyroidism: wasted, fasciculating muscles secondary to a myopathy with brisk reflexes.

Progressive muscular atrophy

Differential diagnoses for PMA include conditions with LMN signs only:

- Postpolio syndrome: progressive weakness and wasting 30 to 40 years after having had polio, which usually affects the limbs involved in the initial disease. The exact cause is uncertain, but it does not involve reactivation of the poliomyelitis virus.

- Multifocal motor neuropathy with conduction block: autoimmune condition with high levels of anti-GM1 antibody. This is treatable with intravenous immunoglobulin and immunosuppression.
- Spinal muscular atrophy: a heterogeneous hereditary condition with anterior horn cell loss.
- Myopathy, e.g., inclusion body myositis, polymyositis (see Chapter 29).
- Lead neuropathy.

Pseudobulbar/bulbar palsy

Differential diagnoses for pseudobulbar palsy include conditions that cause bilateral UMN lesions:

- Cerebrovascular disease can cause pseudobulbar palsy as well as UMN signs in the limbs.
- Multiple sclerosis usually gives a pseudobulbar picture, but this is often in association with cerebellar features, optic atrophy and other brainstem syndromes.
- Kennedy disease (spinal bulbar muscular atrophy): an X-linked recessive hereditary condition giving rise to a slowly progressive LMN syndrome with predominant bulbar and facial muscle involvement as well as axial and limb weakness. Patients might also have sensory symptoms and gynaecomastia and testicular atrophy.

Differential diagnoses for bulbar palsy, i.e., an LMN syndrome with no UMN features, include:

- Myasthenia gravis.
- Multiple lower cranial nerve lesions caused by infiltrating skull base tumours, e.g., nasopharyngeal carcinoma and glomus tumours.
- Rare neuropathies presenting with bulbar weakness, e.g., Guillain–Barré or diphtheria.

DIAGNOSIS

Other conditions that present with mixed UMN and LMN features should be excluded first. This usually requires MRI of the brain and spinal cord. The diagnosis is made clinically (the Gold Coast criteria) and this is supported by electromyography (EMG), which shows the presence of denervation (fibrillation potentials and positive sharp waves) in the muscles supplied by more than one spinal region. The presence of EMG changes in the tongue in association with changes in the limbs is often helpful in confirming the diagnosis. Nerve conduction studies might show a reduction in motor nerve conduction amplitudes (see Chapter 3). Prolonged central motor conduction times are sometimes useful for detecting clinically silent UMN lesions.

TREATMENT

There is no cure for MND. The diagnosis should be carefully and fully discussed with the patient and carers. Ideally, counselling and multidisciplinary support should be made available.

Drug treatment

Riluzole, a glutamate receptor antagonist, has been shown to increase median survival by 2 to 3 months, but it has no effect on disability. It is recommended by the National Institute for Clinical Excellence (NICE) in patients with MND. Liver enzymes should be checked regularly while a patient is taking it. Edaravone is a recently developed drug which acts as an antioxidant and has been approved to treat MND in other countries including Japan, the United States and Canada. It is not approved for use in the United Kingdom.

Symptomatic treatment

Symptomatic treatment is of paramount importance in MND and includes:

- Noninvasive respiratory support (nasal intermittent positive pressure ventilation or continuous positive airway pressure): patients often have nocturnal hypoventilation due to neuromuscular respiratory weakness. This is the only therapy that can significantly improve life expectancy and should be considered when forced vital capacity is less than 50% of that expected on spirometry.
- Speech therapy and communication aids.
- Treatment to reduce or thicken secretions for sialorrhoea caused by dysphagia and weak facial muscles.
- Altered food consistency for safe swallowing and, ultimately in some cases, a percutaneous endoscopic gastrostomy or radiologically inserted gastrostomy.
- Appropriate management of pain, cramps, spasticity and affective symptoms.
- Physiotherapy, splints, walking aids and wheelchairs.
- Full palliative care in the terminal stages.

COMMUNICATION

When assessing a patient for possible motor neurone disease, specific enquiries should be made about breathing difficulties. Often patients might present with subtle features of respiratory muscle/diaphragm weakness and central hypoventilation. These include symptoms such as orthopnoea, morning headaches, daytime somnolence and fatigue.

● Chapter Summary

- Motor neurone disease (MND) is caused by the progressive degeneration of motor neurones in the motor cortex and in the anterior horns of the spinal cord.
- There are a number of presentation subtypes including amyotrophic lateral sclerosis (mixed UMN and LMN), progressive muscular atrophy (mainly LMN), progressive bulbar palsy and primary lateral sclerosis (UMN only).
- Treatment for MND is predominantly supportive, especially with assisted ventilation later in the disease.

UKMLA Conditions
Dementias
Motor neurone disease

UKMLA Presentations
Limb weakness
Neuromuscular weakness
Speech and language problems
Swallowing problems

Radiculopathy and plexopathy

ANATOMY

Thirty paired spinal nerve roots provide the means of entry and exit of information from the central nervous system (CNS). The dorsal root contains the sensory (afferent) fibres arising from sensory receptors in the periphery, as well as a collection of sensory cell bodies, termed the dorsal root ganglion (Fig. 26.1). The ventral (anterior) root contains the motor (efferent) fibres derived from the anterior horn cell bodies in the anterior horn of the spinal cord grey matter (see Fig. 26.1). The dorsal and ventral spinal roots lie within the spinal subarachnoid space and come together at the intervertebral foramen to become a mixed sensorimotor nerve called the spinal root.

The spinal roots are named by the vertebral level at which they emerge from the spinal cord. In the cervical region, the roots exit above each vertebral body and there are therefore eight cervical roots (C1–C8), even though there are only seven cervical vertebrae. By contrast, at all other levels, the roots emerge below the respective vertebral body (i.e., T1–T12, L1–L5) (see Fig. 26.1).

After emerging from the intervertebral foramina, the spinal roots pass into the brachial plexus to supply the upper limb or into the lumbosacral plexus to supply the lower limb. In the thoracic region, they form the intercostal nerves, which supply sensation and motor activity to the chest and upper abdominal wall.

The brachial plexus lies in the posterior triangle of the neck, between scalenus anterior and scalenus medius, and is derived from the C5–T1 spinal roots. At the root of the neck, the plexus lies behind the clavicle. The plexus gives off several motor branches before forming the cords and ultimately becomes the median (C6, C7, C8, T1), ulnar (C8, T1) and radial nerves (C5, C6, C7, C8, T1) (see Chapter 14).

The lumbosacral plexus is subdivided into the lumbar plexus (T12–L5) and the sacral plexus (L4–S3) (see Chapter 14). The lumbar plexus is located in the psoas muscle and forms the femoral nerve (L2, L3, L4), which supplies the anterior thigh muscles and knee extensors. The sacral plexus is on the posterior wall of the pelvis and forms the sciatic nerve (L4, L5, S1, S2, S3), which supplies the hip extensors and knee flexors. The sciatic nerve consists of two parts: those nerves that will form the common peroneal nerve (L4, L5, S1, S2 posterior divisions) and the tibial nerve (L4, L5, S1, S2 anterior divisions), which supplies the ankle invertors and plantar flexors. The common peroneal nerve further divides into the superficial peroneal nerve, which supplies the ankle evertors, and the deep peroneal nerve, which supplies the toe and ankle dorsiflexors.

When a spinal nerve root is damaged, the patient is said to have radiculopathy and when a plexus is damaged, the patient is said to have plexopathy.

RADICULOPATHY (SPINAL NERVE ROOT LESIONS)

Nerve roots can be affected by pathology, causing symptoms and signs referred to that root. Causes of radiculopathy include:

- cervical and lumbar spondylosis (degenerative changes including disc prolapse and osteophytes: see Chapter 24);
- trauma;
- tumours, e.g., neurofibroma, neuroma, lymphoma, metastases;
- herpes zoster virus (shingles);
- meningeal inflammation and infiltration;
- arachnoiditis, e.g., chemical or infections, such as TB;
- the most common cause is degenerative changes affecting the cervical and lumbar regions.

Clinical features

- Pain: severe, sharp, shooting and/or burning pain radiating into the cutaneous distribution (dermatome) or muscle group (myotome) supplied by the root. It can be aggravated

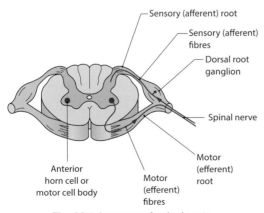

Sensory (afferent) root

Sensory (afferent) fibres

Dorsal root ganglion

Spinal nerve

Motor (efferent) root

Motor (efferent) fibres

Anterior horn cell or motor cell body

Fig. 26.1 Anatomy of spinal roots.

by movement, straining or coughing. Pain may also arise from the soft tissues and joints.

- Neurological signs: lower motor neurone signs, i.e., wasting with or without fasciculations, flaccid weakness and reduced/absent reflexes in the affected myotome and sensory impairment in the affected dermatome.

Specific radiculopathies

Lateral cervical disc protrusion

Lateral disc protrusion in the cervical region often causes severe pain in the upper limb. A C6/C7 disc protrusion causing a C7 radiculopathy is the most common lesion, followed by a C5/C6 disc lesion affecting C6. T1 radiculopathy is rarely caused by spondylotic disease and, if present, should be investigated promptly.

In cervical radiculopathies, there is root pain that radiates into the affected dermatome (into the middle finger with a C7 lesion). Subsequently, there is wasting and weakness of the muscles innervated by the root (triceps and wrist and finger extensors in a C7 lesion) and the reflexes involved in this root will be lost (triceps jerk in a C7 lesion). If the compression is severe, the nerve root might infarct, leading to loss of pain, but the motor features will remain.

Lesions can be visualized on magnetic resonance imaging (MRI). Most cases in which pain is the only symptom recover with rest, the aid of a neck collar and analgesia as the disc prolapse resolves spontaneously. When recovery is delayed, especially if motor neurological signs exist or there is severe intractable pain, surgical spinal root decompression can be performed.

In some cases, the patient might have a central and a lateral disc protrusion, in which case the patient might have cervical cord compression with upper motor neurone signs in the legs and a sensory level as well as the radiculopathy at the level of the lesion and disturbed bladder and bowel function. In older patients, cervical spondylotic changes themselves (see Chapter 24) can compress the nerve roots, spinal cord or both, causing a spondylotic radiculomyelopathy.

Lateral lumbar disc protrusion

The most common lesion in the lumbar region causes compression of L5 and S1 roots due to lateral prolapse of L4/L5 and L5/S1 discs, respectively (Fig. 26.2). This results in low back pain and sciatica, which is pain radiating down the buttock and back of the leg to the foot. Mechanical pain alone without radiculopathy only causes pain to radiate as far as the knee. If the pain is particularly severe or there are atypical features, consider rare causes such as tumours, neoplastic, infectious or inflammatory infiltration or structural causes.

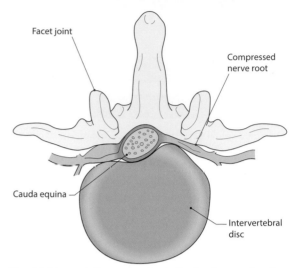

Fig. 26.2 Lateral disc protrusion in the lumbosacral region.

COMMON PITFALLS

Sciatica refers to pain radiating down the buttock and back of leg, usually due to radiculopathy. It is not related to pathology of the sciatic nerve.

In sciatica, raising the affected leg straight is limited due to pain referred in a sciatic distribution. This is caused by root tension that stretches the affected root. This pain may be aggravated by dorsiflexion of the foot. There may be weakness of extension of the big toe (L5) or of plantar flexion (S1). The reflexes may be lost (ankle jerk in an S1 root lesion or, rarely, the knee jerk in an L3/L4 lesion). Sensory loss might develop in the affected dermatome.

Investigations include MRI or myelography if MRI is not available. Most cases of disc protrusion resolve with rest and analgesia, but decompressive surgery may be required.

Central lumbar disc protrusion

The spinal cord ends at L1/L2. A central disc protrusion below this level will result in polyradiculopathy and not myelopathy. Multiple nerve roots (cauda equina) might be involved and will cause lower back pain with radiation down the legs, lower motor neurone weakness of the legs and feet, sacral numbness, retention of urine, bowel dysfunction and impotence (cauda equina syndrome).

The onset can be acute, causing a flaccid paraparesis, or chronic, producing symptoms similar to intermittent claudication caused by vascular insufficiency; this is called neurogenic claudication. A patient with back pain who develops retention of urine should be suspected of having a central lumbar disc protrusion. Urgent imaging and decompression should follow.

> ### HINTS AND TIPS
>
> It is a common mistake to assume that a central lumbar disc protrusion causes spinal cord compression. The spinal cord ends at L1/2 and, therefore, the more common central disc protrusions (L4/5 or L5/S1) cause damage to the cauda equina, which is the loose bundle of nerve roots descending through the lumbosacral canal. Any patient presenting with lumbosacral root symptoms should be questioned about bowel and bladder function and erectile dysfunction in the male. Furthermore, these patients should have a rectal (and pelvic where appropriate) examination to assess anal sphincter tone.

PLEXOPATHIES

Disease of the brachial and lumbosacral plexuses is relatively uncommon. Several specific conditions affect the plexuses. The clinical features of a plexopathy will reflect motor and sensory findings extending over more territory than that of a single nerve root or peripheral nerve.

Brachial plexopathies

Causes of brachial plexopathies include:

- trauma
- neuralgic amyotrophy
- malignant infiltration
- radiotherapy
- compression, e.g., thoracic outlet syndrome (cervical rib or fibrous band)

Trauma

Trauma is the most common cause of a brachial plexus lesion and, in severe cases, early referral to a specialist unit with experience in the surgical repair of plexus injuries is advised as some recovery of function can be obtained even with complete disruption:

- Upper plexus lesion (C5, C6): upper plexus injury is usually caused by falling on the shoulder or traction on the neck and shoulder, which may occur at birth (Erb palsy). It is associated with the characteristic posture of a waiter's tip, i.e., with the arm internally rotated, extended and slightly adducted with loss of shoulder abduction and elbow flexion. Sensory loss occurs in the outer aspect of the shoulder, arm, forearm and thumb in the C5, C6 dermatomes.
- Lower plexus lesion (C8, T1): lower plexus injury is usually caused by forced abduction of the arm, which may occur at birth (Klumpke palsy) or after trauma in later life, e.g., motorcycle accidents. There is characteristically a clawed hand with loss of function of the intrinsic muscles of the hand and long flexors and extensors of the fingers as well as loss of sensation in C8 and T1 dermatomes and Horner syndrome.

Neuralgic amyotrophy (acute brachial neuropathy, brachial neuritis)

Neuralgic amyotrophy is a condition in which severe pain in the muscles of the shoulder is followed 2 to 7 days later, as the pain resolves, by rapid wasting and weakness in the proximal, more commonly than distal, muscles of the arm. It might occur bilaterally and tendon reflexes can be lost in the affected limb. Sensory findings are usually minor. It might follow an infection, inoculation or surgery, but most often a precipitating cause is not found. It is thought to be caused by an inflammatory process affecting the nerve roots and plexus, often causing demyelination and subsequent axonal degeneration. Recovery is gradual over many months but might not be complete. Recurrent episodes can occur, which are either idiopathic or rarely hereditary in nature: hereditary neuralgic amyotrophy and hereditary neuropathy with liability to pressure palsy. A very similar process can affect the lumbosacral plexus.

Malignant infiltration

Invasion of the brachial plexus usually occurs in association with metastatic or locally invasive breast carcinoma and can occur many years after the initial tumour was diagnosed and treated. There is usually severe and intractable pain in the arm.

Pancoast tumour

An apical lung tumour (usually squamous cell carcinoma) can involve the lower brachial plexus by affecting C8/T1-derived roots.

Clinically, the patient has:

- severe pain in the arm
- ipsilateral weak and wasted hand
- sensory loss (C8, T1)
- Horner syndrome

Radiotherapy-induced plexopathy

Irradiation of the brachial plexus following breast carcinoma can lead to damage of the brachial plexus, especially the lower parts. The onset is usually delayed for 5 to 30 months and can be difficult to differentiate from metastatic breast cancer clinically and radiologically.

Compression

A fibrous band or cervical rib extending from the tip of the transverse process of C7 to the first rib can stretch the lower part of the brachial plexus (C8, T1). There is pain along the ulnar border of the forearm and sensory loss initially in the distribution of T1, with wasting of the abductor pollicis brevis more than the interossei or hypothenar muscles (Gilliatt–Sumner hand). There might also be Horner syndrome. Patients often complain of pain in the shoulder and numbness in the forearm, especially on carrying heavy objects.

Some patients also develop a vascular syndrome if there is compression of the subclavian artery or vein by a cervical rib or fibrous band. This will be associated with vascular symptoms, such as an audible bruit in the supraclavicular fossa, unilateral Raynaud phenomenon, pallor of the limb on elevation and loss of the radial pulse on abduction and external rotation of the shoulder. This is known as Adson sign. The vascular and neurological syndromes rarely coexist. Treatment is surgical decompression.

Lumbosacral plexus

Symptoms of a lumbosacral plexus lesion might be unilateral or bilateral. Diabetic amyotrophy and malignant infiltration in the pelvis are the most common causes. Weakness, reflex change and sensory loss depend on the location and extent of plexus damage. In general, the following features are found:

- Upper plexus lesion: weakness of hip flexion and adduction, with anterior leg sensory loss.
- Lower plexus lesion: weakness of the posterior thigh (hamstrings) and foot muscles, with posterior leg sensory loss.

Diabetic amyotrophy

Diabetic amyotrophy is usually seen in older men with mild-to-moderate diabetes and may be associated with periods of poor glycaemic control. The site of the pathology can be in the lumbosacral plexus or in the roots and might have an inflammatory aetiology. Patients present with painful wasting, usually strikingly asymmetrical, of the quadriceps and psoas muscles. There is loss of the knee jerks and extreme tenderness in the affected area. There is usually minimal sensory loss. It resolves with careful control of blood glucose over many months.

Other causes of lumbosacral plexopathy:

- Infiltration by neoplasia, e.g., prostate, ovarian and cervical, can infiltrate or metastasize to the lumbosacral plexus. This is usually associated with severe pain in the pelvis or/and legs.
- Radiotherapy.
- Trauma following abdominal or pelvic surgery, e.g., hysterectomy.
- Compression from an abdominal aortic aneurysm or retroperitoneal haematoma.

● Chapter summary

- The spinal roots are named according to the vertebral level at which they emerge from the spinal cord. In the cervical region, the roots exit above the vertebral body; in the thoracic and lumbar region, the roots exit below the vertebral body.
- There are three main plexuses in the nervous system: the brachial plexus (C5–T1), the lumbar plexus (T12–L5) and the sacral plexus (L4–S3).
- Pain in a specific dermatome/myotome with associated LMN signs suggests radiculopathy. If neighbouring dermatomes are affected, plexopathy or multiple radiculopathies should be considered.
- The most common cause of painful radiculopathy is cervical disc protrusion, usually at the C6/C7 level.

UKMLA Conditions
Peripheral nerve injuries/palsies
Radiculopathies
Spinal cord compression
Spinal cord injury

UKMLA Presentations
Altered sensation, numbness and tingling
Back pain
Limb weakness
Neck pain/stiffness
Neuromuscular weakness
Trauma
Urinary symptoms

Disorders of the peripheral nerves 27

ANATOMY

Peripheral nerves are made up of numerous axons bound together by three types of connective tissue: endoneurium, perineurium and epineurium (Fig. 27.1). The vasa nervorum located in the epineurium provides the blood supply.

Peripheral nerve trunks contain myelinated and unmyelinated fibres. Myelin is a protein–lipid complex that forms an insulating layer around some axons, resulting in increased rates of conduction in these fibres. All peripheral nerves have a cellular sheath, the Schwann cell, but only in some does the membrane of the cell spiral around the axon, forming the multilayered myelin sheath.

Schwann cells of myelinated nerves are separated by Ranvier nodes. At these points, the axons are not surrounded by myelin. During conduction, impulses jump from one node to the next, which is called saltatory conduction. Conduction in unmyelinated nerves is slower and dependent on the diameter of the axon.

Within the peripheral nerve, the axons vary structurally and this is related to function. Three distinct types of fibre can be distinguished (Table 27.1). All are myelinated, apart from the C fibres, which carry impulses from painful stimuli. The function of peripheral nerves can be disrupted by damage to the cell body, the axon, the myelin sheath, the connective tissue or the blood supply.

Two basic pathological processes occur:

1. Wallerian degeneration: the axon and myelin sheath degenerate distal to injury to the axon. The process occurs within 7 to 10 days of the injury and the degenerating portion of the nerve is electrically inexcitable. Regeneration can occur because the basement membrane of the Schwann cell survives and acts as a skeleton along which the axon regrows up to a rate of about 1 mm per day.

2. Demyelination: segmental destruction of the myelin sheath occurs mostly without axonal damage although prolonged

Table 27.1 Fibre types in peripheral nerve

Fibre type	Fibre diameter (µm)	Velocity (m/s)	Function/nerve type
Type A (myelinated); Group I	12–20	90	Vibration and position sense alpha motor neurones
Group II	6–12	50	Touch and pressure afferents
Group III	1–6	30	Gamma afferents
Type B (myelinated)	2–6	10	Autonomic preganglionic
Type C (unmyelinated)	<1	2	Pain and temperature afferents, autonomic postganglionic

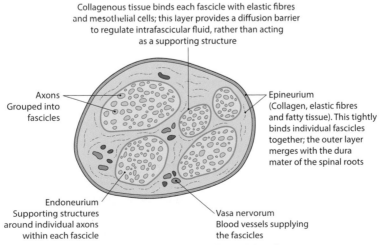

Perineurium
Collagenous tissue binds each fascicle with elastic fibres and mesothelial cells; this layer provides a diffusion barrier to regulate intrafascicular fluid, rather than acting as a supporting structure

Axons
Grouped into fascicles

Epineurium
(Collagen, elastic fibres and fatty tissue). This tightly binds individual fascicles together; the outer layer merges with the dura mater of the spinal roots

Endoneurium
Supporting structures around individual axons within each fascicle

Vasa nervorum
Blood vessels supplying the fascicles

Fig. 27.1 Transverse section of a peripheral nerve.

demyelination can cause secondary axonal damage. The primary lesion affects the Schwann cell and causes marked slowing of conduction or conduction block. Local demyelination is caused by pressure, e.g., entrapment neuropathies, or by inflammation, e.g., Guillain–Barré syndrome.

DEFINITIONS OF NEUROPATHIES

- Neuropathy: a pathological process that affects a peripheral nerve or nerves and might involve axonal degeneration (Wallerian degeneration) or demyelination.
- Mononeuropathy: focal involvement of a single nerve is affected, e.g., the median nerve in carpal tunnel syndrome. If multiple single nerves are affected either simultaneously or sequentially in an asymmetrical pattern, it is termed multifocal neuropathy or mononeuritis multiplex. With time, the pattern might become more symmetrical in appearance and, therefore, difficult to distinguish from a polyneuropathy.
- Polyneuropathy: a diffuse disease process affecting many nerves that is usually distal and symmetrical with some proximal progression. In certain disease processes, there might be a more proximal involvement initially, e.g., demyelinating neuropathies. However, it is most commonly axonal and, therefore, length related, affecting the longest axons first, i.e., the feet, and gradually involving shorter axons in the legs and hands. Depending on the underlying cause, it can be acute, subacute or chronic. It might be progressive, relapsing or transient and can be motor, sensory, autonomic or mixed (sensorimotor ± autonomic).

NEUROPATHY SYMPTOMS

Sensory symptoms and signs

Negative symptoms (loss of sensation)

Large myelinated fibre disease causes loss of touch, vibration and joint-position sense (proprioception), leading to:

- difficulty discriminating textures
- feet and hands feeling like cotton wool
- gait unsteady through loss of position sense, especially at night when vision cannot compensate

Small unmyelinated fibre disease causes loss of pain and temperature appreciation, leading to:

- painless burns and trauma
- damage to joints (Charcot joint), resulting in painless deformity

Positive symptoms

Large myelinated fibre disease can cause paraesthesia (pins and needles). Small unmyelinated fibre disease produces painful positive symptoms:

- Burning sensations.
- Dysaesthesia: pain on gentle touch.
- Hyperalgesia: lowered threshold to pain.
- Hyperpathia: pain threshold is elevated, but pain is excessively felt.
- Lightning pains: sudden, very severe, shooting pains, which can suggest a diagnosis of tabes dorsalis (tertiary syphilis).
- Allodynia: when nonpainful stimuli are perceived as painful.

HINTS AND TIPS

A classic polyneuropathy will produce sensory loss in the characteristic glove-and-stocking distribution. This phenomenon is usually due to a length-related axonal process and signs in the hands will therefore not develop until there is sensory loss up to at least mid-shin level.

Autonomic symptoms

Autonomic symptoms and signs include postural hypotension, impotence, constipation, diarrhoea, loss of bladder control, abnormal sweating and blurring of vision. In any assessment of a neuropathy, it is important to check pupillary responses and to check for postural hypotension.

Motor symptoms

Weakness is usually the main presenting feature. This is usually distal (e.g., difficulty clearing the kerb when walking or unable to open jars) but some neuropathies can be proximal (e.g., difficulty climbing stairs or combing hair). Wasting of the muscles would usually accompany significant weakness. Patients may also complain of cramps and twitching of muscles (fasciculations). When a neuropathy is present during early development, skeletal deformities might be seen. These include clawing of the toes, pes cavus and kyphoscoliosis.

INVESTIGATION OF PERIPHERAL NEUROPATHY

In up to 30% of cases, the cause of a neuropathy might not be identified. The following investigations can be helpful in the diagnosis:

- Blood tests: routine blood tests to exclude certain causes of peripheral neuropathy should include full blood count, erythrocyte sedimentation rate, C-reactive protein, urea and electrolytes (especially renal function tests), liver function tests, glucose, vitamin B_{12} and serum protein electrophoresis.
- Nerve conduction studies: these can differentiate axonal degeneration (reduced amplitude of electrical impulse) from demyelination (reduced conduction velocity) and can characterize whether sensory and/or motor fibres are involved. They can also localize the sites of abnormality, e.g., in entrapment neuropathies.
- Electromyography: use of a fine needle inserted into the muscle can discern whether complete or partial denervation is present and whether reinnervation is occurring. This can help in localization, depending on the distribution of muscles affected.
- Nerve biopsy: the sural nerve is the most commonly biopsied because it is purely sensory and the small resulting clinical deficit is therefore trivial. Pathological information can be gained from light and electron microscopy. Nerve biopsies can be useful to confirm the presence of vasculitis or other inflammatory infiltration, when the cause of a progressive neuropathy has not been revealed by other investigations. In addition, small punch biopsies of the skin are being increasingly used to help diagnose small-fibre neuropathies.
- Cerebrospinal fluid (CSF) examination: this might be helpful, for example, in inflammatory demyelinating neuropathies such as Guillain–Barré syndrome or chronic inflammatory demyelinating polyradiculoneuropathy (CIDP), when the protein content is usually elevated, without inflammatory cells.

SPECIFIC NEUROPATHIES

Mononeuropathies

Peripheral nerve compression and entrapment neuropathies

Nerves can be damaged by compression either acutely (e.g., by a tourniquet or a tight-fitting cast over the leg) or chronically (e.g., carpal tunnel syndrome). This usually causes localized demyelination, although, if prolonged, it might lead to axonal degeneration.

Acute compression tends to affect nerves that lie superficially to the skin (e.g., the common peroneal nerve at the fibular head by prolonged knee crossing or the radial nerve as it passes around the humerus, causing Saturday-night palsy). Chronic compression causes entrapment neuropathies, which occur when the nerve passes through tight anatomical spaces (e.g.,

the median nerve in the carpal tunnel). A history of recurrent compressive neuropathic lesions should raise the possibility of an underlying hereditary neuropathy with a liability to pressure palsies.

The most common nerves to be involved by compression are described below.

Carpal tunnel syndrome

The median nerve is supplied from the C6, C7, C8 and T1 nerve roots. The median nerve can become compressed in the fibro-osseous carpal tunnel at the wrist, in which case the C8/T1 small muscles of the hand are affected. Carpal tunnel syndrome is usually idiopathic but can be associated with:

- hypothyroidism
- pregnancy
- diabetes mellitus
- rheumatoid arthritis
- renal dialysis

It presents with tingling, pain and numbness in the hand, which tends to wake the patient from sleep or in the morning. The pain might extend up the arm to the shoulder and be relieved by shaking of the arm and hand. In some cases, there is weakness of the thenar muscles (first lumbrical, opponens pollicis, abductor pollicis brevis and flexor pollicis brevis), especially abductor pollicis brevis. Sensory loss affects the palm and the lateral three-and-a-half digits. If it is long-standing and severe, there might be wasting of the abductor pollicis brevis. The Tinel sign may be present – tapping on the carpal tunnel reproduces tingling and pain. In the Phalen test, forced wrist flexion might provoke similar sensory symptoms.

Diagnosis is clinical and by electrophysiology, confirming slowing of the impulse across the wrist with a reduced amplitude in some cases. Surgical decompression is the definitive procedure, although splints and steroid injections into the carpal tunnel sometimes provide temporary relief (Fig. 27.2A).

Ulnar nerve compression

The ulnar nerve arises from the roots of C8 to T1. Ulnar nerve compression is less common than carpal tunnel syndrome. Entrapment typically occurs at the elbow, where the nerve is compressed in the olecranon groove within the cubital tunnel, which lies behind the medial epicondyle. It can follow fracture of the ulna or prolonged/recurrent pressure at this site. The ulnar nerve might be compressed at other sites within the cubital tunnel, such as between the two heads of flexor carpi ulnaris.

In an ulnar neuropathy, a patient might complain of tingling or numbness affecting the little finger, part of the ring finger and, sometimes, the ulnar side of the hand distal to the wrist. Sensory loss extending to the medial side of the forearm indicates a more proximal lesion, such as a brachial plexus or

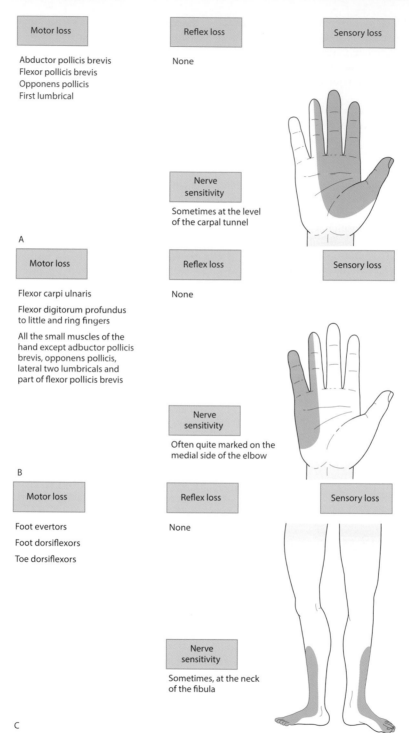

Motor loss

Abductor pollicis brevis
Flexor pollicis brevis
Opponens pollicis
First lumbrical

Reflex loss

None

Sensory loss

Nerve sensitivity

Sometimes at the level of the carpal tunnel

A

Motor loss

Flexor carpi ulnaris

Flexor digitorum profundus to little and ring fingers

All the small muscles of the hand except adbuctor pollicis brevis, opponens pollicis, lateral two lumbricals and part of flexor pollicis brevis

Reflex loss

None

Sensory loss

Nerve sensitivity

Often quite marked on the medial side of the elbow

B

Motor loss

Foot evertors

Foot dorsiflexors

Toe dorsiflexors

Reflex loss

None

Sensory loss

Nerve sensitivity

Sometimes, at the neck of the fibula

C

Fig. 27.2 Sensory loss associated with (A) carpal tunnel, (B) ulnar nerve compression and (C) common peroneal nerve compression.

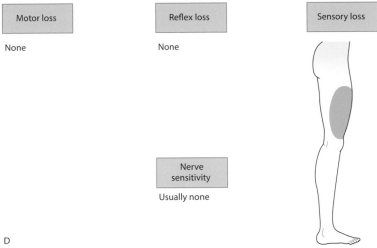

Motor loss	Reflex loss	Sensory loss
None	None	

Nerve sensitivity
Usually none

D

Fig. 27.2, cont'd, (D) meralgia paraesthetica.

C8 root lesion. In severe cases, there might be wasting of the hypothenar muscles and weakness of ulnar-innervated muscles of the forearm and hand. The patient might develop an ulnar claw hand due to involvement of the medial two lumbricals, especially when the nerve is affected at the wrist, leaving the long ulnar flexors unopposed. Weakness of the adductor pollicis (which adducts the thumb), abductor digiti minimi (which abducts the little finger) and the interossei (which abduct and adduct the fingers) muscles is sometimes present.

Electrophysiology may localize the lesion. Surgical decompression or anterior transposition can be performed, but results from the latter procedure are generally poor and these days it is seldom performed.

A more distal ulnar compression neuropathy can occur in the deep motor branch as it passes across the palm. This is due to regular pressure from tools, e.g., screwdrivers, crutches or cycle handlebars (Fig. 27.2B). The deep palmar branch is purely motor and, therefore, damage will cause wasting and weakness of the interossei muscles and adductor pollicis, but sensation will be spared. The hypothenar muscles are also typically spared.

Radial nerve compression

The radial nerve is supplied by C5, C6, C7, C8 and T1 roots. It supplies the triceps, brachioradialis, supinator, wrist and finger extensors and long thumb abductor. Radial nerve compression occurs when the radial nerve is compressed against the humerus, e.g., when the arm is draped over the back of a chair for several hours (Saturday-night palsy), and results in wrist drop and weakness of finger extension and brachioradialis. Sensation is lost in the region of the anatomical snuffbox on the dorsum of the hand over the base and shafts of the first two metacarpals. Recovery is usually spontaneous but can take up to 3 months (Fig. 27.2).

More proximal lesions can cause impaired sensation on the posterolateral aspect of the forearm.

Common peroneal nerve palsy

The common peroneal nerve is supplied by L4, L5, S1 and S2 nerve roots. It has two branches: the superficial branch supplies the ankle evertors and skin on the lateral side of the lower leg; the deep branch supplies the toe and ankle dorsiflexors and a small area of skin on the dorsum of the foot between the first and second toes. Common peroneal nerve palsy occurs when the nerve is compressed at the fibular head and can result from prolonged squatting or leg crossing, wearing a tight plaster cast, prolonged bed rest or coma. It results in a foot drop and weakness of eversion and dorsiflexion, with sensory loss on the anterolateral border of the shin and dorsum of the foot. Recovery is usual, but not invariable, within a few months (Fig. 27.2C).

Lateral cutaneous nerve of the thigh (meralgia paraesthetica)

The sensory lateral cutaneous nerve of the thigh is supplied by L2 and L3 roots. This nerve might be compressed beneath the inguinal ligament, which causes burning, tingling and numbness on the anterolateral surface of the thigh. There is no weakness or reflex change. It usually occurs in overweight patients and weight loss often helps (Fig. 27.2D).

Multifocal neuropathy (mononeuritis multiplex)

Certain systemic illnesses are associated with multiple mononeuropathies. They can be caused not only by preferential sites of entrapment but also by a focal pathological process in a nerve(s) (e.g., infarction in diabetes). These include:

- diabetes mellitus
- connective tissue disease, e.g., systemic lupus erythematosus (SLE), rheumatoid arthritis
- vasculitis, e.g., polyarteritis nodosa, pANCA/cANCA vasculitis
- sarcoidosis
- amyloidosis
- leprosy

HINTS AND TIPS

Small vessel vasculitic neuropathy can occur in isolation or in association with other connective tissue diseases, e.g., systemic lupus erythematosus, rheumatoid arthritis. Characteristically, it is associated with severe pain in the affected nerves and multiple mononeuropathy. It often affects muscle as well and, therefore, a combined biopsy of both muscle and nerve is often performed if the diagnosis is suspected. It is an important cause not to miss as a delay in diagnosis and treatment can lead to severe neurological deficits.

Polyneuropathies

Polyneuropathies can be classified according to their mode of onset, functional or pathological type, distribution or causation. The classification used as follows is based on causation.

Systemic disease

Diabetic neuropathy

Neuropathies found in diabetes mellitus are often related to poor glycaemic control. The exact cause of the nerve damage is uncertain but might relate to sorbitol accumulation or to vascular disease in both large and small vessels.

A number of different types of neuropathy complicate diabetes:

- Distal symmetrical polyneuropathy: most commonly sensory but might be sensorimotor and have autonomic features. Improving glycaemic control has been demonstrated to reduce the risk of developing peripheral neuropathy.
- A painful small fibre neuropathy affecting the feet is common in diabetes and is often the presenting feature of the disease.
- Proximal asymmetrical motor neuropathy: a lumbosacral radiculoplexus neuropathy, also known as diabetic

amyotrophy, acutely painful and occurs in older men. There is lumbar or proximal leg pain from the outset, followed by asymmetric proximal leg weakness and wasting.
- Autonomic neuropathy: with gastroparesis and resultant diarrhoea, arrhythmias and postural hypotension. This neuropathy is also length dependent and loss of sweating in the feet is often an early feature.
- Mononeuropathies can be single or multiple, especially entrapment.
- Cranial nerve lesions: especially isolated third (usually pupil sparing) and sixth nerve palsies.

Renal disease

Chronic renal failure produces a progressive sensorimotor neuropathy. The response to dialysis is variable, but the neuropathy usually improves after renal transplantation.

Paraneoplastic polyneuropathy

Malignant disease, especially small-cell carcinoma of the bronchus, can produce a pure sensory neuropathy affecting the large fibres, leading to a sensory ataxic neuropathy. It is often associated with antineuronal antibodies, such as anti-Hu antibodies. The neuropathy might predate the appearance of the malignancy by months or years.

Haematological malignancies such as multiple myeloma and other monoclonal gammopathies characteristically produce peripheral neuropathies that resemble CIDP or vasculitic neuropathies.

Connective tissue diseases and vasculitides

Connective tissue diseases and vasculitides classically produce a very painful mononeuritis multiplex, although individual diseases might produce a symmetrical sensorimotor neuropathy (especially SLE), entrapment neuropathy (rheumatoid arthritis) or trigeminal neuropathy (Sjögren syndrome). With progression, mononeuritis multiplex can resemble a polyneuropathy with a glove-and-stocking distribution. Factors suggestive of vasculitic aetiology include subacute onset, asymmetrical distribution, pain, leg involvement and systemic symptoms. Treatment is with steroids and immunosuppressants.

Porphyria

Acute intermittent porphyria produces a predominantly axonal motor neuropathy/polyradiculopathy in addition to abdominal pain, psychosis and seizures. The onset is usually acute or subacute, similar to Guillain–Barré syndrome, and often presents with asymmetrical proximal weakness. Like Guillain–Barré syndrome, respiratory, facial, ocular, bulbar and autonomic function can be affected.

Amyloidosis

Amyloid is deposited around the vessels in the nerve, causing distortion. The neuropathy is characterized by predominantly sensory, painful, dysaesthetic features. Autonomic features are common.

BOX 27.1 DRUGS THAT CAN CAUSE PERIPHERAL NEUROPATHY

Sensory axonal	Motor axonal	Sensorimotor axonal	Sensorimotor demyelinating
Chloramphenicol	Amphotericin	Chlorambucil	Amiodarone
Isoniazid	Dapsone	Cisplatin	
Phenytoin	Gold	Disulfiram	
Paclitaxel		Nitrofurantoin	
		Vincristine	

Neuropathies caused by drugs and toxins

Drugs

A wide variety of drugs are known to cause a peripheral neuropathy. Most produce a chronic, progressive, sensorimotor polyneuropathy and are generally reversible. Examples of the most common are given in Box 27.1.

Toxins

A wide variety of metals and industrial toxins have been shown to cause polyneuropathy. Peripheral nerve involvement is often accompanied by other systemic features. For example:

- Lead causes a motor neuropathy.
- Arsenic and thallium cause a painful peripheral sensory neuropathy.
- Acrylamide, trichloroethylene and fat-soluble hydrocarbons, e.g., as in glue sniffing, cause a progressive polyneuropathy.

Alcoholic neuropathy

Alcohol is the most common toxin associated with peripheral neuropathy (up to 30% of all cases of neuropathy) and is primarily axonal.

It progresses slowly, with distal sensory loss, paraesthesia and burning pains. Distal muscle weakness might occur and spread proximally, with muscle cramps and gait disturbance.

The cause can be primarily due to alcohol toxicity but also to a secondary deficiency of vitamins, particularly in thiamine and other B vitamins, as well as often having an inadequate general dietary intake.

Abstinence from alcohol, supplementation of thiamine and a balanced diet constitute the principal therapy. The painful symptoms might be eased with the use of neuropathic pain medications, such as antidepressants (e.g., amitriptyline or duloxetine) or antiepileptics (e.g., gabapentin or pregabalin).

Neuropathies caused by nutritional deficiencies

Thiamine (vitamin B_1) deficiency (beriberi)

Thiamine deficiency is strongly implicated in the causation of alcoholic neuropathy. In addition to the peripheral neuropathy, deficiency can cause Wernicke–Korsakoff syndrome (see Chapter 34).

Pyridoxine (vitamin B_6) deficiency

Pyridoxine deficiency causes a mainly sensory neuropathy. It might be precipitated by isoniazid therapy for tuberculosis and pyridoxine is, therefore, given in association with this drug.

Vitamin B_{12} deficiency

Peripheral neuropathy can occur in association with subacute combined degeneration of the cord (spastic paraparesis, loss of proprioception, paraesthesia); vitamin B_{12} deficiency is also linked to optic neuropathies and dementia. Treatment involves intramuscular replacement injections (see Chapter 24).

Vitamin E deficiency

Vitamin E deficiency occurs in the context of fat malabsorption. The onset of neurological symptoms takes many years. It involves a large-fibre sensory neuropathy with spinocerebellar degeneration.

Inflammatory neuropathies

Guillain–Barré syndrome

Guillain–Barré syndrome is also called acute inflammatory demyelinating polyradiculoneuropathy. It occurs worldwide, with an annual rate of 1.5 cases per 100,000. It can appear 1 to 3 weeks after a respiratory infection or diarrhoea. *Campylobacter jejuni* has been particularly implicated as a cause of the diarrhoea and is associated with a more severe form. It might also follow other infections such as HIV seroconversion or following vaccines.

The classic presentation is with distal paraesthesia, often with little sensory loss, and weakness tends to occur in a patchy manner (proximal, distal to proximal or generalized). The symptoms ascend up the lower limbs and body over days to weeks and at this point tendon reflexes are usually lost. Facial weakness is present in 50% of cases and is often asymmetrical. Lower back pain is also a common symptom. Ophthalmoparesis occurs in 15% of patients with typical Guillain–Barré syndrome. In patients with cranial nerve involvement, bulbar weakness or neck and proximal arm weakness, there is a significant risk of intercostal muscle and diaphragmatic weakness leading to respiratory failure. If the vital capacity drops to 1 L or below, artificial ventilation is often necessary. Autonomic dysfunction might also occur in 60% of patients and causes arrhythmias, urinary retention and constipation. Clinically, symptoms usually reach their peak within 6 weeks of the onset of symptoms.

A proximal variant of Guillain–Barré syndrome exists, with an associated triad of signs including ophthalmoparesis, areflexia and ataxia (Miller–Fisher syndrome).

Diagnosis is usually clinical, supported by slowed conduction velocities on nerve conduction studies and a raised CSF protein with a normal cell count or mild lymphocytosis. Both these investigations might be normal early in the disease. Patients with Miller–Fisher variant have anti-GQ1b ganglioside antibodies.

Differential diagnoses include other paralytic illnesses, such as poliomyelitis, myasthenia gravis, botulism and primary muscle disease.

Patients with Guillain–Barré syndrome should be monitored for cardiac and respiratory function. They should have continuous heart monitoring and regular vital capacity and oxygen saturation assessments. The use of intravenous immunoglobulin has been shown to produce significant improvement in the course of the disease and is equivalent to the more invasive plasmapheresis. Corticosteroids and immunosuppressive agents have not been successful in acute Guillain–Barré syndrome. Careful management of the paralyzed patient and ventilation as indicated is also essential. Recovery, although gradual over many months, is usual in 80% of patients. Approximately 10% to 15% of patients might have a prolonged stay in an intensive care unit, with a recovery period extending up to 2 years. Mortality of 5% is associated with inadequate ventilatory support, complications of immobility (aspiration, pulmonary embolism) and arrhythmias. By definition, the symptoms and signs cease to progress after 8 weeks or the disease becomes termed CIDP.

Acute motor axonal neuropathy

Acute motor axonal neuropathy is clinically very similar to Guillain–Barré and is an immune-mediated disorder directed against axonal function rather than causing demyelination. It can be associated with anti-GM1 antibodies. Nerve conduction studies show an axonal picture of reduction in impulse amplitude and conduction block. The prognosis is usually worse than Guillain–Barré with a much longer recovery time. Variations include acute sensory axonal neuropathy and acute motor and sensory axonal neuropathy.

COMMON PITFALLS

In the differential diagnosis of Guillain–Barré syndrome, the following atypical features suggest an alternative diagnosis:

- Significant asymmetry: vasculitis.
- Marked cerebrospinal fluid lymphocytosis: infectious, e.g., HIV; malignancy, e.g., lymphoma.
- Sensory level: spinal cord syndrome.

Chronic inflammatory demyelinating polyradiculoneuropathy

CIDP represents an often-milder syndrome that is related to Guillain–Barré syndrome but has a more protracted clinical course. The clinical, diagnostic features and pathology are similar to those of Guillain–Barré syndrome, although it is rarely associated with a preceding infection. It is usually a symmetrical, progressive, polyradiculoneuropathy with symptoms of weakness, sensory loss and paraesthesia. The weakness can be both proximal and distal and facial weakness is rare although neck weakness is common. The sensory loss is typically glove-and-stocking, with marked large-fibre loss leading to a sensory ataxia. CSF protein is elevated with a normal cell count. A nerve conduction study will show demyelination.

Drug treatment includes corticosteroids, with or without other immunosuppressive agents such as azathioprine or cyclophosphamide, or recurrent intravenous immunoglobulin infusions/plasmapheresis.

Multifocal motor neuropathy

This is an uncommon disorder, but an important differential for the lower motor neurone variant of motor neurone disease. It is characterized by progressive, asymmetrical weakness without sensory involvement. Cranial nerve and respiratory involvement are rare and nerve conduction studies show multifocal conduction block. There are usually high levels of anti-GM1 ganglioside antibodies. It is potentially treatable with intravenous immunoglobulin.

Neuropathies caused by infection

In the developed world, the most relevant infections that can cause a peripheral neuropathy are HIV and Lyme disease; worldwide diphtheria and leprosy are also important. HIV can cause a variety of peripheral nerve syndromes, either directly or indirectly through immune suppression and comorbid infections, or the side effects of medications. Lyme disease can cause a cranial neuropathy, radiculopathy or an asymmetric peripheral neuropathy.

Hereditary neuropathies

The field of hereditary neuropathies is a complex one, with clinically and genetically heterogeneous conditions. This section will consider the group of conditions known as the hereditary motor sensory neuropathies (HMSN), also known as Charcot–Marie–Tooth (CMT) disease. Other less common types of hereditary neuropathy are not discussed.

The number of CMT types is expanding rapidly due to advances in genetic analysis. The most common mutations associated with CMT are PMP22 and MPZ and the most common types are:

- CMT type I: most common form, autosomal dominant demyelinating neuropathy with hypertrophy of nerves (onion bulb formation on electron microscopy); onset at age between 5 and 15 years.

- CMT type II: mostly autosomal dominant inheritance, axonal neuropathy; onset between 10 and 20 years.
- CMT type III (Dejerine–Sottas disease): autosomal dominant or recessive demyelinating neuropathy, variant of type I but more severe with earlier onset, gross hypertrophy of peripheral nerves and often the CSF protein is elevated due to hypertrophied nerve roots.
- X-linked CMT: the second most common form and clinically similar to CMTI although there is no male-to-male transmission, demyelinating in males and axonal in females.
- Complex forms of HMSN: additional features such as optic atrophy, retinitis pigmentosa, deafness and spastic paraparesis can coexist.

General characteristics of hereditary motor sensory neuropathies

All forms of HMSN are characterized by distal wasting of the lower limbs, which progresses, often over many years, and might involve the upper limbs. When the wasting in the legs is severe, they resemble inverted champagne bottles (Fig. 27.3A). The wasting is accompanied by reduced or absent reflexes and a variable loss of sensation. Pes cavus (loss of lateral arch) with clawing of the toes is almost invariable and reflects early onset of disease (Fig. 27.3B). These features might be the only signs in mild cases. Clawing of the hands is also sometimes seen. One-third of patients might have a postural tremor and half have palpable thickening of peripheral nerves. Sensory features are not as marked as the motor features.

The age of onset varies from childhood to middle age. There is variability within subgroups and within families.

Critical illness polyneuropathy

This is an axonal sensorimotor polyneuropathy that can occur in patients who are critically ill in intensive care units with multiorgan failure and infection. It can cause significant problems in weaning from artificial ventilation and its pathogenesis is unknown. In some patients, the weakness is muscular, i.e., they have a critical illness myopathy.

The causes of peripheral neuropathies are summarized in Table 27.2.

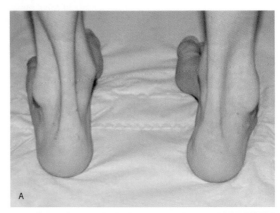

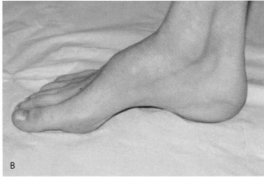

Fig. 27.3 (A) Inverted-champagne-bottle legs; (B) pes cavus, associated with hereditary motor sensory neuropathy. (From Kulshrestha R, Burton-Jones S, Antoniadi T, et al. Deletion of P2 promoter of GJB1 gene: a cause of Charcot-Marie-Tooth disease. *Neuromuscul Disord*. 2017 Aug;27(8):766–770.)

Table 27.2 Summary of causes of peripheral neuropathies

Cause	Notable examples
Inflammatory	Guillain–Barré syndrome CIDP Multifocal motor neuropathy with conduction block
Metabolic	Diabetes Renal disease Porphyria
Nutritional deficiencies	Vitamin B_1 Vitamin B_6 Vitamin B_{12} Vitamin E

Continued

Table 27.2 Summary of causes of peripheral neuropathies—cont'd

Cause	Notable examples
Toxic	Drugs: isoniazid, vincristine, nitrofurantoin Alcohol Lead
Vasculitis/connective tissue disease	Primary vasculitis, e.g., polyarteritis nodosa, Wegener granulomatosis, Churg–Strauss syndrome, microscopic polyangiitis Secondary vasculitis, e.g., connective tissue disorders (rheumatoid arthritis, SLE, Sjögren syndrome), drugs, viral infections (hepatitis C, HIV, CMV), malignancy
Malignancy (paraneoplastic)	Bronchus Breast, ovarian, uterus Haematological malignancies including lymphoma, myeloma and MGUS
Infection	HIV Lyme disease Leprosy
Hereditary	CMT syndromes
Trauma	Often mononeuropathies or multiple mononeuropathies: crush, section, avulsion
Miscellaneous	Critical illness neuropathy

CIDP, *Chronic inflammatory demyelinating polyradiculoneuropathy;* CMT, *Charcot–Marie–Tooth;* CMV, *cytomegalovirus;* MGUS, *monoclonal gammopathy of undetermined significance;* SLE, *systemic lupus erythematosus.*

● Chapter Summary

- There are three types of peripheral nerve, characterized by the speed of their conduction; Type A is the fastest and responsible for proprioception and Type C is the slowest and responsible for pain and temperature sensation.
- Peripheral neuropathy can be described by the distribution of nerves affected; a mononeuropathy affects one nerve, polyneuropathy usually progresses in a symmetrical length manner and multifocal neuropathy affects a number of single nerves in an asymmetrical pattern.
- Symptoms associated with peripheral neuropathy can be divided into negative (e.g., loss of sensation, unsteadiness) and positive (e.g., pins and needles, burning).
- Causes of a peripheral neuropathy can be grouped into inflammatory (e.g., CIDP), nutritional (e.g., B_6 deficiency), toxic (e.g., alcohol excess), vasculitic/connective tissue (e.g., SLE), malignancy (e.g., small cell lung), infection (e.g., leprosy) and hereditary (e.g., Charcot–Marie–Tooth).

UKMLA Conditions
Diabetic neuropathy
Peripheral nerve injuries/palsies
Wernicke encephalopathy

UKMLA Presentations
Altered sensation, numbness and tingling
Back pain
Facial weakness
Limb weakness
Unsteadiness

Disorders of the neuromuscular junction 28

The normal anatomy and physiology of the neuromuscular junction are outlined in Fig. 28.1. An action potential passes down the motor axon towards skeletal muscle. Each motor axon divides up into a number of terminal branches just before it reaches the muscle. Each one of these branches ends at the presynaptic nerve terminal. The action potential is sensed by presynaptic calcium sensors, causing calcium to enter into the terminal via voltage-gated calcium channels, promoting acetylcholine-containing vesicles to fuse with the nerve membrane, thereby releasing acetylcholine into the synaptic cleft. The acetylcholine crosses the synaptic cleft and binds to acetylcholine receptors (AChRs) on the postsynaptic muscle end-plate membrane. This results in depolarization of the muscle fibre and subsequent contraction of the muscle. The acetylcholine is then broken down by acetylcholinesterase, which is bound to the basement membrane in the synaptic folds.

Two main diseases of neuromuscular transmission will be discussed in this chapter–myasthenia gravis and Lambert–Eaton myasthenic syndrome (LEMS).

MYASTHENIA GRAVIS

Myasthenia gravis is an often acquired (with rare young-onset inherited exceptions) autoimmune disorder, in which antibodies are directed against the postsynaptic AChR. This results in weakness and fatigability of skeletal muscle groups. The most commonly affected muscles are the proximal limbs, the ocular and bulbar muscles.

There is often an associated abnormality of the thymus in patients with myasthenia gravis. Thymic hyperplasia is found in 70% of patients below the age of 40 years. In 10% of all patients with myasthenia gravis, a benign thymic tumour (thymoma) is found, the incidence of which increases with age.

There appear to be two distinct groups of patients who develop myasthenia gravis, split by age and sex:

- Young women (20–35 years), who tend to have an acute, severely fluctuating, more generalized condition.
- Older men (60–75 years), who tend to have a more oculobulbar presentation.

Clinical features

The clinical features of myasthenia gravis are listed in Table 28.1. The most important characteristic of myasthenia gravis is fatigability. All the features listed may present with fluctuating weakness, which is worse after exercise and at the end of the day. Ptosis and ophthalmoplegia are the presenting features in 50% of patients.

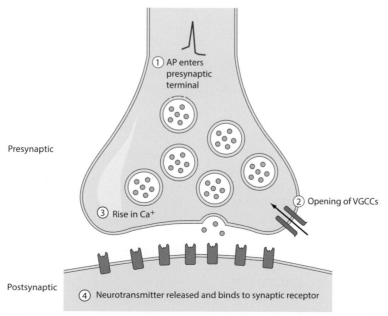

Fig. 28.1 The neuromuscular junction. Antibodies directed against acetylcholine receptors cause myasthenia gravis, whereas antibodies against the presynaptic voltage-gated calcium channels *(VGCCs)* cause Lambert–Eaton myasthenic syndrome. *AP,* Action potential.

Table 28.1 Symptoms of myasthenia gravis – all these features show fatigability

System affected	Associated symptoms
Ocular	Ptosis Diplopia
Other cranial muscles	Weak face and jaw Dysarthria Dysphonia Dysphagia
Limb weakness	Usually proximal – shoulder and hips
Neck weakness	Neck flexion and extension – patients can present with difficulty lifting head up
Respiratory muscle weakness	Shortness of breath

Fatigability of the levator palpebrae superioris can be demonstrated by asking a patient to look downwards for a period, before instructing them to look up. In this situation the eyelid may twitch (Cogan lid twitch) as elevation is initially normal, before fatigue occurs due to myasthenia. Alternatively, the affected muscles can be exercised by making a patient, in whom ptosis is sometimes apparent, look upwards for 1 to 2 min. The ptosis will become more severe and the eyes may drift to the primary position. Similar manoeuvres can be carried out for the proximal limb muscles by testing power before and after repeated contractions such as shoulder abduction.

Limb reflexes are normal or hyperactive but fatigue on repeated testing. Muscle wasting is rare, occurring at a late stage in only a minority of more severe cases. It is rarely as severe as in disorders affecting the motor cell body or nerve. Sensory examination is normal.

> **HINTS AND TIPS**
>
> Any young woman with a complex ophthalmoplegia is likely to have myasthenia, multiple sclerosis (MS) or thyroid eye disease. With bilateral ptosis in addition to ophthalmoplegia, myasthenia is probable and, very rarely, ocular myopathies occur. In thyroid eye disease there will typically be proptosis, not ptosis, and in MS usually there will be other brainstem symptoms or signs.

Investigations

Serum acetylcholine receptor and muscle-specific kinase antibodies

The highly specific AChR antibody is present in the serum of up to 85% of patients with generalized myasthenia gravis. About 50% of patients with ocular myasthenia gravis have the antibody. About 50% of patients who are seronegative for AChR test positive for muscle-specific kinase antibodies (anti-MUSK).

Electromyography

There are two classic electromyographic findings in myasthenia gravis:

- A decrement in amplitude (progressive 'fatigue') of the compound muscle action potential following repetitive stimulation.
- Increased jitter using a single-fibre electrode.

Thymus imaging

It is essential to image the chest with computed tomography or magnetic resonance imaging for the presence of thymic hyperplasia or tumour, as removal of a hyperplastic thymus improves the condition in some patients and removal of thymomas prevents malignant transformation.

Tensilon (edrophonium) test

This is rarely performed nowadays due to the sensitivity of other tests, e.g., AChR antibodies, and potential cardiac complications. Edrophonium is a fast-acting anticholinesterase (i.e., it antagonizes the action of acetylcholinesterase and thus prevents the breakdown of acetylcholine). This enables more acetylcholine to stimulate the reduced numbers of AChRs. When edrophonium is given as an intravenous bolus, usually with atropine to prevent cardiac side effects, ptosis, diplopia and proximal limb fatigability improves within seconds and for only 2 to 3 minutes.

Spirometry

The patient's vital capacity (both standing and lying) needs to be checked. A vital capacity falling below 1.5 L requires transfer of the patient to intensive therapy unit/high dependency unit before potential ventilatory failure occurs.

> **COMMON PITFALLS**
>
> Any known myasthenic with new-onset bulbar dysfunction should have their vital capacity (VC) carefully monitored. There can often be very few other features of myasthenia at the start of a relapse and neuromuscular respiratory weakness can be missed. Patients may complain that their breathing is difficult lying flat or that their voice is getting weaker. It is critical that this is checked with urgency if a patient with myasthenia is admitted to hospital or if a patient develops symptoms or signs of breathing impairment.

Management

The illness may have a protracted and fluctuating course. Acute exacerbations may be unpredictable or may follow infections or treatment with certain drugs. It is important to recognize respiratory involvement, as assisted ventilation may be required. However, patients may remit permanently, especially after thymectomy or with immunosuppressive treatment.

Oral acetylcholinesterases

Pyridostigmine is the most widely used drug; it has a time of onset of less than 60 min and a duration of action of about 3 to 5 hours. The patient's response will determine the dosage required.

Overdosage, usually early on in its use, may precipitate a cholinergic crisis with severe weakness, which may be difficult to differentiate from the myasthenic weakness. Colic and diarrhoea may also occur. Acetylcholinesterases are excellent symptomatic drugs but do not alter the natural history of the disease.

Thymectomy

In patients with thymic hyperplasia, thymectomy, for likely immunological reasons, improves the prognosis of the disease, especially in those under 40 years of age and in those who have had the disease for less than 10 years.

In patients with a thymoma, surgery is essential to remove a potentially malignant tumour, but this rarely results in improvement of the myasthenia.

Immunosuppression

Corticosteroids provide the mainstay of immunosuppressive treatment. An excellent response is seen in 70% of patients but the dose must be increased slowly, preferably in hospital, as there is often a temporary exacerbation of symptoms before the therapeutic effect. Azathioprine is most commonly used as a steroid-sparing agent, though many other immunosuppressants are also used, e.g., methotrexate, ciclosporin and mycophenolate.

Plasmaphercsis or intravenous immunoglobulin may sometimes be used during an acute exacerbation or when there is bulbar or respiratory involvement. The effects are usually short-lived and therefore must be repeated if required.

LAMBERT–EATON MYASTHENIC SYNDROME

LEMS is a rare condition associated with antibodies that are directed against the presynaptic voltage-gated calcium channels at the neuromuscular junction. This results in a failure of acetylcholine release from the presynaptic nerve terminal. In many cases, it is a nonmetastatic manifestation of malignancy, especially small-cell carcinoma of the lung.

LEMS is characterized by weakness of the proximal limb muscles, especially in the lower limbs. Ocular and other cranial muscles are typically spared. There may be fatigability but, characteristically, there is a paradoxical initial improvement in power after exercise, followed by sustained weakness. Reflexes are usually absent, but then return following use of the muscle (posttetanic potentiation). Autonomic involvement is especially common in cases associated with an underlying malignancy.

The diagnosis can be confirmed electromyographically by an 'incremental' increase of the compound muscle action potential after repetitive stimulation (the opposite to myasthenia gravis). AChR antibodies and edrophonium testing are negative. Voltage-gated calcium channel antibodies are usually positive. A search should be made for malignancy, especially small-cell carcinoma of the lung; although the tumour may not be found initially, it may appear several years later or be seen only on positron emission tomography scanning.

Guanethidine hydrochloride and 4-aminopyridine may enhance acetylcholine release. Intravenous immunoglobulin and plasmapheresis may also help. The prognosis for those with a primary lung tumour is usually poor.

OTHER MYASTHENIC SYNDROMES

Drugs

There are a number of drugs thought to worsen symptoms in myasthenia gravis or even induce a myasthenic syndrome. These include penicillamine (used to treat rheumatoid arthritis, Wilson disease) and antibiotics such as ciprofloxacin, quinine and phenytoin.

Congenital myasthenia

A number of mutations affecting proteins involved in the synaptic cycle have been identified to cause myasthenia gravis. They tend to present in early life, either from birth (causing breathing difficulty, feeding problems), early childhood (causing delay in developmental milestones) or adolescence (causing proximal muscle weakness and eye symptoms).

BOTULINUM TOXIN

Clostridium botulinum is a bacterium that can make a preformed toxin, which can enter the body through food poisoning or wounds (e.g., intravenous drug users). This toxin rarely can damage the neuromuscular junction, resulting in a paralytic condition resembling severe, acute myasthenia gravis, often starting with cranial pathology such as double vision and difficulty swallowing. The autonomic system is also affected. Treatment is usually supportive with delivery of a botulism antitoxin.

● Chapter Summary

- The neuromuscular junction is the connection between the peripheral nerve and target muscle. Electrical signal from the nerve is converted to a chemical signal in neurotransmitter release, which effects an electrical signal in the muscle.
- Myasthenia gravis is the common condition that affects the neuromuscular junction and can affect the ocular, bulbar limb and respiratory muscles.
- Myasthenia gravis can be investigated by electromyography (demonstrating a decrement in compound muscle action potential on repetitive testing) and serum antibody test to the acetylcholine receptor.

UKMLA Condition
Myasthenia gravis

UKMLA Presentations
Breathlessness
Facial weakness
Limb weakness
Ptosis
Speech and language problems
Swallowing problems

ANATOMY

Skeletal muscle is made up of large numbers of multinucleated muscle fibres, which have an outer membrane (sarcolemma) and cytoplasm (sarcoplasm) and in which lie the contractile components of the muscle (myofibrils). The fibres are separated by connective tissue (endomysium) and arranged in bundles (fasciculi). Each fasciculus has a connective tissue sheath (perimysium). The muscle is made up of a number of fasciculi bound together and surrounded by a connective tissue sheath (epimysium; Fig. 29.1).

There are two broad types of muscle fibre, which are functionally different:

1. Type I: rich in myoglobulin, with low metabolism (aerobic) and rich in sarcoplasm.
2. Type II: low in myoglobin, with high metabolism (aerobic or anaerobic) and little sarcoplasm.

CLINICAL FEATURES OF MUSCLE DISEASE (MYOPATHY)

Muscle has a uniform structure and function and thus diseases of muscles from a variety of causes can produce similar clinical features.

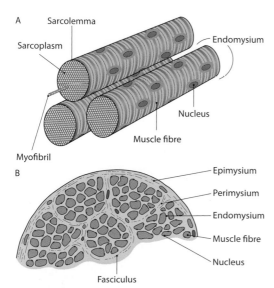

Fig. 29.1 Normal skeletal muscle morphology: (A) longitudinal muscle fibres; (B) cross-section of muscle.

Weakness

Myopathies are characterized by weakness of muscles. Each muscle disease exhibits a particular pattern of involvement (e.g., proximal limb, facial and dysphagia), which is an important diagnostic clue. Proximal muscle wasting and weakness is common in inflammatory myopathies. In one of the hereditary forms, facioscapulohumeral dystrophy, muscle wasting and weakness are often asymmetrical and can affect the face, proximal upper limbs and distal lower limbs. By contrast, inclusion body myositis causes focal wasting and weakness in the flexor compartment of the forearm and thighs in an asymmetrical pattern. Careful examination of all muscle groups is important to classify a myopathy and to differentiate it from a lower motor neurone (LMN) disorder or a disorder of the central nervous system.

Changes in muscle tone

There may be a loss of tone (hypotonia) secondary to disease of muscle, although this sign can be difficult to differentiate from normal tone.

Changes in muscle bulk

Wasting of the affected muscles is distinctive in contrast to the distal wasting of most neuropathies.

Enlargement of muscle may be the result of overactivity or an early sign in certain dystrophies, caused by infiltration of fat, exacerbating the weakness (pseudohypertrophy).

Changes in reflexes

These are usually preserved in muscle disorders, at least until wasting and weakness are severe, which help to distinguish myopathies from LMN syndromes.

Changes in muscle contractility

Myotonia (i.e., persistence of contraction, often for several seconds, during attempted relaxation) is found in myotonic dystrophy, paramyotonia congenita, hyperkalaemic periodic paralysis and congenital myotonia. On electromyography (EMG), the characteristic findings consist of rhythmic discharges. This phenomenon may also be elicited by a sharp tap on the muscle belly (percussion myotonia). Myotonia must be differentiated from fasciculations (muscle twitching) and myokymia (rippling of the muscle), which are typically due to denervation of muscle. Contractures indicate long-standing muscle weakness and can be seen in several dystrophies.

Pain

Pain is a rare complaint in primary muscle disease except in deficiencies of certain enzymes of the carbohydrate or lipid pathways or in severe inflammatory myopathy (e.g., polymyositis, vasculitis). It is important to ask about a change in the colour of urine, as this may indicate myoglobinuria secondary to rhabdomyolysis, which can occur in some metabolic disorders.

HINTS AND TIPS

The pattern of wasting and weakness of muscles in muscle disease and presenting symptoms:

- Proximal weakness – difficulty standing up from chairs, getting out of bed, climbing stairs, hanging clothes on the washing line and storing items in overhead cupboards.
- Distal weakness – difficulty with writing, doing up buttons, opening bottles and tripping over feet/toes.
- Facial weakness – expressionless/myopathic facies, drooling and difficulty whistling.
- Eyes – ptosis, diplopia and ophthalmoplegia (rare).
- Bulbar muscle weakness – dysarthria and dysphagia.
- Neck and spine – 'dropped' head and scoliosis.
- Respiratory musculature weakness – breathlessness, especially lying flat.
- Heart – exercise intolerance, palpitations and blackouts.

Onset of muscle weakness and family history

Many muscle diseases are inherited, and the onset of muscle weakness can typically be traced back to early childhood with delayed motor milestones (sitting, walking, feeding) or difficulty keeping up with peers and playing sports. A full family history is essential. Inherited muscle diseases include:

- X-linked: Duchenne muscular dystrophy, Becker muscular dystrophy and Emery–Dreifuss dystrophy.
- Autosomal dominant: facioscapulohumeral dystrophy, scapuloperoneal dystrophy and myotonic dystrophy.
- Autosomal recessive: limb-girdle dystrophy, all deficiencies of enzymes of glycolytic and lipid metabolism.

- Mitochondrial: complex inheritance pattern as DNA found in mitochondria (maternally inherited) and somatic; chronic progressive external ophthalmoplegia and Kearns–Sayre syndrome.

INVESTIGATION OF MUSCLE DISEASE

The diagnosis may be possible from the clinical features in some causes of muscle disease. Other helpful tests include:

- Serum creatine phosphokinase (creatine kinase [CK]): this can be raised in dystrophies and in inflammatory muscle disorders (e.g., polymyositis).
- EMG: needle examination will reveal 'myopathic units' (small, short-duration, spiky polyphasic units). There may be evidence of myotonic discharges in myotonias and an increase in spontaneous activity (fibrillation potentials and positive sharp waves) in primary myopathies and inflammatory muscle disease.
- Muscle biopsy: this can yield information about fibre type (type I or II), inflammation and dystrophic and histochemical changes. Electron microscopy is sometimes required.
- Magnetic resonance imaging: this is now used to demonstrate the patterns of muscle involvement, which may be helpful in differentiating the dystrophies and selecting a muscle for biopsy.
- Genetic testing: an increasing number of the hereditary myopathies (Table 26.1) can be diagnosed by a genetic test.

SPECIFIC DISEASES

Myopathies can be subdivided as in Table 26.1. Important examples are discussed in the following subsections.

Hereditary myopathies

Muscular dystrophies

Duchenne muscular dystrophy

Duchenne muscular dystrophy is an X-linked recessive disease caused by an absence of dystrophin, a protein that is vital for connecting the cytoskeleton of muscle cells to the extracellular matrix through the membrane. It occurs in 1 in 4000 liveborn males. It also affects skeletal and cardiac muscles.

Clinical features—Patients with Duchenne muscular dystrophy display no abnormality at birth, but the condition is apparent by the fourth year. The child is usually wheelchair bound by 10 years. Death used to be commonplace by the age of 20

Table 29.1 Hereditary and acquired myopathies

Myopathy	System/pathway affected	Notable examples
Hereditary myopathies	Muscular dystrophies	Duchenne, Becker, facioscapulohumeral, limb-girdle, Emery–Dreifuss, oculopharyngeal
	Myotonic disorders	Myotonic dystrophy, myotonia congenita
	Metabolic myopathies	Glycogen storage diseases (most common is McArdle disease) Defects of fatty acid metabolism
	Channelopathies	Periodic paralysis
	Mitochondrial myopathies	Chronic progressive external ophthalmoplegia; Kearns–Sayre syndrome; myopathy, encephalopathy, lactic acidosis and stroke-like episodes Myoclonic epilepsy with red ragged fibres
Acquired myopathies	Inflammatory	Polymyositis, dermatomyositis, inclusion body myositis
	Metabolic or endocrine myopathies	Cushing syndrome, hyperthyroidism or hypothyroidism, hypokalaemia, vitamin D deficiency
	Drug induced	Zidovudine (azidothymidine), steroids, statins, amiodarone, alcohol
	Paraneoplastic	Often necrotizing
	Critical illness	Multifactorial

years, from respiratory failure or cardiac complications including cardiomyopathy and arrhythmias; however, with improved surveillance, life expectancy has significantly improved.

There is initially proximal muscle weakness with pseudohypertrophy of the calves caused by the accumulation of fat and connective tissue. The weakness then spreads. When rising to an erect position, there is a characteristic manoeuvre in which the patient has to 'climb' his legs with his hands (Gower sign; Fig. 29.2). The gait is waddling, and patients can have difficulty rising from sitting, crouching or lying.

Diagnosis. The diagnosis of Duchenne muscular dystrophy is often made clinically. The CK is grossly elevated (often 10,000 U/L). The EMG is myopathic and muscle biopsy shows fatty infiltration and absence of staining for dystrophin. An accurate and rapid DNA diagnosis is now available, allowing reliable identification of carrier status and prenatal diagnosis if required.

Management. There is no cure for Duchenne muscular dystrophy, so the management is supportive. Steroids may provide short-term improvement. Genetic counselling is important. Carrier females may have a raised CK and mildly myopathic EMG, but with minimal clinical symptoms or signs.

Becker muscular dystrophy

Becker muscular dystrophy is also an X-linked recessive condition, with similar characteristics to Duchenne muscular dystrophy, but it has a much milder course. Dystrophin is altered rather than absent. It occurs in approximately 1 in 20,000 live male births.

Clinical features. The symptoms of Becker muscular dystrophy begin in the first decade, although often are not noticed until later. Children continue to walk into their teens and early adult life. Cramps associated with exercise are common. The effects of the cardiomyopathy can be worse than the skeletal weakness and patients are predisposed to developing arrhythmias. These patients often succumb to the cardiac effects before the skeletal muscle problems.

Other muscular dystrophies

Other muscular dystrophies include facioscapulohumeral dystrophy (autosomal dominant), limb-girdle dystrophy (autosomal recessive or dominant), Emery–Dreifuss (X-linked, autosomal dominant or recessive) and oculopharyngeal dystrophy (autosomal dominant).

Myotonic disorders

Myotonic dystrophy (dystrophia myotonica)

Myotonic dystrophy type 1 is the most common adult muscle disease, with a prevalence of 1 in 7000 in the United Kingdom. It is an autosomal dominant inherited condition, caused by an expanded trinucleotide repeat (CTG) within the myotonin protein kinase gene on chromosome 19. This trinucleotide repeat disorder exhibits 'anticipation', whereby successive generations are more severely affected. Myotonic dystrophy is unusual in that it is the female transmission of the mutation that results in more severely affected offspring rather than paternal transmission, which is seen in other forms of anticipation. The features may be very mild in some cases if the length of the expanded repeat is only just above normal.

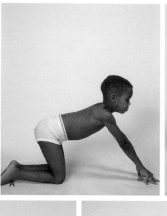
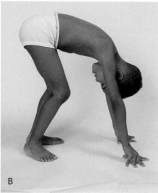
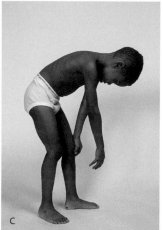
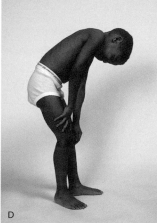
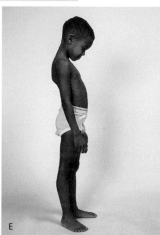

Fig. 29.2 Gower sign. This involves having to 'climb up' the legs with the hands to overcome pelvic muscle weakness. It is found in any condition with pelvic muscle weakness. (From Ball JW, Bindler R. Pediatric Nursing: Caring for Children. 4th ed. Upper Saddle River, NJ: Prentice Hall Health; 2008.)

It is a multisystem disease resulting in (Fig. 29.3):

- Progressive proximal and distal muscle weakness especially in the upper limbs.
- Myotonia (worse in the cold): this can be elicited either through voluntary contraction or through percussion myotonia; tapping the thenar eminence with a tendon hammer causes the thumb to be drawn across the palm, followed by slow relaxation.
- Myopathic facies: weakness and thinning of the face and sternomastoids.
- Ptosis.
- Cataracts.
- Frontal balding.
- Dysarthria and dysphagia: caused by bulbar muscle weakness.
- Apathy and sleep disturbance.
- Cardiomyopathy and conduction defects.
- Nocturnal hypoventilation.

- Impaired gastrointestinal motility due to smooth muscle involvement.
- Gynaecomastia and testicular atrophy.
- Glucose intolerance/diabetes mellitus.

The features usually develop between the ages of 20 and 50 years and progress gradually. Diagnosis is based on genetic testing and management includes treatment of the associated disorders.

COMMON PITFALLS

Patients with myotonic dystrophy are often hypersomnolent. It is important to ask about and investigate for nocturnal hypoventilation as a cause of fatigue and sleepiness. Patients are also prone to cardiac conduction deficits and therefore require regular electrocardiograms (at least yearly or when symptomatic).

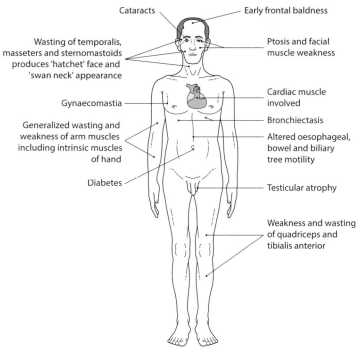

Cataracts

Early frontal baldness

Wasting of temporalis, masseters and sternomastoids produces 'hatchet' face and 'swan neck' appearance

Ptosis and facial muscle weakness

Gynaecomastia

Cardiac muscle involved

Generalized wasting and weakness of arm muscles including intrinsic muscles of hand

Bronchiectasis

Altered oesophageal, bowel and biliary tree motility

Diabetes

Testicular atrophy

Weakness and wasting of quadriceps and tibialis anterior

Fig. 29.3 Clinical features of myotonic dystrophy.

Metabolic myopathies

Any disturbance of the biochemical pathways that support adenosine triphosphate levels in muscle will cause exercise intolerance, with pain during exercise and extreme fatigue. Continued exercise will lead to destruction of muscle (rhabdomyolysis) and the release of myoglobin, which may cause the patient's urine to turn red-orange. There are a large number of specific enzyme deficiencies that are classified as either glycogen storage diseases or defects of fatty acid metabolism (Table 29.1).

Periodic paralyses

The periodic paralyses are rare and belong to a group of disorders known as 'channelopathies' (conditions caused by channel dysfunction). They are characterized by episodes of sudden weakness with alterations in serum potassium levels.

Hypokalaemic periodic paralysis. Hypokalaemic periodic paralysis is an autosomal dominant condition that is most commonly caused by abnormalities in L-type calcium channels due to mutations in the *CACNA1S* gene. Patients present between 10 and 20 years of age and may remit after 35 years of age. Attacks of generalized weakness develop after a heavy carbohydrate meal or after a period of rest following strenuous exertion (e.g., the following morning). During an attack, the serum potassium falls to below 3.0 mmol/L. Attacks may last from 4 to 24 hours. The weakness responds to treatment with potassium replacement. Prophylactic treatment involves the

use of potassium supplements or potassium-sparing diuretics. Some older patients can develop a permanent weakness that progresses slowly over years.

The condition is rarely fatal, as the respiratory and bulbar muscles tend to be spared. Cardiac and eyelid involvement are also rare. Similar weakness with hypokalaemia may occur in thyrotoxicosis.

Hyperkalaemic periodic paralysis. Hyperkalaemic periodic paralysis is an autosomal dominant condition that is caused by abnormalities of voltage-gated sodium channels SCN4A.

It becomes apparent between 5 and 15 years of age and tends to remit after 20 years of age; however, a chronic proximal myopathy may persist. The attacks of weakness, especially of proximal muscles, become apparent 30 minutes to 2 hours after exercise and during fasting. They tend to be less severe than in hypokalaemic periodic paralysis and last less than an hour.

During an attack, the serum potassium is raised above 5.0 mmol/L. Attacks may be terminated by intravenous calcium gluconate or by salbutamol.

Mitochondrial myopathies

The final oxidative pathway involves the respiratory chain in mitochondria, which have their own DNA. Abnormalities of mitochondrial DNA (maternally inherited) cause a wide range of different conditions affecting muscles, the central nervous system, peripheral nervous system and other systems within the body. Mutations in nuclear genes encoding mitochondrial proteins are also described and present with a muscle disorder.

Inflammatory myopathies

Polymyositis and dermatomyositis

Polymyositis and dermatomyositis are conditions in which there is inflammation within the muscle. There may be associated connective tissue disease (25%) or underlying carcinoma usually lung carcinoma (10%), especially if skin changes are present (dermatomyositis).

Clinical features

Polymyositis and dermatomyositis are usually present in the fourth to fifth decade, with women more commonly affected than men. Proximal muscle weakness is the cardinal symptom (difficulty rising from a chair or climbing stairs). Pain and tenderness of the muscles occur in less than half the patients.

The associated skin changes (dermatomyositis) include:

- Macular erythema on the face, especially in the periorbital area, where it is heliotrope (blue-violet) in colour.
- Erythematous plaques over the dorsal aspects of the fingers (Gottron papules).
- Nail-fold haemorrhages.
- Photosensitivity.

As the disease progresses, there may be widespread wasting and weakness, with bulbar dysfunction and respiratory muscle weakness. Patients with polymyositis can also develop interstitial fibrosing lung disease.

Investigations

Investigations for polymyositis and dermatomyositis include the following:

- Erythrocyte sedimentation rate: raised.
- CK: usually highly raised.
- EMG: myopathic picture, but may include fibrillations.
- Muscle biopsy: muscle fibre necrosis with an inflammatory infiltrate, which is distinct for polymyositis and dermatomyositis.
- Autoantibodies (anti-Jo, antinuclear antibodies, rheumatoid factor, extractable nuclear antigen): present in up to 25% of patients.
- Investigation for underlying carcinoma (chest X-ray as a minimum).

Treatment

Corticosteroids and other immunosuppressive drugs (e.g., azathioprine, cyclophosphamide) reduce the symptoms in about 75% of cases of polymyositis and dermatomyositis that are not associated with malignancy. Removal of an associated tumour may cause complete remission. Intravenous immunoglobulin may be useful in patients with severe dermatomyositis.

There is full recovery in about 10% of patients. The remainder of patients have varying degrees of disability and the disease may become inactive or 'burnt out' after a few years. When associated with connective tissue disease, the prognosis is linked to the course of this disease.

Inclusion body myositis

This disorder is the most common cause of muscle disease in people aged over 50 years, occurs more frequently in men and often presents with weakness and wasting of the flexor muscles of the forearm and hand, causing difficulty grasping objects. The proximal muscles can also become involved, particularly the quadriceps (difficulty climbing stairs), and the oesophagus may be affected as the disease progresses. Extraocular and cardiac muscle involvement are rare, though respiratory muscles may be affected in approximately 10% of patients. There is an association with diabetes, but not with an underlying malignancy.

The investigation of choice is the muscle biopsy as characteristic inclusions are seen in muscle fibres, along with features of an inflammatory myopathy. There is no definitive treatment for the condition, and the disease is progressive, with death from respiratory compromise or an aspiration pneumonia.

Acquired electrolyte and endocrine myopathies

A wide range of diseases (especially endocrinological), acquired biochemical abnormalities and drugs can result in myopathy (Table 29.1). The weakness tends to be proximal. Most cases are reversible with treatment of the primary condition or removal of the drug.

Drug-induced myopathies

Statins are increasingly recognized to be associated with a variety of muscle disorders, ranging from asymptomatic raised CK through to muscle pain and overt myopathy. The causative statin should be stopped in all but in the mildest cases and a different statin commenced and monitored. Other drugs are mentioned in Table 29.1. Again, improvement of symptoms occurs with cessation of drug.

Paraneoplastic myopathy

A necrotizing myopathy can occur with malignancies, especially colorectal, lung and breast, independent of either polymyositis or dermatomyositis.

Critical illness myopathy

Patients who are ventilated can sometimes develop a severe myopathy. It can present as an inability to wean off the ventilator and may be associated with prolonged use of paralyzing agents. It is a symmetric proximal myopathy, but the neck flexors may be involved and respiratory failure occurs in 80% of cases. Patients often show a slow improvement. Muscle biopsy shows myosin loss in muscle fibres and the cause of this remains uncertain.

● **Chapter Summary**

- The pattern of weakness is key in diagnosing muscle disorders; weakness can be proximal (e.g., Duchenne), asymmetrical (e.g., facioscapulohumeral dystrophy) or part of a multisystem disorder (e.g., myotonic dystrophy).
- Investigations that can aid diagnosis of a muscle disorder include blood tests and in particular creatine kinase level, electromyography looking for abnormal spontaneous activity or small unit potentials and in selected cases muscle biopsy and genetic tests.
- In inherited myopathies, it is important to consider other muscle that can be affected, such as respiratory or cardiac muscle, as dysfunction is usually associated with significant mortality.
- Secondary muscle disorders such as complications of drug use (e.g., statin) or systemic disease (e.g., hypothyroidism, vitamin D deficiency) should be initially ruled out as they are easily treatable.

UKMLA Condition
Muscular dystrophies

UKMLA Presentations
Abnormal development/developmental delay
Facial weakness
Limb weakness
Muscle pain/myalgia
Urinary symptoms

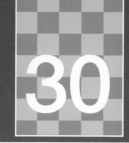
CEREBROVASCULAR DISEASE

Cerebrovascular disease is a significant cause of mortality and morbidity in the developed world. Strokes of all types rank third as a cause of death and are surpassed only by heart disease and cancer. Stroke is a syndrome of clinical features, but an accurate diagnosis requires the localization of the anatomical territory involved, the underlying pathology (infarction or haemorrhage), the mechanism (e.g., embolism), the underlying aetiology (e.g., atherosclerosis) and contributing risk factors (e.g., smoking).

Stroke

Stroke is a focal, neurological deficit caused by a compromise of the cerebral circulation. The onset is sudden and the symptoms last longer than 24 hours, if the patient survives.

Transient ischaemic attack

A transient ischaemic attack (TIA) is a focal, sudden-onset, neurological deficit lasting less than 24 hours, with complete clinical recovery, caused by focal hypoperfusion within the brain. The distinction of a TIA from a stroke is largely arbitrary, as the mechanisms underlying both may be identical, and the main difference is that of duration. However, the differential diagnosis of transient events encompasses other causes of transient neurological symptoms (Table 30.1).

Up to 10% of patients with TIA may suffer a stroke within the following week. It is therefore essential that assessment and investigation occur within 48 hours of a TIA.

Types of stroke

The main subdivisions of stroke (Table 30.2) are cerebral infarction (ischaemic stroke) and intracranial haemorrhage (haemorrhagic stroke). About 80% of strokes are caused by infarction, which may affect all or a part of a vascular territory, occupy the border zone between arterial supplies or occupy only a small area of brain supplied by a penetrating vessel (lacunar stroke). Ischaemic and infarcted brain can occasionally become haemorrhagic. 'Haemorrhagic transformation' is important to recognize because it is a cause of later deterioration in a patient with an ischaemic stroke. In 12% of cases, stroke is caused by primary haemorrhage (intracerebral haemorrhage) within the brain that may affect deep structures or more superficial lobes of the brain. In 8% of stroke cases, bleeding occurs primarily within the subarachnoid space (subarachnoid haemorrhage (SAH)). Sometimes an SAH can be complicated by cerebral infarction due to vasospasm. Cerebral venous thrombosis is a rare cause of stroke but can present with either cerebral infarction or haemorrhage or both in venous territories of the brain.

Incidence of stroke

The incidence of stroke is approximately 150 to 200 cases per 100,000 persons per annum in the United Kingdom, and approximately 20% of patients will die within 30 days. The incidence of TIA is 30 cases per 100,000 persons per annum, although many probably go unreported. The rates increase markedly with advancing age and 20% to 25% of individuals over the age of 45 years will have a stroke.

Table 30.1 Differential diagnoses of transient ischaemic attacks (TIAs)/stroke mimics

Differentials	Notes
Hypoglycaemia	Can present with focal neurology including hemiparesis
Mass lesions (e.g., abscess, tumour)	Can present acutely
Benign positional vertigo	Vertigo affected by head position
Epilepsy	Postictal paralysis, history of seizure
Migraine	Aura consists of positive symptoms, evolves over minutes, lasts < 1 hour, associated with headache. TIAs consist of negative symptoms and reach maximum deficit within 1 minute
Multiple sclerosis	Can present acutely with focal neurology
Transient global amnesia acute disorientation typically lasting < 24 hours	

Table 30.2 Types of stroke and relative frequency

Type	Frequency	Subtype
Cerebral infarction	About 80%	Territorial Border zone Lacunar
Intracerebral haemorrhage	About 12%	Lobar Deep Posterior fossa
Subarachnoid haemorrhage	About 8%	
Cerebral venous thrombosis	Rare	

Aetiology of stroke

The causes of stroke are:

- Atherosclerosis: this causes thrombotic stroke in large extracranial arteries, most commonly the bifurcation of the carotid arteries or intracranial arteries arising from the circle of Willis, especially the origin of the middle cerebral artery.
- Cardiac or carotid embolism: embolic stroke usually arises from pieces of ruptured atherosclerotic plaques or cardiac thrombus. The bifurcation of the common carotid and the akinetic segments of myocardium (e.g., after a heart attack or in atrial fibrillation) are the most common sources of emboli. Valvular heart disease is another important cause.
- Arterial dissection: in the younger population, dissection of either the carotid or vertebral arteries is a relatively common cause of stroke. This may occur spontaneously or there may be a history of injury to the neck such as sudden twisting movements or flexion–extension injuries such as 'whiplash'. Emboli from mural thrombosis associated with the dissection are a common mechanism of stroke in this setting.
- Intracerebral haemorrhage: this is most often secondary to chronic untreated hypertension, but can be caused by other factors (e.g., trauma, anticoagulant therapy, neoplasia) and coagulation disorders (e.g., haemophilia or abnormalities of platelet number or function).
- Lipohyalinosis of small arteries: this degenerative process especially affects small perforating arteries that supply structures deep to the cortex (e.g., basal ganglia, internal capsule and pons). It usually occurs in patients with chronic untreated hypertension. Occlusion of these penetrating arteries causes subcortical infarcts, less than 1.5 cm in diameter, which are called 'lacunes'. Occasionally, their rupture can lead to a small but clinically devastating haemorrhage.
- Nonatherosclerotic diseases of the vessel wall and haematological conditions: these are rarer than the above causes but should always be considered, especially in young patients who present with stroke. Causes include cerebral vasculitis and temporal arteritis in the elderly. Infections involving the base of the brain, such as tuberculous meningitis, can occlude large blood vessels. Any prothrombotic haematological condition such as protein C deficiency can cause a thrombotic stroke.

Risk factors

- Hypertension: this is a major factor in the development of ischaemic and haemorrhagic stroke.
- Diabetes mellitus: this increases the risk of cerebral infarction twofold and should be treated aggressively because it is a recognized risk factor for atherosclerosis.
- Cardiac disease: in addition to cardiac causes of embolic strokes (e.g., atrial fibrillation, cardiomyopathy, arrhythmias and valve disease), the presence of coronary artery disease is a marker for atherosclerosis elsewhere and is therefore a marker for stroke.
- Hyperlipidaemia: this is less significant for stroke than for coronary artery disease.
- Smoking: cessation of smoking lowers the risk of ischaemic stroke.
- Family history: close relatives are at slightly greater risk than nongenetically related family members of a stroke patient.
- Obesity and diet: these are probably less significant for stroke than for coronary artery disease.
- Oral contraceptive: this may increase risk of thromboembolic stroke, cerebral venous sinus thrombosis and SAH in individuals with other risk factors.

Vascular anatomy

A knowledge of the arterial blood supply to the brain and of the common sites for atheromatous plaque formation is important for an appreciation of the various presentations and significance of cerebrovascular disease.

The circle of Willis (Fig. 30.1) is supplied anteriorly by the two carotid arteries and posteriorly by the basilar artery, which is formed by the union of the two vertebral arteries (Fig. 30.2). It is therefore common to classify strokes into those affecting the anterior (carotid) and posterior (vertebrobasilar) circulations.

The most common sites for atheromatous plaques are:

- the origin of the internal carotid arteries
- the origin of the vertebral arteries

The anterior, middle and posterior cerebral arteries arise from the circle of Willis. These supply specific portions of the cerebral hemispheres (Figs. 30.3–30.5); thus reduction in perfusion in each territory will cause different and specific deficits.

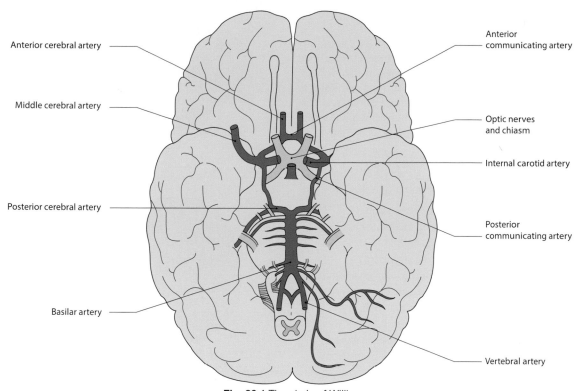

Fig. 30.1 The circle of Willis.

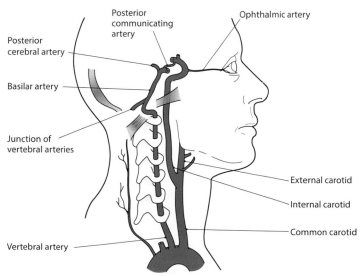

Fig. 30.2 The vertebrobasilar and carotid arteries. The vertebral and basilar arteries give off three cerebellar arteries, which supply the brainstem and cerebellum.

Clinical syndromes

Transient ischaemic attacks

Examples of the types of deficits that can occur in TIAs are listed in Box 27.1. The symptoms typically represent loss of function (negative symptoms), are maximal at onset and last 5 to 30 minutes. Any cause of an ischaemic stroke can cause a TIA, although rarely microhaemorrhages can cause TIA-like symptoms. The most common cause is embolic.

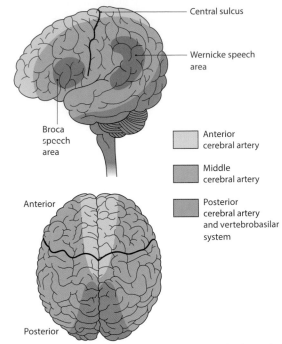

Fig. 30.3 The distribution of the three major cerebral arteries (lateral and tomographic views).

HINTS AND TIPS	
Clinical features of transient ischaemic attacks:	
Anterior circulation (carotid arteries)	Posterior circulation (vertebrobasilar arteries)
Amaurosis fugax	Diplopia, vertigo
Dysphasia	Dysarthria/dysphagia
Contralateral hemiparesis	Unilateral/bilateral or alternating paresis or sensory loss
Contralateral homonymous visual field loss	Binocular visual loss
	Ataxia
	Loss of consciousness (rare)
Any combination of the above	Any combination of the above

Middle cerebral artery occlusion

The middle cerebral artery is the largest branch of the internal carotid artery and supplies the largest area of the cerebral cortex (see Fig. 30.3). It is the most commonly involved artery in stroke. As well as supplying the motor and sensory cortices, the middle cerebral artery supplies the areas of the cortex pertaining to the comprehension (Wernicke area) and expression (Broca area) of speech (see Figs. 30.3 and 30.4). These areas are found in the dominant hemisphere only, and thus in the majority of right-handed individuals, speech production will be affected only when there is occlusion of the left middle cerebral artery. Nondominant lesions often cause visuospatial problems (e.g., inattention). Lesions of either side can be associated with a hemianopia.

The signs of a middle cerebral artery occlusion are listed in Box 27.2. Initially, the limbs are flaccid and areflexic. After a variable period, the reflexes recover and become exaggerated, and the plantar responses become extensor, with spastic limb tone. There is variable recovery of weakness over the course of days, weeks or months. The most common cause of occlusion is thromboembolism or, in Asians/Africans, stenosis, at the origin of the middle cerebral artery. Total occlusion can lead to severe malignant oedema, which may need surgical decompression with a hemicraniectomy.

HINTS AND TIPS
Signs of middle cerebral artery occlusion:
• Contralateral hemiplegia (including the lower part of the face and relative sparing of the leg)
• Contralateral cortical hemisensory loss
• Dominant hemisphere (usually left): aphasia
• Nondominant hemisphere: neglect of contralateral limb and dressing apraxia
• Contralateral homonymous hemianopia
• Conjugate eye deviation (towards the side of the lesion)

Anterior cerebral artery occlusion

The anterior cerebral artery is a branch of the internal carotid artery and runs above the optic nerve to follow the curve of the corpus callosum. The two arteries are linked by the anterior communicating artery and thus the effect of occlusion depends on the relation with respect to the anterior communicating artery (see Figs. 30.1 and 30.5). Occlusion proximal to the anterior communicating artery is normally well tolerated because of adequate cross-flow and thus few symptoms result. Occlusion distal to the anterior communicating artery causes contralateral weakness

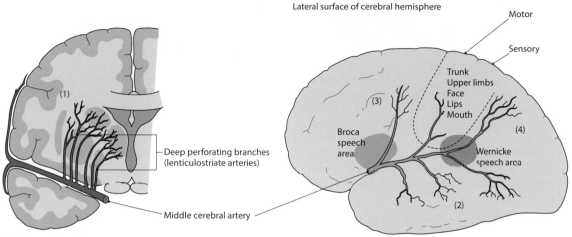

Fig. 30.4 The middle cerebral artery is the largest branch of the internal carotid artery. It gives off *(1)* deep branches (perforating vessels – lenticulostriate), which supply the anterior limb of the internal capsule and part of the basal nuclei. It then passes out to the lateral surface of the cerebral hemisphere at the insula of the lateral sulcus. Here it gives off cortical branches: *(2)* temporal, *(3)* frontal and *(4)* parietal.

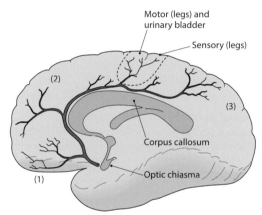

Fig. 30.5 Medial surface of the right cerebral hemisphere. The anterior cerebral artery is a branch of the internal carotid and runs above the optic nerve to follow the curve of the corpus callosum. Soon after its origin, the vessel is joined by the anterior communicating artery. Deep branches pass to the anterior part of the internal capsule and basal nuclei. Cortical branches supply the medial surface of the hemisphere: *(1)* orbital, *(2)* frontal and *(3)* parietal.

and cortical sensory loss in the leg (see Chapters 14 and 15). It is relatively uncommon for the anterior cerebral artery to be purely involved in stroke; it is often due to occlusion more proximally in the internal carotid, or unusual aetiologies such as vasospasm.

Posterior cerebral artery occlusion

The posterior cerebral arteries are the terminal branches of the basilar artery. In addition to cortical branches to the medial inferior temporal lobes and occipital and visual cortices, there are perforating branches that supply the midbrain and thalamus. Occlusion is typically embolic and most patients are in atrial fibrillation.

The effect of occlusion depends on the site:

- Proximal occlusion: which includes midbrain syndrome (Weber syndrome), third nerve palsy and contralateral hemiplegia.
- Thalamic or temporal lobe involvement may cause confusion, memory impairment and hemisensory disturbance.
- Cortical vessel occlusion: homonymous hemianopia with macular sparing (the macular area is additionally supplied by the middle cerebral artery).
- Bilateral occlusion: Anton syndrome (cortical blindness) is rare. The patient is blind but lacks insight into the degree of visual loss and often denies it.

Carotid artery occlusion

Often an internal carotid artery occlusion does not present as a stroke due to the presence of a collateral blood supply from the circle of Willis. A stroke will only occur if the collateral supply is inadequate or thrombosis spreads or embolizes to involve the middle cerebral artery or its branches. Thus, clinically, carotid artery occlusion may present similarly to a middle cerebral artery stroke.

Lacunar stroke

Lacunar infarction is caused by occlusion of small penetrating vessels to the subcortical deep white matter, internal capsule, basal ganglia or pons (see Fig. 30.4). Although these vessels supply a very small area, a number of extremely important structures pass through this space. A very small lesion can cause a marked neurological deficit. Lacunar infarcts are most commonly caused by lipohyalinosis and microatheroma affecting the small perforating vessels, as opposed to embolic disease. Most patients have hypertension, diabetes or hypercholesterolaemia. Clinically, patients present with unilateral weakness and/or sensory loss affecting at least two of the face, arm or leg. There are no cortical signs (e.g., dysphasia, neglect, apraxia, hemianopia, conjugate eye deviation). A computed tomography (CT) brain may not detect lacunar infarcts, and magnetic resonance imaging (MRI) is more sensitive. Multiple lacunar infarcts in multiple domains can cause vascular dementia (see Chapter 21).

Vertebral and basilar artery occlusion – brainstem stroke

Vertebral and basilar artery occlusion are typically due to atheromatous disease. Multiple patterns of deficit can arise depending on the exact location of the lesion with respect to the long tracts (i.e., corticospinal, medial and lateral lemnisci, brainstem connections to the cerebellum and cranial nerve nuclei). Possible clinical features are summarized in Table 30.3.

Specific brainstem syndromes

Lateral medullary syndrome (posterior inferior cerebellar artery syndrome; Wallenberg syndrome): lateral medullary syndrome (Fig. 30.6) is the most widely recognized brainstem syndrome. Clinical features comprise sudden-onset vertigo, vomiting, nystagmus, ipsilateral ataxia (cerebellar connections), ipsilateral facial numbness (fifth cranial nerve descending tract), ipsilateral Horner syndrome (sympathetic tract), contralateral loss of pain and temperature sensation in the limbs (ascending spinothalamic tract) and dysarthria and dysphagia (tenth nerve). See also Chapter 15.

Locked-in syndrome: this is caused by a bilateral infarction in the ventral pons, with or without medullary involvement. The patient is conscious (intact brainstem reticular formation), but is mute and paralysed. Patients can often move their eyes because of sparing of the third and fourth cranial nuclei in the midbrain.

Weber syndrome: Weber syndrome is caused by a lesion in one-half of the midbrain, resulting in an ipsilateral third nerve palsy (III nucleus) and contralateral hemiplegia (descending pyramidal tract above the decussation).

Border zone ischaemia

Hypoperfusion of the brain (e.g., hypovolaemia due to blood loss or hypoxia due to cardiac arrest) can cause border zone or 'watershed' infarction in terminal areas of arterial supply. The parieto-occipital cortex between the middle and posterior cerebral artery territories is especially vulnerable, as is the area between the anterior and middle cerebral arteries, hippocampi and basal ganglia.

Investigation of stroke and transient ischaemic attack

Initial investigations

The following routine investigations should be performed:

- Full blood count: polycythaemia; infection.
- Renal function and electrolytes: patients with electrolyte disturbances may rarely present as stroke mimics with focal or global dysfunction.

Table 30.3 Features of brainstem infarction

Clinical features	Structures involved
Upper motor neurone hemiparesis or tetraparesis	Corticospinal tracts (pyramidal tracts)
Hemisensory or bilateral sensory impairment	Medial lemniscus or spinothalamic tracts
Diplopia	Third, fourth (midbrain) and/or sixth (pons) cranial nerves or nuclei or their connections (e.g., medial longitudinal fasciculus)
Facial sensory loss	Fifth cranial nerve nucleus (midbrain, pons, medulla)
Lower motor neurone facial weakness (upper and lower face)	Seventh nerve nucleus (pons)
Nystagmus, vertigo	Vestibular nuclei (pons and medulla) and connections
Dysphagia, dysarthria	Ninth and tenth cranial nerve nuclei (medulla)
Dysarthria, ataxia, vomiting, hiccoughs	Cerebellum and cerebellar brainstem connection
Horner syndrome (meiosis, ptosis, enophthalmos and disturbed sweating)	Sympathetic fibres in lateral brainstem
Altered consciousness	Reticular formation

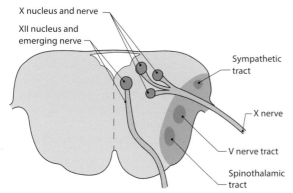

Fig. 30.6 Posterior inferior cerebellar artery syndrome (lateral medullary syndrome).

- Clotting screen: all patients with haemorrhagic stroke and those on anticoagulants.
- Erythrocyte sedimentation rate (ESR), C-reactive protein (CRP): inflammatory disease.
- Thyroid function tests: all patients with atrial fibrillation.
- Blood sugar: hypoglycaemia and diabetes mellitus.
- Fasting lipids.
- Blood culture: if endocarditis or a superadded infection is suspected.
- Autoantibodies and coagulation studies in young patients: connective tissue or vasculitic disease or prothrombotic disorder.
- Electrocardiography (ECG): atrial fibrillation, arrhythmia, myocardial ischaemia/infarction and left ventricular hypertrophy secondary to hypertension.
- Chest X-ray: neoplasia and enlarged heart.

Special investigations

Imaging
All patients should have a CT or an MRI of the brain (Fig. 30.7). CT is more commonly available acutely and can differentiate between an ischaemic and a haemorrhagic stroke. It can also reveal stroke mimics such as subdural haematomas or tumours. CT may appear normal, depending on the time from onset of the stroke to imaging and the size and severity of the infarct. Only approximately 75% of infarcts are ever visible on CT. CT is a critical tool in determining a patient's suitability for thrombolysis.

MRI should be considered if the clinical signs localize to the posterior fossa (i.e., brainstem and cerebellum) because these regions are poorly visualized by CT due to artefacts caused by the surrounding bone. MRI should also be considered in patients who may have had a small stroke, which may not be visible on CT, or where the diagnosis is uncertain. Sophisticated sequences such as diffusion-weighted imaging can differentiate acute from chronic infarcts, while T2* sequences can detect microhaemorrhages. Vascular reconstructive imaging using CT angiography

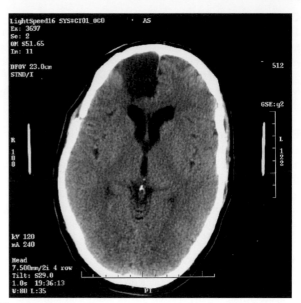

Fig. 30.7 Computed tomography scan showing right frontal ischaemic stroke.

(CTA) and MR angiography (MRA) is helpful in visualizing the intracranial and extracranial carotids and the posterior circulation to look for atheromatous disease, dissections and aneurysms.

HINTS AND TIPS

The UK National Stroke Strategy calls for the urgent imaging of stroke patients who satisfy the criteria for thrombolysis, with a maximum 'door-to-needle time' of 60 minutes. 'Door-to-needle' time should be less than 30 minutes. In high-risk transient ischaemic attacks, investigations should be completed within 24 hours.

Carotid Doppler
The carotid Doppler is an extremely effective, noninvasive means of demonstrating internal carotid artery stenosis when carotid thromboembolism is suspected. A carotid endarterectomy is considered if there is greater than 50% to 70% stenosis in the vessel and a history of a nondisabling ischaemic stroke or TIA within the last 6 months. The longer the period free of symptoms, the smaller the overall benefit from surgery and the National Institute for Health and Care Excellence (NICE) recommends that suitable patients undergo surgery within a maximum of 2 weeks of onset of stroke or TIA symptoms. If the patient is left with a very dense hemiplegia and other cortical problems (e.g., dysphasia), there is little value in performing carotid Doppler as there is little functional brain left to protect.

Cerebral angiography

The advent of carotid Doppler and MRA has meant that conventional cerebral angiography is used infrequently in stroke patients, primarily to locate intracerebral aneurysms, and for the diagnosis of cerebral vasculitides, which are both still poorly detected with MRA. In patients with a recent completed stroke, angiography should not be considered until 1 to 2 weeks have elapsed.

Echocardiography and Holter monitoring

Echocardiography is useful in patients with suspected cardiogenic embolism and may define wall motion abnormalities or the presence of atrial or ventricular thrombus. Holter monitoring or more prolonged monitoring using a Reveal device may confirm paroxysmal atrial fibrillation in patients with suspected cardiogenic embolic stroke, but who have normal ECG.

Management of stroke

The management of stroke can be divided into the management of acute stroke in hyperacute stroke units and thrombolysis in appropriate cases. Beyond this, admission to an organized stroke unit is critical, for the prevention of secondary complications, risk factor management, secondary prevention of stroke and rehabilitation.

Thrombolysis

Thrombolysis is the first treatment that has been shown to be effective in acute stroke. Trials have shown that intravenous recombinant tissue plasminogen activator given within 4.5 hours of onset of ischaemic stroke confers a 1 in 8 chance of a significant recovery, but a 1 in 18 chance of symptomatic intracranial haemorrhage. Knowing the time of onset of stroke is, therefore, crucial and there is a linear decline in functional recovery as the stroke-to-needle time extends, even within the window of 4.5 hours. Patients who wake up with stroke may be eligible for thrombolysis, depending on the duration of time since the midpoint of sleep. Contraindications to thrombolysis include recent major surgery or previous stroke in the last 3 months. Patients on anticoagulants can sometimes receive thrombolysis depending on levels of prethrombolysis coagulation tests.

Thrombectomy

In a number of specialized stroke centres, mechanical removal of a clot from the anterior circulation (usually proximal middle cerebral artery) and occasionally posterior circulation (basilar artery) is attempted in the acute phase. Evidence suggests this should occur within 6 hours of the start of the stroke syndrome, although in some specific cases this window can be extended. In addition, patients in whom thrombolysis is contraindicated (e.g., on anticoagulants) may be suitable candidates for thrombectomy.

Other management aims

- NICE now recommends the use of clopidogrel or, in those intolerant to it, the combination of aspirin and dipyridamole. Antiplatelet treatment helps prevent early stroke recurrence, and reduces death and disability at follow-up.
- Prevent development of complications (e.g., aspiration pneumonia, pressure sores, dislocated shoulders, thromboembolism and depression).
- Rehabilitate the patient (e.g., physiotherapy, occupational therapy and speech therapy).
- Control hypertension only if it is severely elevated (i.e., systolic > 170 mmHg and diastolic > 120 mmHg). An acute drop in blood pressure can reduce perfusion to an already ischaemic brain.
- Risk factor management – encourage the patient to stop smoking, correct lipid abnormalities with statins and ensure good glycaemic control in diabetic patients.
- Remove or treat embolic source (e.g., anticoagulation, antibiotics for endocarditis or endarterectomy). Note: anticoagulation is indicated for cardiac embolus, but only once a cerebral haemorrhage has been excluded and not for at least 7 days after an acute event, to prevent haemorrhagic transformation.

Management of transient ischaemic attacks

The management of TIAs is based on the secondary prevention of stroke and risk factor management. NICE recommends that all patients who have had a TIA should be treated with clopidogrel. In those with a contraindication or intolerance to clopidogrel, aspirin or dipyridamole is recommended as a treatment option. The management of other risk factors such as hypertension is equally important. Anticoagulants are indicated in patients with a known cardiac source of embolus and atrial fibrillation, once a scan has excluded haemorrhage. Those patients with significant carotid stenosis should be treated with a carotid endarterectomy within 48 hours.

> **HINTS AND TIPS**
>
> The risk of recurrence after stroke is 5% to 15% in the first year, and by 5 years 30% would have had a recurrence. For this reason, a key component of the management of patients who have had strokes or transient ischaemic attacks is the management of modifiable risk factors, and secondary prevention with antiplatelet drugs, anticoagulants and carotid endarterectomy where appropriate.

Prognosis

The mortality of stroke is approximately 12% and 19% at 7 and 30 days after stroke, respectively. In the first few days, death is usually the result of cerebral oedema from a large infarction or mass effect from haemorrhage causing brainstem compression, coma and death. Subsequently, mortality results from complications (e.g., chest infection, pulmonary embolus) and from other atherosclerotic disease (e.g., myocardial infarction). There is a significant risk of depression following stroke that requires monitoring.

Among the survivors, gradual improvement usually occurs most rapidly in the first 4 to 6 weeks, although it may continue for as long as rehabilitation input continues. Approximately 50% of survivors remain dependent at 1 year, and about one-third of patients may return to independent mobility, but even these patients often have subtle-to-overt cognitive deficits (e.g., poor memory or concentration).

CEREBROVASCULAR INVOLVEMENT IN VASCULITIS

Vasculitis causing stroke may be secondary to infections (e.g., meningitis) or connective tissue disorders (e.g., systemic lupus erythematosus, polyarteritis nodosa), or rarely may be caused by a primary angiitis of the central nervous system (CNS), without systemic or extracranial features. All of these conditions rarely present solely as a stroke, and there may be other neurological or systemic features. However, they should always be considered in young patients or in patients with unusual features.

Investigations

Investigations should include ESR, CRP, autoantibodies, imaging (MRI), cerebral angiography, cerebrospinal fluid (CSF) analysis and, if appropriate, biopsy of the skin, muscle, kidney or other affected organ. If there is a strong suspicion of vasculitis confined to the CNS and angiography shows no diagnostic features, a biopsy of the brain and meninges may be necessary to make the diagnosis.

Treatment

Treatment is with steroids and other immunosuppressive drugs such as cyclophosphamide.

INTRACRANIAL HAEMORRHAGE

Intracranial haemorrhage can be subdivided by site:
- primary intracerebral haemorrhage
- SAH
- subdural and extradural haemorrhage

Primary intracerebral haemorrhage

The most common nontraumatic causes include chronic hypertension, ruptured intracranial aneurysms and vascular malformations. Cerebral amyloid angiopathy is an important cause of superficial, lobar haematomas in older patients. When in conjunction with chronic hypertension, primary intracerebral haemorrhage often occurs in the internal capsule and/or basal ganglia, but it can occur in any part of the cortex, as well as in the pons and cerebellum. The clinical signs depend on the location, but are often associated with mass effect and, therefore, reduced conscious level. It is otherwise very difficult to clinically differentiate a haemorrhage from an infarct.

Subarachnoid haemorrhage

SAH is caused by spontaneous (rather than traumatic) arterial bleeding into the subarachnoid space. The incidence of SAH is 10 to 15 cases per 100,000 persons per year and the average age of onset is 50 years.

Causes
- Intracranial aneurysms: 85%.
- Nonaneurysmal perimesencephalic haemorrhage (haemorrhage into basal cisterns): 10%.
- Arteriovenous malformation: 5%.

Risk factors
- Family history/genetic factors.
- Smoking.
- Hypertension.

Clinical features
- Patients complain of a severe headache of instantaneous onset (like a sudden 'blow to the head'). The patient often describes it as the worst headache they have ever had. Some patients may report acute headaches just prior to presentation and these 'warning' headaches may represent aneurysmal enlargement or minor rupture.
- Transient or prolonged loss of consciousness or seizure may follow immediately.
- Nausea and vomiting often occur due to raised intracranial pressure.
- Drowsiness or coma may continue for hours to days.
- Signs of meningism occur after 3 to 12 hours: neck stiffness on passive flexion; positive Kernig sign (lifting the leg and extending the knee with the patient lying supine stretches the nerve roots and causes meningeal pain).

- Focal signs due to intraparenchymal extension of blood or vasospasm causing ischaemia and infarction may be present (e.g., limb weakness, dysphasia).
- Papilloedema may be present and may be accompanied by subhyaloid and vitreous haemorrhage visible on fundoscopy.

Investigation

CT scanning is the investigation of choice and shows sub-arachnoid or intraventricular blood in up to 95% of patients who present within 24 hours. Beyond that, the sensitivity of CT decreases to 80% at 3 days, 50% at 1 week and 30% at 2 weeks. A lumbar puncture should be carried out if the clinical suspicion of an SAH is high but CT is normal, only if the patient is alert and orientated without focal signs (i.e., no evidence of raised intracranial pressure). In a patient with a mass lesion, lumbar puncture can precipitate transtentorial herniation or 'coning' and should not be performed. The diagnosis of SAH can be made when the CSF is uniformly bloodstained or xanthochromic (straw-coloured supernatant), due to breakdown products of haemoglobin accumulating over a period of 6 hours or more. Xanthochromia determined by spectrophotometry will be positive in all patients between 12 hours and 2 weeks. An extra 5% of cases of SAH can be diagnosed after lumbar puncture.

Angiography is carried out at the earliest convenience in most patients, but is delayed in patients with a poor clinical condition. Angiograms are required to localize aneurysms and arteriovenous malformations prior to intervention and to confirm the cause of the diagnosis. Formal cerebral angiography provides better resolution than CTA.

Immediate management

- General supportive care: regular neurological observations, bedrest and fluid replacement, analgesia for headache and avoidance of hypotension and hypertension.
- Nimodipine (a calcium-channel blocker): reduces risk of delayed ischaemia secondary to vasospasm.

Subsequent management

Berry aneurysms are the most common finding at angiography. These can be dealt with neurosurgically by clipping of the aneurysm neck or by endovascular coiling. Arteriovenous malformations can be treated conservatively, or with direct surgery, radiosurgery, endovascular embolization or a combination of these.

Prognosis

SAH has a poor prognosis, with an overall mortality rate of almost 50%, and 30% of survivors have major neurological deficits. The risk of rebleeding from aneurysms is high in the first 2 weeks, and then declines. In arteriovenous malformations the risk is lower but persists, while perimesencephalic bleeds carry the lowest risk of rebleeding.

Subdural haematoma

Subdural haematoma occurs as a result of rupture of cortical veins bridging the dura and brain. It is usually caused by trauma to the head in a patient with brain atrophy (e.g., elderly and alcoholics).

In an acute subdural haemorrhage, there can be rapid accumulation of blood with a space-occupying effect, leading to rapid transtentorial 'coning'.

With a chronic subdural haematoma, the initial injury may be minor and there may be a latent interval, from days to months, between injury and symptoms. Symptoms can be indolent and fluctuating and include headache, drowsiness (a key feature) and confusion. However, focal deficits (usually hemiparesis), seizures, stupor and coma can occur.

Extradural haemorrhage

Extradural haemorrhage is caused by a traumatic tear in the middle meningeal artery, usually associated with a temporal or parietal skull fracture.

Blood accumulates rapidly in the extradural spaces, over minutes to hours. After a lucid period, the patient may then develop focal signs, coma and transtentorial coning, leading to death.

Management

Diagnosis is by CT scan (Fig. 30.8).

Urgent surgical drainage is undertaken for acute subdural or extradural haematoma. Chronic subdural haematoma is often evacuated through burr holes as an elective procedure.

CEREBRAL VENOUS THROMBOSIS

Blood from the brain is drained by cerebral veins, which empty into dural sinuses, which subsequently drain into the internal jugular veins.

Venous sinus thrombosis is associated with:

- Pregnancy, puerperium, oral contraception.
- Haematological diseases (e.g., polycythaemia, thrombophilia).
- Dehydration (e.g., prolonged vomiting).
- Infection: the middle ear, paranasal sinuses and face all drain into the dural sinuses.
- Inflammatory disorders (e.g., Behçet disease, systemic lupus erythematosus).

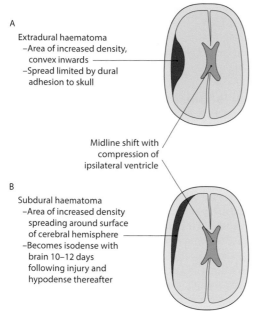

A

Extradural haematoma
–Area of increased density, convex inwards
–Spread limited by dural adhesion to skull

Midline shift with compression of ipsilateral ventricle

B

Subdural haematoma
–Area of increased density spreading around surface of cerebral hemisphere
–Becomes isodense with brain 10–12 days following injury and hypodense thereafter

Fig. 30.8 (A) Extradural haematoma: biconvex, high-density lesion abutting the inner margin of the skull. Midline ventricular shift and sulcal effacement can occur in both subdural and extradural haematomas if they are sufficiently large. (B) Subdural haematoma: crescent-shaped, high-density lesion lying adjacent to the inner margin of the skull. As the haematoma ages, it can become isodense with the brain substance.

- meningitis
- brain malignancy.

The superior sagittal sinus is most commonly involved, followed by the lateral sinus and cavernous sinus, although all are uncommon.

Clinical features

The clinical features of thrombosis in the major sinuses and cerebral veins are variable. The most common presentations are acute headache, motor and sensory deficit, seizures, altered consciousness and papilloedema. The thrombosis within the sinus may lead to venous infarction, which is often haemorrhagic, in the territory draining into the affected sinus.

Cavernous sinus thrombosis

Cavernous sinus thrombosis has a distinctive clinical picture. The cavernous sinus drains venous blood from the eye and many important structures run by or through it, including the carotid artery and the third, fourth, fifth (ophthalmic division) and sixth cranial nerves. In classic, acute cases of cavernous sinus thrombosis, there is proptosis, chemosis and painful ophthalmoplegia.

Diagnosis

Diagnosis can be made with CT angiogram or MRI supplemented with MR venography images.

Treatment

NICE recommends that anticoagulation is used and it is safe even in those with haemorrhagic infarction. Symptomatic treatments include anticonvulsants, antibiotics (if associated with infection) and methods to reduce intracranial pressure.

DISSECTION

Arterial dissection should always be considered as a cause of stroke in young patients. Dissection is due to a tear in the intima of the vessel wall, which causes development of a subintimal or intraluminal haematoma. The haematoma can embolize to produce a stroke and most cases involve the extracranial carotid or vertebral arteries. Although there may be an underlying connective tissue disorder, the majority of these patients develop dissections either spontaneously or secondary to trivial neck trauma or manipulation. Clinically, patients present with a history of minor neck trauma and pain, preceding development of a stroke. The association of Horner syndrome with stroke should alert one to the possibility of carotid dissection. CTA or MRA is diagnostic, and dissection is typically treated with antiplatelet medication. There is no evidence for the use of anticoagulants.

VASCULAR DISEASE OF THE SPINAL CORD

The blood supply to the spinal cord is complex. The main vessels are the paired posterior spinal arteries, which run down the posterior surface of the cord, and the single anterior spinal artery, which runs down the median fissure anteriorly (Fig. 30.9).

During development, five to eight radicular arteries become predominant and provide most of the flow to the spinal cord through the anterior spinal artery. The largest is the artery of Adamkiewicz, which enters at the T9–T11 level and supplies the major portion of blood to the lower thoracic cord and lumbar enlargement.

The midthoracic region is most vulnerable because the supply to the anterior spinal artery often consists of only one significant radicular artery and because there is a poor anastomotic network at this level.

The posterior spinal arteries have a rich collateral supply and, therefore, the posterior part of the cord is relatively protected from the effects of vascular disease, including the dorsal columns.

Fig. 30.10 shows the vascular supply of the cord in cross-section and indicates the supply of the major pathways.

Anterior spinal artery syndrome

If the anterior spinal artery becomes occluded, the supply to the anterior two-thirds of the cord is disrupted, causing anterior spinal artery syndrome, resulting in disruption of the corticospinal and spinothalamic tracts bilaterally (see Fig. 30.10).

Causes

- Small vessel disease (e.g., diabetes, hypertension, angiitis).
- Arterial compression or occlusion (e.g., disc fragments, extradural mass, dissecting aortic aneurysm, aortic surgery).

- Embolism (e.g., aortic angiography, decompression sickness).
- Hypotension: the arterial watershed at the midthoracic region is especially susceptible to hypoperfusion (e.g., pericardiac arrest).

Clinical features

The clinical features of anterior spinal artery syndrome are dependent on the level of the lesion and include:

- Segmental pain at onset: usually in the back and around the trunk.
- Sphincter disturbance: usually urinary retention, but incontinence of bladder and bowel can occur.
- Flaccid paraparesis, which progresses to spasticity over days (corticospinal tracts). Tetraparesis is less common because the thoracic cord is most vulnerable.
- Areflexia below the level of the lesion, which progresses to hyperreflexia and extensor plantar responses over days.
- Loss of pain and temperature sensation up to the dermatome level at which the lesion occurred (spinothalamic tracts).

COMMON PITFALLS

Vibration and joint position sense are not affected as the dorsal columns are supplied by the posterior spinal artery.

Management

Treatment is symptomatic. The prognosis for recovery is variable but usually poor.

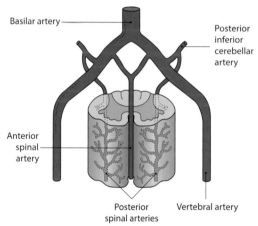

Fig. 30.9 Vascular supply of the spinal cord.

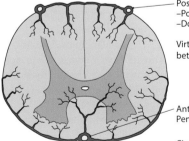

Fig. 30.10 Cross-sectional view of the vascular supply of the spinal cord.

● Chapter Summary

- Stroke and transient ischaemic attack (TIA) are defined as a focal neurological deficit caused by a compromise of the cerebral circulation. TIA lasts less than 24 hours and stroke lasts longer than 24 hours.
- The vascular supply to the brain can be divided into anterior circulation (anterior cerebral arteries and middle cerebral arteries) and posterior circulation (posterior cerebral arteries and basilar artery). Their occlusion produces clinically distinct syndromes.
- The most commonly affected artery is the middle cerebral artery; signs associated with its occlusion are contralateral hemiplegia (including the lower part of the face and relative sparing of the leg), contralateral cortical hemisensory loss, contralateral homonymous hemianopia, aphasia (dominant hemisphere), neglect (nondominant).
- Subarachnoid haemorrhage (SAH) is caused by spontaneous arterial bleeding into the subarachnoid space; 85% of cases as a result of an intracranial aneurysm. Clinically SAH presents as a severe headache of instantaneous onset (like a sudden 'blow to the head').

UKMLA Conditions
Extradural haemorrhage
Migraine
Spinal cord injury
Stroke
Subarachnoid haemorrhage
Subdural haemorrhage
Transient ischaemic attacks

UKMLA Presentations
Altered sensation, numbness and tingling
Dizziness
Facial weakness
Fits/seizures
Head injury
Headache
Limb weakness
Neck pain/stiffness
Speech and language problems
Swallowing problems
Trauma
Urinary symptoms
Vertigo

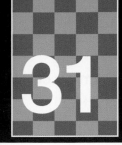
Intracranial tumours can be defined as benign or malignant lesions within the cranial cavity. They can be:

- Primary: primary intracranial tumours account for approximately 10% of all neoplasms and represent 60% of all intracranial neoplasms. They can be derived from neuroepithelial cells (primarily gliomas), the meninges (meningiomas), nerve sheath cells (schwannomas), the anterior pituitary (adenomas) or blood vessels (haemangiomas).
- Secondary: metastatic carcinoma (e.g., lung, breast) or lymphoma.

The relative frequencies of the most common intracranial tumours are shown in Table 31.1. Epidemiologically there are two peaks in the incidence of brain tumours: childhood and in the eighth decade of life.

TYPES OF INTRACRANIAL TUMOUR

Gliomas

Gliomas are malignant, intrinsic brain tumours originating from astrocytes and oligodendrocytes. They virtually never metastasize outside the central nervous system (CNS) and spread only by direct extension. The most common types are described in the following sections.

Table 31.1 Relative frequencies of the most common intracranial tumours

Tumour	RF (%)
Metastases	40
Gliomas	33
Meningiomas	8
Pituitary adenomas	8
Schwannomas	3
Haemangioblastomas	3
Others (include primitive neuroectodermal tumours, primary central nervous system lymphoma, germ cell tumours, craniopharyngiomas, chordomas and chondrosarcomas)	5

RF, Relative frequency.

Astrocytoma

Astrocytomas arise from astrocytes and are the most common primary brain tumour. They can be separated histologically into four grades dependent on the degree of malignancy (grade I, slow-growing over years; grade IV, death within months).

Oligodendroglioma

Oligodendrogliomas arise from oligodendrocytes and form slow-growing, sharply defined tumours that may become calcified. Variants include an anaplastic form and a mixed astrocytoma/oligodendroglioma (oligoastrocytoma).

Glioblastoma multiforme

A glioblastoma multiforme is a highly malignant tumour with no cell differentiation, preventing identification of its tissue of origin. Life expectancy is usually less than a year.

Ependymoma

Derived from ependymal cells and choroid plexus, ependymomas can arise anywhere throughout the ventricular system or spinal canal, but usually in the fourth ventricle or cervical spine or conus medullaris. They are divided into three grades, depending on histology. They spread through cerebrospinal pathways and infiltrate surrounding tissue. Overall, in adults, they have a better survival rate than other gliomas.

Medulloblastoma

Medulloblastoma or primitive neuroectodermal tumours occur in children usually between the ages of 3 and 8 years. They originate in the posterior fossa, either at the cerebellum or at the brainstem and can cause an obstructive hydrocephalus as a result. Medulloblastomas are malignant and treated with surgery in the first instance to debulk the tumour and relieve associated hydrocephalus. Radiotherapy is often used after surgery to target remaining malignant cells.

Meningiomas

Meningiomas are mostly benign tumours that arise from the arachnoid membrane and granulations and may grow to a large size, usually over many years. They peak in the sixth decade of life and are more common in women. They tend to compress adjacent brain structures rather than infiltrate. Calcification is common and they may erode adjacent bone. They are rare below the tentorium cerebelli. The most common sites are parasagittal, olfactory groove, tuberculum sellae and sphenoidal wing.

Primary central nervous system lymphoma

This is a rare form of B-cell non-Hodgkin lymphoma accounting for about 5% of all primary brain tumours. It is more common in male patients over 60 years of age, and especially in immunosuppressed patients, such as those with HIV. It arises in the brain, spinal cord and leptomeninges, and 20% of patients can have intraocular involvement at diagnosis. Lesions are typically multifocal and enhance on imaging. Treatment options include chemotherapy and radiotherapy, but surgery has no role.

> **COMMON PITFALLS**
>
> Steroid treatment of central nervous system lymphomas usually causes a marked reduction in mass effect, contrast enhancement and can cause temporary regression of the tumour. This can confuse the radiological diagnosis and biopsy targeting. Where possible, steroid treatment should be avoided prior to biopsy.

Pituitary tumours

Pituitary tumours are benign and may cause endocrine dysfunction that is not always apparent to the patient. They may also present with visual symptoms due to chiasmal compression and can result in bitemporal hemianopia (see Chapter 43). The visual failure may progress and become irreversible if the tumour is left untreated.

The most common types of pituitary tumour include:

- Prolactinomas: usually microadenomas.
- Nonfunctioning adenomas (Fig. 31.1).

- Growth hormone-secreting adenomas (causing acromegaly and usually macroadenomas).
- Craniopharyngiomas in children.
- Adrenocorticotrophic hormone-secreting adenomas or hyperplasia: Cushing disease.

> **HINTS AND TIPS**
>
> Pituitary apoplexy occurs when there is acute infarction or haemorrhage into the pituitary in the presence of tumour, causing a sudden headache, diplopia, visual loss and reduced conscious level. It is more common in pregnancy, trauma and diabetic ketoacidosis. Management includes steroids and decompressive surgery.

Nerve sheath tumours – neurofibromas and schwannomas

Schwannomas arise from Schwann cells; neurofibromas arise from nonmyelinating Schwann cells and other cells in the peripheral nerves such as fibroblasts. The principal intracranial site of schwannomas is in the cerebellopontine angle, where they arise from the vestibular portion of the eighth cranial nerve sheath. They are a common finding in neurofibromatosis type 2, when they can be bilateral, although they are usually sporadic and unilateral. Clinical features of a vestibular schwannoma (also known as an acoustic neuroma) include ipsilateral sensorineural deafness and fifth nerve involvement (sometimes only loss of the corneal reflex, with no sensory symptoms), then later facial weakness (seventh nerve) and ipsilateral cerebellar signs. Ultimately, contralateral pyramidal signs and hydrocephalus may develop. In general, these tumours are more common arising from spinal nerve roots.

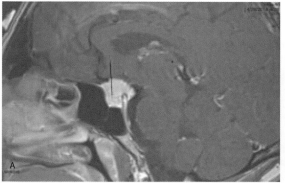 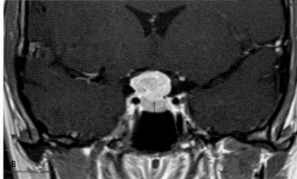

Fig. 31.1 Sagittal (A) and coronal (B) magnetic resonance images of a pituitary adenoma. (From Pressman BD. Pituitary imaging. *Endocrinol Metab Clin North Am.* 2017;46:713–740.)

Haemangioblastomas

Haemangioblastomas are derived from blood vessels and occur within the cerebellar parenchyma or spinal cord. They are found in von Hippel–Lindau disease in association with similar tumours in the retina and cystic lesions in the pancreas and kidney.

Metastases

Metastases are the most common intracranial tumour, especially in the elderly. The most common primaries are from the lung, breast and melanomas. More than half are solitary lesions at presentation, but there are usually many micrometastases that cannot be seen with magnetic resonance imaging (MRI) or computed tomography (CT) scanning.

CLINICAL FEATURES OF INTRACRANIAL TUMOURS

Mass lesions or space-occupying lesions within the cranium may present with one or more of the following features:

- Effects of raised intracranial pressure.
- Focal neurological signs occurring in isolation or in various combinations, caused by the direct effects of the tumour.
- Diffuse cerebral symptoms: seizures and cognitive impairment.

Primary and secondary intracranial tumours are the most common cause of these symptoms, but any space-occupying lesion can present similarly (e.g., cerebral abscess, tuberculoma, subdural or intracerebral haematoma).

Raised intracranial pressure

Raised intracranial pressure can be due to mass effect (direct tumour infiltration and vasogenic oedema), haemorrhage into the tumour or obstruction of cerebrospinal fluid pathways. It produces the classic triad of headache, vomiting and papilloedema. However, these features, especially papilloedema, are relatively infrequent early presentations, as the symptoms usually imply obstruction to the cerebrospinal fluid pathways. The full picture is more common early in posterior fossa tumours, when the flow of cerebrospinal fluid is disrupted and lesions are usually within a very confined space. Early morning headache, which improves with an upright posture, is a common first symptom of intracranial tumours, although focal neurological signs and symptoms often occur without headache.

The raised pressure can also cause symptoms and signs distant to the tumour, including:

- herniation
- false localizing signs

Herniation

There may be compression of the medulla by herniation of the cerebellar tonsils through the foramen magnum (coning), which leads to impairment of consciousness, respiratory depression, bradycardia, decerebrate posturing and death (Fig. 31.2). This is called 'tonsillar herniation'. Similarly, the uncus of the temporal lobe may herniate through the tentorial opening (see Fig. 31.2). This is called 'uncal herniation' and the resulting compression of the third nerve is the cause of the dilating pupil on the side of the tumour, then later bilaterally. There may also be ipsilateral hemiparesis (see below).

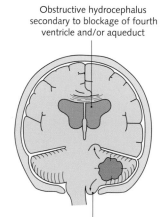

Fig. 31.2 Herniation of (A) the temporal lobe (supratentorial tumours) and (B) the cerebellar tonsils (infratentorial tumours; coning).

False localizing signs

These are 'false' in that they are distant to the site of the mass and caused by the raised pressure. They include:

- Sixth nerve palsy: this is caused by compression of the nerve during its long intracranial course. It is often unilateral initially, then bilateral.
- Third nerve palsy: caudal herniation of the uncus of the temporal lobe causes pupillary dilatation and then later ophthalmoplegia.
- Hemiparesis on the same side as the tumour: this is caused by compression of the brainstem on the free edge of the tentorium in uncal herniation.

False localizing signs are very important because they indicate an increase in pressure with brain shift and require urgent investigation and treatment, which may include surgery.

Focal neurological signs

Focal neurological signs may be caused by direct effects of the tumour (compression, infiltration or oedema) or be false localizing signs (as discussed earlier). The direct effects will depend on the site of the tumour.

Seizures

Focal seizures, whether accompanied with loss of awareness or not, are characteristic of many focal hemispheric lesions. They may then secondarily generalize to a tonic–clonic seizure. The seizures caused by tumours are often difficult to control with drugs but are often helped by steroids in the acute setting.

INVESTIGATIONS

Imaging of the head is essential if an intracranial tumour is suspected. However, as many intracranial tumours are metastatic, more systemic investigations may also be necessary (e.g., chest X-ray; CT scan of chest, abdomen and pelvis; and mammography).

Computed tomography

CT scans should be carried out with contrast, as enhancement of a lesion (which may not be visible precontrast) adds to the discriminating ability.

However, CT scans show only the presence and site of a mass, and whether there is oedema, shift or hydrocephalus; they do not provide much information about the type of tumour. Different intracranial masses (i.e., tumours (benign and malignant), cerebral abscesses and tuberculomas) all have characteristic, but not entirely diagnostic, appearances (Fig. 31.3).

Magnetic resonance imaging

MRI usually provides more anatomical information about soft tissue and tumour delineation than CT scanning, and is always the investigation of choice for suspected posterior fossa mass lesions and pituitary tumours. Small metastases and meningeal lesions may also be missed by CT scans. CT provides more information about calcification and bony abnormalities.

Specialized neuroradiology

Modern imaging techniques such as magnetic resonance spectroscopy, MRI perfusion techniques, diffusion-weighted imaging and positron emission tomography are able to provide complementary biological information about blood flow and cellular ultrastructure that can guide the choice of treatments and assessment of response. They can be particularly helpful in tumour grading and the distinction between tumour recurrence and radiation necrosis.

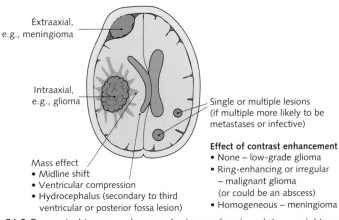

Fig. 31.3 Computed tomography scan features of various intracranial tumours.

COMMON PITFALLS

Lumbar puncture is contraindicated in any case of suspected or definite intracranial mass because it can lead to herniation (coning) and prove fatal.

Stereotactic brain biopsy

A frame is positioned on the head with identifiable external reference (fiducial) markers. CT or MRI can then be used to place a biopsy needle into the precise coordinates of the lesion. The subsequent histological findings help determine further management.

TREATMENT

A multidisciplinary approach is critical to the management of patients with brain tumours.

Cerebral oedema and raised intracranial pressure

The oedema around the tumour can be reduced with the use of oral corticosteroids (usually dexamethasone). In a neuro-surgical emergency setting, raised intracranial pressure can be rapidly reduced with the use of intravenous corticosteroids or intravenous mannitol. Raised intracranial pressure due to hydrocephalus may be treated with insertion of a ventriculo-peritoneal shunt or third ventriculostomy.

Seizures

Seizures are treated with anticonvulsants, but are often difficult to control and the patient may be left with mild ongoing focal seizures and/or secondary generalized seizures.

Surgery

The location of benign tumours (e.g., meningiomas) is critical to likelihood of complete resection, especially if it is in a diffi-cult anatomical position (e.g., near the premotor cortex, speech areas). Malignant tumours cannot be totally removed and, therefore, they are usually only debulked for palliation, if they are in an amenable position.

Radiotherapy and chemotherapy

Radiotherapy is usually recommended for gliomas and radio-sensitive metastases to provide palliation. Chemotherapy can be curative or palliative and is combined with surgery and/or radiotherapy.

PROGNOSIS

The prognosis for brain tumours depends on tumour type and grade, tumour location and size and patient age and perfor-mance status at diagnosis. There is an overall 1-year survival of less than 50% for high-grade malignant tumours. Benign tumours, especially meningiomas, neurofibromas and pitu-itary tumours, can often be removed entirely and therefore cured.

NEUROLOGICAL COMPLICATIONS OF CANCER

The neurological complications of cancer are the second most common cause of admission to hospital for oncology patients. Neurological complications arise for a number of reasons:

- Direct or indirect (metastatic) invasion of the brain or spinal cord.
- Leptomeningeal metastases – these are most commonly associated with breast, small-cell lung cancer, lymphoma and melanoma. They can present with multifocal symptoms and meningism, without obvious masses on brain imaging. Cytological examination of cerebrospinal fluid is the most valuable diagnostic test but should be carried out at least three times with at least 10 mL of fluid each time for adequate sensitivity.
- Delirium – this can be caused by many different factors, including direct effects of the tumour, toxic/metabolic encephalopathy or drug effects.
- Vascular disorders – patients with cancer are at increased risk of both ischaemic and haemorrhagic strokes.
- Infections – patients with cancer may be immunosuppressed and may be susceptible to infection of the CNS by atypical organisms.
- Paraneoplastic disorders – paraneoplastic disorders are rare neurological complications of cancer and discussed in Chapter 35.
- Neurotoxicity of chemotherapy and radiotherapy – chemotherapeutic agents can affect all levels of the nervous system. Many cause a peripheral neuropathy, which is usually sensory and axonal in nature. Radiotherapy to the brain can also give rise to neurological toxicity and predispose patients to secondary tumours, sometimes many years after treatment.

● Chapter Summary

- As with any other organ malignancy, intracranial tumours can either be primary, including gliomas, meningiomas and schwannomas, or secondary with brain metastases commonly originating from lung, breast or renal tumours.
- The clinical presentation of brain tumours is either related to high intracranial pressure (e.g., headache, false lateralizing signs) or location of the tumour (e.g., focal neurology, focal seizures).
- The management of brain tumours includes surgical debulking (sufficient alone for the majority of meningiomas), radiotherapy (for gliomas) and chemotherapy in combination with radiotherapy/surgery. Antiepileptic medication may be required to treat seizures associated with the tumour and oral steroids for associated cerebral oedema.

UKMLA Conditions
Acoustic neuroma
Brain metastases
Metastatic disease
Raised intracranial pressure

UKMLA Presentations
Confusion
Decreased/loss of consciousness
Diplopia
Facial weakness
Fits/seizures
Headache

Infections of the nervous system 32

GENERAL CONDITIONS

Meningitis

The term 'meningitis' typically refers to inflammation of the meninges caused by an infective agent, but meningeal inflammation may be caused by malignancy, granulomatous disease (e.g., sarcoidosis), drugs and blood (following sub-arachnoid haemorrhage). All of these causes can have a similar presentation to infective causes of meningitis. Infective agents can reach the meninges from direct spread (e.g., from sinuses, the nasopharynx or the inner ear), through fractures of the skull or, more commonly, from the bloodstream (haematogenous).

Causative agents

Infective meningitis can be caused by a variety of organisms, including bacteria, viruses, fungi and parasites.

Bacteria

The incidence of bacterial meningitis is 2–6/1,000,000 with peaks in infancy and the elderly. The organisms causing bacterial meningitis vary with age and the predisposing factors of the host (Table 32.1). The three most common meningeal pathogens accounting for more than 80% of cases are:

- *Haemophilus influenzae*
- *Neisseria meningitidis*
- *Streptococcus pneumoniae*

Clinical features

The classic clinical triad of 'meningism' is:

- headache
- photophobia
- neck stiffness

Patients with bacterial meningitis classically present with fever, headache, neck stiffness and signs of cerebral dysfunction (confusion, delirium, decreasing consciousness). Symptoms have typically developed over the course of hours or days. Neck stiffness or meningism may be subtle or marked and may be accompanied by Kernig or Brudzinski signs. Kernig sign is positive when there is painful extension of the knee with the hip flexed at 90 degrees and Brudzinski sign is positive when there is involuntary lifting of the legs with the patient supine and the neck flexed passively.

The absence of any of these findings does not exclude a diagnosis of bacterial meningitis. The clinical picture may change quickly, with rapid clinical decline seen over the course of a few hours. In a severe infection there may be cerebral oedema and raised intracranial pressure, leading to confusion, fluctuating conscious levels, seizures and cranial nerve palsies. In the elderly or immunocompromised patient, signs may be subtle,

Table 32.1 Causes of bacterial meningitis depending on specific age groups and risk factors

Age group	Organism
Neonate <1 month	Group B streptococcus, *Escherichia coli*, *Listeria monocytogenes*, *Klebsiella* species
1–23 months	Group B streptococcus, *E. coli*, *Streptococcus pneumoniae*, *Neisseria meningitidis*, *Haemophilus influenzae*
2–50 years of age	*S. pneumoniae*, *N. meningitidis*
Over 50 years of age	*S. pneumoniae*, *N. meningitidis*, *L. monocytogenes*, aerobic gram-negative bacilli
Immunocompromised	*S. pneumoniae*, *N. meningitidis*, *L. monocytogenes*, aerobic gram-negative bacilli (including *Pseudomonas aeruginosa*)
Risk factor	
Pregnancy	*L. monocytogenes*
Diabetes	*S. pneumoniae*, *Staphylococcus aureus*, gram-negative bacilli
Alcoholism	*S. pneumoniae*, *L. monocytogenes*
Head trauma; postneurosurgery	*S. aureus*, coagulase-negative staphylococci, aerobic gram-negative bacilli (including *P. aeruginosa*)

and patients may present with fever and confusion, but with no specific evidence of meningeal irritation. In all subgroups of patients presenting with acute confusion or altered mental state, it is essential to exclude bacterial meningitis before ascribing to another cause (i.e., urinary sepsis).

COMMON PITFALLS

In cases of meningococcal septicaemia with (or without) meningitis, a rapidly progressive petechial/purpuric nonblanching rash may be present on the extremities. The rash may be absent or atypical on presentation. All cases require urgent treatment and input from critical care. Treatment should be started urgently and not delayed by waiting for a lumbar puncture.

Viral meningitis

Viruses are the major cause of aseptic meningitis syndromes (predominant cerebrospinal fluid (CSF) lymphocytosis and negative routine stains and culture). At presentation, it is often difficult to differentiate from bacterial meningitis as patients typically present with similar symptoms of headache, fever, neck stiffness and photophobia. Where there is any doubt, treatment for bacterial meningitis should be instituted and changed accordingly once results are known. Viral meningitis can be acute or subacute and is usually self-limiting, lasting between 4 and 10 days. Headaches may persist for some weeks, but serious sequelae are rare. If the virus proceeds to affect the brain substance, the patient can become very unwell with meningoencephalitis/encephalitis (see below).

Enteroviruses are the leading cause of viral meningitis, accounting for 85% to 95% of all cases in which a pathogen is identified. This encompasses a large group of viruses including echoviruses and coxsackieviruses. Other common viral pathogens causing meningitis include mumps virus and the herpesviruses including herpes simplex virus (HSV) types 1 (HSV-1) and 2 (HSV-2) and varicella zoster virus (VZV). HSV meningitis is most commonly associated with primary genital infection with HSV-2. In any sexually active individual presenting with aseptic meningitis it is important to consider HIV, which can be seen as part of the primary infection or in already infected individuals. In the immunocompromised, cytomegalovirus (CMV), Epstein–Barr virus, human herpesvirus-6 (HHV-6) and HHV-7 are important pathogens. It is important to take a good travel history as travels abroad will change the viral differential.

BOX 32.1 WHO SHOULD UNDERGO COMPUTED TOMOGRAPHY PRIOR TO LUMBAR PUNCTURE?

- Immunocompromised.
- History of central neurological disease.
- New-onset seizures.
- Papilloedema.
- Abnormal level of consciousness.
- Focal neurological deficit.

Tuberculous meningitis

Tuberculosis meningitis (TBM) typically causes a chronic meningitis, developing over a few weeks to months. Symptoms are initially nonspecific, with gradual onset of headache and malaise. Meningeal symptoms follow, progressing to seizures, cranial nerve palsies and cerebral dysfunction. About 50% of patients will have an abnormal chest X-ray, so look for evidence of tuberculosis (TB) elsewhere. Cerebral imaging with computed tomography (CT) or magnetic resonance imaging (MRI) may reveal associated hydrocephalus, basal meningeal enhancement, infarcts or tuberculomas.

Fungal meningitis

Cryptococcal meningitis is the most common fungal meningitis in Europe and is associated with immunocompromised individuals, particularly those with advanced HIV. The presentation is similar to TBM.

Diagnosis

Lumbar puncture (LP) is the gold-standard diagnostic tool. This should be carried out immediately to prevent delay in treatment. If there are signs of raised intracranial pressure, a CT scan should be carried out first so that the risk of coning can be assessed. Box 32.1 lists the patients that should undergo CT prior to LP.

The diagnosis of bacterial meningitis depends on the CSF examination performed after LP. Normal CSF opening pressures are between 10 and 18 mmHg. Pressures are typically elevated in bacterial meningitis and may be grossly elevated in cases of tuberculous or cryptococcal meningitis. Table 32.2 gives the typical CSF findings in meningitis.

The appearance of the CSF also gives important clues. A cloudy CSF is due to presence of significant concentrations of white blood cells, red blood cells, bacteria and/or protein and is always abnormal.

Table 32.2 Cerebrospinal fluid findings in meningitis

	Normal	Bacterial	Viral	Tuberculous
Appearance	Clear	Turbid/pus	Clear/turbid	Turbid/viscous
Neutrophils	Nil	200–10,000/mm^3	Nil/few	0–200/mm^3
Lymphocytes	<5/mm^3	<5/mm^3	10–100/mm^3	100–300/mm^3
Protein	0.2–0.4 g/L	0.5–2.0 g/L	0.4–0.8 g/L	0.5–3.0 g/L
Glucose	>1/2 blood glucose	<1/3 blood glucose	<1/2 blood glucose	<1/3 blood glucose

Staining of cerebrospinal fluid

- A Gram stain should be performed immediately to diagnose bacterial meningitis. The higher the concentration of bacteria in the CSF, the more likely the Gram stain will yield a positive result. Typical Grams seen in bacterial meningitis include gram-positive diplococci (*S. pneumoniae*), gram-negative diplococci (*N. meningitidis*), gram-negative coccobacilli (*H. influenzae*) and gram-positive rods (*Listeria monocytogenes*).
- Request a Ziehl–Neelsen stain when TBM is suspected. Acid-fast bacilli are visualized in only 20% of cases of TBM.
- Request an Indian-ink stain when cryptococcal meningitis is suspected.

Cerebrospinal fluid culture

- CSF cultures are positive in 70% to 85% of patients who have not received prior antimicrobial therapy, but cultures may take up to 48 hours for organism identification.
- When TBM or fungal meningitis is suspected, dedicated TB and fungal cultures should be set up.
- In the case of TBM, a positive culture is achieved in less than 50% of cases and can take up to 6 weeks to grow. It is especially important that sufficient quantities are put up for TB culture (approximately 10 mL) and repeated LPs are almost always required.

Polymerase chain reaction

- Polymerase chain reaction (PCR) can be carried out on CSF, and ethylenediaminetetraacetic acid (EDTA) blood and throat swabs in cases where bacterial meningitis is suspected. When PCR is used results can be available in hours.
- CSF PCR is the gold-standard test for viral meningitis. A typical viral panel would include testing for enterovirus, HSV and VZV.

Serology

Since the advent of PCR, this has been used much less frequently. However, serology performed on blood is a useful way of diagnosing cases of HIV, mumps and enterovirus meningitis.

Imaging

Chest X-rays, CTs or MRIs may be necessary to define the extent of spread or other involved areas.

Complications

Complications of meningitis often require urgent imaging and discussion with a neurosurgical unit and admission to critical care. Complications include:

- Hydrocephalus due to obstruction of CSF outflow, leading to raised intracranial pressure: this is especially common in TB meningitis.
- Cerebral oedema.
- Venous sinus thrombosis.
- Subdural empyema.
- Cerebral abscess.
- Arteritis and endarteritis: TB can often inflame the origin of the cerebral vasculature as it rises from the base of the brain. In severe cases, this can lead to occlusion of the artery causing a large-vessel stroke. Meningitis can also inflame the smaller arteries within the meninges, causing further damage from ischaemia.

Treatment

Bacterial meningitis is a medical emergency. Each hour of delay increases the likelihood of a fatal outcome or permanent neurological deficit.

The empirical treatment of community-acquired meningitis is with a third-generation cephalosporin (either cefotaxime or ceftriaxone). Cover with ampicillin ± gentamicin can be added in cases where *Listeria* is suspected.

In more complicated circumstances, for example, if the patient is immunocompromised, postneurosurgery, has recently travelled abroad or has been recently hospitalized, cases should be discussed urgently with the on-call microbiologist as treatment regimens will differ depending on the presumed pathogen. Once the results of the LP are known, treatment can then be tailored appropriately.

Role of adjunctive dexamethasone in adults with bacterial meningitis

Steroids may be useful in decreasing the inflammatory response during bacterial meningitis, which is a major factor contributing to morbidity (e.g., deafness) and mortality. Current evidence suggests that adjunctive dexamethasone should be initiated in all adult patients with suspected or proven pneumococcal meningitis (*S. pneumoniae*). Dexamethasone should only be continued if the CSF Gram stain reveals gram-positive diplococci, or if blood or CSF cultures are positive for *S. pneumoniae*. There is no evidence to recommend adjunctive dexamethasone in adults with meningitis caused by other bacterial pathogens.

Tuberculous meningitis

Tuberculous meningitis is treated for 12 months usually with a combination of isoniazid, rifampicin, pyrazinamide and ethambutol with pyridoxine for 2 months (to protect against the peripheral nerve side effects of isoniazid) and with isoniazid and rifampicin for a further 10 months. Adjunctive dexamethasone has been shown to reduce mortality by 30%. Treatment is highly specialized and always requires the involvement of an infection expert.

Viral meningitis

The treatment of viral meningitis is supportive. Aciclovir is used in cases of confirmed HSV meningitis.

Infection control, notification and chemoprophylaxis of contacts

Bacterial meningitis, suspected or confirmed, is a notifiable disease. Patients with suspected bacterial meningitis should be nursed in respiratory isolation, with staff and visitors using masks, gloves and gowns until 48 hours after initiation of antibiotics. Chemoprophylaxis should be offered to household, school or work contacts and medical staff involved in the initial resuscitation of patients with *H. influenzae* (rifampicin) or *N. meningitidis* (ciprofloxacin). Liaison with infection control, occupational health and the health protection agency is essential.

Encephalitis

Definition

- Encephalitis is characterized by inflammation of the brain parenchyma in association with clinical evidence of neurological dysfunction. Traditionally a pathological diagnosis, CSF and parenchymal changes on imaging are now used as surrogate markers.
- 'Meningoencephalitis' is a term used to describe the encephalitic component with associated meningeal inflammation.

- 'Encephalopathy', by contrast, is defined by a disruption of brain function in the absence of a direct inflammatory process in the brain parenchyma. Causes include metabolic disturbances, hypoxia, drugs, organ dysfunction or systemic infections.

Aetiology

The causes of encephalitis comprise:

- Direct infection of the central nervous system (CNS)
- Postinfectious/postimmunization causes
- Noninfectious causes (such as paraneoplastic antibody-associated encephalitis)

The reported incidence in developed country settings ranges from 0.7 to 12.6 cases per 100,000 adults. In the United Kingdom less than half of patients presenting with encephalitis had an infectious cause. In immunocompetent individuals the top five causes of encephalitis were HSV, acute disseminated encephalitis and encephalomyelitis (see Chapter 33), antibody-associated encephalitis, *Mycobacterium tuberculosis* and VZV. In the immunocompromised, VZV followed by HSV were the main causes. Viruses can enter the CNS either via the bloodstream or via peripheral nerves (HSV, VZV, polio, rabies; Table 32.3).

Clinical features

Encephalitis can be difficult to differentiate from acute meningitis, as patients with each syndrome will often present with fever, headache and altered conscious levels. Focal neurological signs and seizures are common. Disturbance of consciousness ranges from stupor, to confusion and coma.

Diagnosis

- CSF examination is essential. A lymphocytosis usually predominates (10–2000 cells/mm^3), but the CSF may be acellular or contain neutrophils. The CSF protein is usually mildly or moderately elevated, with a normal CSF-to-serum glucose ratio. In cases of haemorrhagic encephalitis, red blood cells may be detected in the CSF.
- All patients with suspected encephalitis should have a CSF PCR test for HSV (1 and 2), VZV and enteroviruses as this will identify 90% of cases due to known viral pathogens. In HSV encephalitis, HSV PCR may be negative in the first few days of illness, but a second CSF taken 3 to 7 days later will often be positive, even if aciclovir has been started.
- Further testing should be directed towards specific pathogens as guided by clinical features. An HIV test (blood serum) should be performed on all patients with encephalitis or suspected encephalitis, regardless of risk factors.
- MRI is the imaging of choice in encephalitis, being more sensitive and specific than CT. Temporal lobe changes are

Table 32.3 Infective causes of encephalitis

	Viruses
Herpes viruses	Herpes simplex virus (HSV) 1 and 2 Varicella zoster virus, Epstein–Barr virus, cytomegalovirus (mainly immunocompromised) Human herpesvirus (HHV) 6 and 7 (immunocompromised and children)
Enteroviruses	Enterovirus 70 and 71 Poliovirus Coxsackieviruses Echoviruses Parechovirus
Paramyxoviruses	Measles virus Mumps virus
Others	Influenza viruses Adenoviruses Rubella virus
Associated with travel	West Nile virus Japanese encephalitis Tick-borne encephalitis virus Dengue viruses Rabies
Bacteria	
	Mycobacterium tuberculosis, Mycoplasma pneumoniae, Chlamydophila

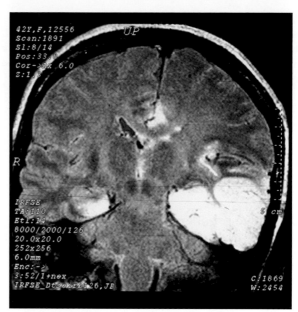

Fig. 32.1 Unilateral temporal changes associated with herpes simplex virus encephalitis. (From Walters RJL, Wills A, Smith P. *Specialist Training in Neurology*. Edinburgh: Mosby; 2007.)

virtually pathognomonic for HSV encephalitis (Fig. 32.1) but are a late development.

- Electroencephalogram (EEG) is a sensitive indicator of cerebral dysfunction and may uncover concomitant nonconvulsive seizures. In HSV encephalitis, there may be a temporal lobe focus demonstrating stereotypical sharp and slow wave complexes occurring at intervals of 2 to 3 s.
- A septic screen with blood and CSF cultures is also essential in excluding other pathogens such as bacterial and fungi.
- Brain biopsy may be considered in cases where the diagnosis remains unknown and the clinical situation continues to deteriorate despite aciclovir.

Treatment

- Intravenous (IV) aciclovir should be initiated if the initial CSF and/or imaging suggests viral encephalitis, or within 6 hours of admission if these results are not yet available, or if the patient is very unwell or deteriorating. This can be continued or stopped according to later CSF PCR results.
- In patients with proven HSV encephalitis, IV therapy should be continued for 14 to 21 days, and a repeat LP performed at

this time to confirm that the CSF is negative for HSV by PCR. If the PCR is still positive, aciclovir should be continued.

- Institute other antivirals/antibiotics as per presumed/confirmed aetiologies. Treatment is otherwise supportive, including seizure control and intubation with sedation if necessary.

Prognosis

Prognosis, in terms of neurological sequelae and death, is dependent on the aetiological cause. The overall mortality rate is 7% to 10% in industrialized countries. Even if not fatal, individuals often have severe physical, cognitive, emotional, behavioural and social difficulties.

HSV causes the most severe viral encephalitis in the United Kingdom, with high mortality and morbidity rates. Early treatment with aciclovir improves outcome in adults with HSV encephalitis, reducing mortality from 70% to 20%–30%.

Cerebral abscess

Definition

A cerebral abscess is a focal encapsulated area of infection within the cerebrum or cerebellum. The abscess passes through several stages, from localized suppurative cerebritis to complete encapsulation. There may be solitary or multiple abscesses.

Aetiology

Infection can reach the brain by local spread, via the blood-stream or by being directly inoculated (i.e., through trauma or neurosurgery). Disease states that predispose to cerebral abscess formation include:

- otitis media/mastoiditis
- sinusitis
- bacterial endocarditis
- dental sepsis
- chronic lung infections
- trauma or neurosurgery
- infections in immunocompromised patients

Causative organisms

Bacteria are the usual causative organisms; however, in immunocompromised patients, other organisms (e.g., fungi and parasites) are more common. Anaerobic and microaerophilic organisms are the main pathogens:

- *Streptococcus* species, especially *S. viridans* and *S. milleri*
- *Bacteroides* species
- *Fusobacterium*
- Enterobacteriaceae (e.g., *Escherichia coli* and *Proteus* species)
- *Staphylococcus aureus*

The following organisms are important in immunocompromised patients:

- *Toxoplasma*
- *Aspergillus*
- *Candida*
- *Listeria*
- *Cryptococcus*

Clinical features

The history in patients with cerebral abscess is usually short (less than 1 month) and progressive. Brain abscesses present as space-occupying lesions with features of raised intracranial pressure:

- headache
- vomiting
- deterioration in conscious level
- papilloedema

There may also be focal features associated with the space occupation:

- seizures (occur in 30% of cases)
- focal neurological signs, depending on location of abscess

There may also be symptoms of systemic infection (e.g., pyrexia, malaise) or of focal infection (e.g., cough, earache), but these may not be present, particularly in immunocompromised patients.

Diagnosis

CT scanning or, if available, MRI is the investigation of choice. LP is contraindicated in the presence of a mass lesion because of the risk of herniation. Other investigations include X-rays/CT of the chest, sinuses and middle ear, which may reveal the primary source of the infection. A full septic screen, including blood cultures, is essential. The classic appearance seen on a CT scan with contrast comprises:

- 'Ring enhancement' of the lesion, which is usually spherical
- Central area of low density
- Surrounding area of oedema

In addition, there may be ventricular compression and midline shift due to a mass effect.

Treatment

- Discuss all cases with the regional neurosurgical centre: a diagnostic aspirate with or without surgical drainage will likely be required.
- Commence empirical antibiotics based on the most likely pathogen; all cases should be discussed with the microbiology team. A third-generation cephalosporin with metronidazole would be appropriate for community-acquired infections, pending rationalization, once antimicrobial sensitivities are known.
- Treat any source of infection (e.g., drainage of chronic sinus infection, mastoiditis, dental abscess).
- Exclude risk factors for immunosuppression and perform an HIV test if appropriate.
- Adjunctive corticosteroid therapy in those with significant oedema and mass shift.
- Antiepileptics where appropriate.

Prognosis

Mortality rates have vastly improved since the advent of CT scanning, surgical drainage and antimicrobial therapy. However, even with appropriate therapy, the mortality rate can range from 0% to 24%. Poor prognostic indicators include:

- Reduced preoperative level of consciousness
- Rupture of the abscess into the ventricles or subarachnoid space
- Immunocompromised patient

Of survivors, 25% to 50% have neurological sequelae, 30% to 50% have persistent seizures, 15% to 30% have a persistent hemiparesis and 10% to 20% have disorders of speech and language.

SPECIFIC ORGANISMS AND THEIR ASSOCIATED DISEASES

Tuberculosis

TB is caused by the bacterium *M. tuberculosis*. It is spread via the respiratory route, and coughed or sneezed out by someone with infectious TB. TB in organs other than the lungs is rarely infectious to others. Neurological TB results from haematogenous spread of TB from other sites, principally the lungs.

Diagnosis
- TB is diagnosed in a number of ways. A definite diagnosis of neurological TB requires culturing the TB bacterium from CSF or other samples.
- Tuberculin testing and/or interferon-γ immunological testing is used for diagnosing latent TB and should not be used to diagnose active cases of TB. They may be helpful in proving past exposure to TB in suspected cases.
- Imaging is an essential part of the diagnosis. A chest X-ray may show signs of associated pulmonary involvement. Spinal/brain CT or MRI are favoured when there are signs of neurological involvement.

Neurological complications of tuberculosis
- Tuberculous meningitis complicated by hydrocephalus, cranial nerve palsies and cerebral infarcts (see above).
- Tuberculoma (brain and spine).
- Spinal TB (Pott disease of the spine).
- Spinal arachnoiditis causing myelopathy and radiculopathy.

Tuberculoma
Tuberculomas are inflammatory masses in the brain, which can be present at diagnosis or develop during treatment. They may produce focal neurological symptoms and signs.

Spinal tuberculosis (Pott disease)
Spinal TB accounts for half of all the sites of bone and joint TB seen in England and Wales. Symptoms include back pain, fever, night sweats and weight loss. Spinal cord compression can result from extradural abscesses and/or vertebral collapse. Aspiration of paraspinal abscesses and/or biopsy from spinal sites may be required to obtain material for diagnosis, culture and sensitivity.

Spinal arachnoiditis
Spinal arachnoiditis may result from downwards spread of intracranial infection or from direct spread from epidural infection. The presentation is of a spreading myelitis with root involvement, that is, weakness (pyramidal and radicular), root pain, sensory loss and sphincter disturbance.

Treatment
Treatment for spinal TB comprises conventional antituberculous therapy for a minimum of 6 months. If there is direct parenchymal or spinal cord involvement (i.e., spinal cord tuberculoma), management should be as for meningeal TB. Spinal decompression may be required in cases of severe spinal cord compression.

Neurocysticercosis

Neurocysticercosis is caused by *Taenia solium*, a pork tapeworm, that infects the CNS. Transmission is via contaminated water and food containing tapeworm eggs. These then reside in the intestine of the carrier and then spread haematogenously to other organs including the nervous system.

Clinical features
The main clinical feature is epilepsy caused by calcified cysts in the brain. Indeed, it is the most common cause of epilepsy in the developing world. A cyst can on occasion block the fourth ventricle causing an obstructive hydrocephalus with its associated symptoms.

Diagnosis
Brain imaging such as MRI or CT can show cysts at various stages of their life cycle, from viable cysts in the early stage (fluid circles with a dot in the middle) to contracted calcified nodules in the late stage.

Treatment
The treatment of patients with cystic brain disease is usually with albendazole. This will kill the parasites and decrease the potential severity of subsequent epilepsy.

Syphilis

Syphilis is caused by the motile spirochaete *Treponema pallidum*. Transmission occurs from direct contact with an infectious lesion (usually through sexual contact), during pregnancy from mother to child or via infected blood products. Syphilis is divided into acquired or congenital cases. Acquired syphilis is classified into early and late stages.

Early:
- primary
- secondary
- early latent less than 2 years of infection

Late:
- late latent over 2 years of infection
- tertiary (including gummatous, cardiovascular and neurological)

Conditions associated with neurosyphilis

The main syphilitic syndromes that affect the nervous system are described in the following subsections.

Asymptomatic neurosyphilis (early/late)

Up to 30% of patients with primary and secondary syphilis may have abnormalities of their CSF, but no neurological symptoms or signs. The clinical significance of this is unknown.

Meningovascular (2–7 years)

Patients may present in a number of ways:

- Acute basal meningitis associated with hydrocephalus, cranial nerve palsies and papilloedema.
- Focal meningitis: when a gumma (granulomatous mass) presents as an expanding intracranial mass, favouring the meninges rather than parenchyma.
- Meningovascular meningitis causing an obliterative endarteritis and presenting as a 'stroke', most often in a young person.

Tabes dorsalis (15–20 years)

Tabes dorsalis is a late presentation of syphilis, causing a meningoradiculitis with degeneration of the dorsal columns and pupillary involvement. The classic features include:

- Lightning pains: irregular, severe, sharp stabbing pains, usually in the lower limb, chest or abdomen, caused by dorsal root involvement.
- Visceral crises: abdominal pain, diarrhoea and tenesmus.
- Argyll Robertson pupils: small, irregularly shaped pupils that do not react to light but do accommodate.
- Impaired vibration and joint position sense and reduced deep pain. This results in a sensory ataxia, trophic skin lesions and Charcot joints (painless joint damage).
- Extensor plantar responses despite absent ankle jerks: caused by the combination of radiculopathy and upper motor neurone involvement.

General paralysis of the insane (10–20 years)

General paralysis of the insane develops 10 to 20 years after primary infection and, as its historical name indicates, involves psychiatric abnormality and weakness. There are two phases:

- Preparalytic: with progressive dementia
- Paralytic: with involvement of the corticospinal tracts and extrapyramidal system

  Clinical features include:

- Dementia: usually similar to that associated with Alzheimer's disease, but occasionally involves manic behaviour or delusions of grandeur
- Seizures and incontinence

- Pupil abnormalities: pupils are large, unequal and unreactive in 75% of cases; the remainder have Argyll Robertson pupils.
- Tremor of tongue ('trombone' tongue).
- Hypertonia with brisk reflexes and extensor plantar responses.

Diagnosis

In late syphilis a thorough clinical examination should be undertaken, especially of the cardiovascular and neurological systems.

Serological testing

Serological diagnosis for syphilis consists of treponemal and nontreponemal tests. Specific (treponemal) tests include:

- Treponemal enzyme immunoassay (EIA) to detect immunoglobulin (Ig; IgG or IgM)
- *T. pallidum* haemagglutination assay
- *T. pallidum* particle agglutination assay (TPPA)
- Fluorescent treponema antibody absorbed test
- Cardiolipin tests (venereal disease research laboratory/rapid plasma reagin (VDRL/RPR))

A treponemal test, most commonly the EIA or TPPA, is used for screening. A quantitative VDRL/RPR should be performed when treponemal tests are positive, as this helps diagnose the stage of disease and indicates the need for treatment. A VDRL/RPR titre of >16 and/or a positive IgM test indicates active disease and the need for treatment. The VDRL/RPR and EIA-IgM are often negative in late syphilis.

Evaluation of neurological syphilis

CSF examination is recommended only when neurological or ophthalmic signs or symptoms are present and syphilis serological tests are positive:

- The white cell count (>5 cells/mm^3) is usually raised in symptomatic neurosyphilis.
- A positive treponemal test on CSF is highly sensitive for neurosyphilis but lacks specificity.
- A positive CSF VDRL/RPR is diagnostic of neurosyphilis.

Neurological imaging should be performed on all patients who have symptoms/signs consistent with neurosyphilis.

Treatment

Procaine penicillin intramuscularly od plus probenecid is given for 17 days. Established neurological disease can be arrested, but may not be reversed. Alternative agents include doxycycline, amoxicillin and ceftriaxone. Treatment of all cases should be discussed with infectious diseases or genitourinary medicine team.

Table 32.4 Approach to patient with HIV and neurological features

CD4 cell count	Differentials
>500/μL	Benign and malignant brain tumours
200–500/μL	HIV-associated cognitive and motor disorders
<200/μL	Opportunistic infections and acquired immune deficiency syndrome-associated tumours: • *Toxoplasma* encephalitis • Primary central nervous system lymphoma • Progressive multifocal leucoencephalopathy • HIV encephalopathy • Cytomegalovirus encephalitis • Cryptococcal meningitis

Jarisch–Herxheimer reactions (severe allergic reactions) may occur following treatment and high-dose steroid cover is often given with the penicillin. All patients diagnosed with syphilis should have partner notification discussed at the time of treatment by a trained healthcare professional.

HIV

HIV is a retrovirus that invades the nervous system early in the infection. HIV can also cause neurological involvement via induced immunosuppression, resulting in opportunistic infections or acquired immune deficiency syndrome (AIDS)-related malignancies. Both the central and peripheral nervous system can be affected.

Central nervous system involvement

The most important feature in determining the differential diagnosis when evaluating a neurological complaint in an HIV-infected individual is the degree of immunosuppression in the host (Table 32.4). Central lesions can further be classified according to whether there is associated mass effect.

Central nervous system lesions with mass effect

The two leading diagnoses associated with mass effect in developed countries are *Toxoplasma* encephalitis and primary CNS lymphoma:

- CNS toxoplasmosis is the most commonly encountered neurological opportunistic infection. Patients present with fever, headache, altered mental state and focal neurological complaints or seizures. The CD4 cell count is often <100 cells/μL. Lesions are often multiple, with ring enhancement present in approximately 90%. Surrounding oedema with

mass effect is often seen. It can uncommonly present with diffuse encephalitis not associated with focal abscess formation.
- Primary CNS lymphoma is similar in presentation to, and can often be very difficult to initially distinguish from, CNS toxoplasmosis.
- Other rarer infections that can cause lesions with mass effect include bacterial brain abscesses, cryptoccomas, neurocysticercosis, TB or fungal infections.

CNS lesions without mass effect

- Progressive multifocal leucoencephalopathy (PML) is caused by John Cunningham (JC) virus, a papovavirus that reactivates in the setting of advanced immunosuppression. PML causes a relentlessly progressive central demyelination with a poor prognosis. Differentials include HIV encephalopathy, CMV encephalitis and primary CNS lymphoma.
- HIV encephalopathy typically presents with memory and psychomotor speed impairment, depressive symptoms and movement disorders. Although it rarely presents with mass lesions, it can be similar in presentation to PML.

Dementia in HIV-infected patients

As life expectancy of patients with HIV in developed countries has increased, cognitive impairment in HIV has also increasingly been seen.

Neurological impairment has recently been classified into three conditions:

- Asymptomatic neurocognitive impairment (ANI): individuals who score one standard deviation below the mean on at least two areas of a standardized neuropsychological test.
- HIV-associated mild neurocognitive disorder: individuals who in addition to meeting the criteria for ANI demonstrate some mild impairment in daily functioning. The prevalence is estimated at 20% to 30% of patients with HIV who have no specific neurological symptoms and may be missed without formal neuropsychological testing.
- HIV-associated dementia (HAD): individuals who show marked impairment on neuropsychological testing and in daily functioning. The incidence of HAD has declined since the introduction of highly active antiretroviral therapy (HAART), from 20%–30% to 10%–15% of those with advanced HIV infection.

Peripheral nervous system involvement

HIV may be associated with the following peripheral neuropathies:

- Distal symmetrical polyneuropathy: the most common type of neuropathy. It is usually a late feature, with pain and paraesthesia of the feet. Treatment is symptomatic.
- Chronic inflammatory demyelinating polyradiculoneuropathy (CIDP): an early feature. It comprises a subacute, predominantly motor polyneuropathy, affecting proximal muscles more than distal, without painful dysaesthesia.
- Guillain–Barré syndrome (GBS): the acute counterpart of CIDP. This is an early feature that can occur at seroconversion. It has the same clinical features as seronegative GBS, but with a high CSF lymphocyte count. Plasmapheresis may help.
- Multifocal neuropathy: nerve infarction leads to sudden-onset sensory and motor deficits. Herpes zoster and CMV radiculitis must be excluded.
- Mononeuritis/mononeuritis multiplex: asymmetrical mix of motor and sensory defects occurring over several weeks. Exclude CMV infection if CD4 cell count <50 cells/μL.
- Antiretroviral toxic neuropathy: associated with didanosine and stavudine, which are now rarely used.

Myopathy

Myopathies caused by HIV include:

- Polymyositis: indistinguishable from seronegative polymyositis. Immunosuppressive treatment results in improvement.
- Type 2 fibre muscle atrophy: frequent finding on biopsy in patients with proximal weakness and normal creatine kinase levels.
- Drug-induced myopathy, especially from zidovudine.

Poliomyelitis

Poliovirus is an enterovirus that is transmitted via the oral–faecal route. It has an incubation period of 7 to 14 days. In a small minority of patients, poliovirus causes a selective destruction of anterior horn cells/motor neurones, characterized by severe back, neck and muscle pain.

Europe has been declared officially polio-free since 2001. In 2010 there were 1300 cases worldwide, with the major foci of disease in South Asia, West and Central Africa and the Horn of Africa.

Clinical features

There is considerable variation in symptoms:

- Asymptomatic (95%): with resultant immunity.
- Abortive poliomyelitis (4%–5%): a self-limiting illness with gastrointestinal and mild upper respiratory symptoms and pyrexia.
- Nonparalytic poliomyelitis (0.5%): features of abortive poliomyelitis with meningism. Recovery is complete.

- Paralytic poliomyelitis (0.1%): initially there are features of abortive poliomyelitis, which subside and then recur with meningism and myalgia. There is subsequent asymmetrical paralysis with no sensory involvement. Respiratory failure is due to paralysis of the respiratory muscles. The lower limb or limbs are most commonly affected, especially in children. Bulbar symptoms can occur with cranial nerve involvement. When paralytic poliomyelitis occurs before puberty, the patient is often left with a wasted, shortened limb.

Diagnosis of paralytic poliomyelitis

Poliomyelitis is suspected based on the clinical presentation and CSF findings. Paralytic poliomyelitis is distinguished clinically from GBS by the lack of sensory signs and the asymmetry.

CSF findings are similar to those in other viral meningitides (raised protein, increased number of lymphocytes and normal glucose), but there are usually increased numbers of polymorphs initially. The virus may be grown from throat swabs and stool. It is rarely isolated from CSF. The diagnosis can also be confirmed by PCR amplification of poliovirus RNA from CSF or serologically.

Treatment of paralytic poliomyelitis

Treatment is supportive. Patients with paralytic poliomyelitis should be isolated and contacts immunized. Respiratory failure may develop, requiring mechanical ventilation. Patients with bulbar involvement require close monitoring of cardiovascular status because of the association with blood pressure fluctuations, circulatory collapse and autonomic dysfunction.

Prognosis

Lack of ventilatory support for respiratory paralysis is the usual cause of death, but otherwise mortality rates are very low. Improvement in muscle power can commence a week after paralysis and continue for up to 1 year. Bulbar palsies usually recover well. Some muscles may remain permanently paralysed and fasciculations may persist. In affected limbs in children, bone growth is retarded, resulting in a wasted, shortened limb.

Vaccination

Routine immunization from 2 months of age occurs in the United Kingdom. In areas of the world where polio is endemic, primary immunization is performed with the Sabin oral poliovirus vaccine (live attenuated). Live virus will be excreted in the stool after immunization and therefore great care must be taken to avoid transmission of infection to immunocompromised and nonvaccinated individuals. The Sabin vaccine causes polio in 1 of 2.5 million cases and thus has been replaced by the Salk vaccine (inactive) in nonendemic countries such as the United Kingdom.

Postpolio syndrome

A deterioration in function with atrophy in the affected as well as the unaffected limbs can occur many years after the primary infection (usually between 20 and 40 years). The cause is uncertain, but theories include progressive degeneration of reinnervated motor units, persistence of poliovirus in neural tissue and induction of autoimmunity with subsequent destruction of neural structures.

Lyme disease

The causative agent in Lyme disease is the spirochaete (spiral bacteria) *Borrelia burgdorferi,* which is transmitted by the bite of infected ticks of the *Ixodes ricinus* complex. It is acquired in temperate regions of the northern hemisphere, usually forested, woodland or heathland areas. The organism is prevalent throughout Europe and North America (e.g., Lyme, Connecticut, where the disease was first recognized).

Clinical features

There is evidence for variation in the types of clinical presentation caused by different genospecies of the ticks. The most common manifestation of Lyme disease is a slowly expanding rash called 'erythema migrans', which spreads out from a tick bite, after 5 to 14 days (range 3–30 days). It is not usually painful or itchy and may enlarge over several weeks if not treated with antibiotics, but will eventually disappear without treatment. Other symptoms may include tiredness, headaches and muscle or joint aches and pains.

If the infection is untreated, organisms may spread in the bloodstream and lymphatics to other parts of the body, including the nervous system. In the United Kingdom the most common complications are neurological, which occur in 10% to 15% of untreated individuals. These include:

- Cranial nerve palsies, particularly uni/bilateral facial palsy
- Lymphocytic 'viral-type' meningitis
- Meningoencephalitis
- Radiculopathy causing pain, altered sensation or weakness of a limb

A small number of untreated patients may progress to late neuroborreliosis, with brain and spinal cord damage. Treatment given at an early stage will minimize progression to this unusual, but serious, complication.

> ### HINTS AND TIPS
>
> A patient who presents with a unilateral or bilateral Bell palsy, a rash and a systemic upset (e.g., fever) should always be considered to have possible Lyme disease.

Diagnosis

It is important that a patient's risk of exposure to ticks is properly assessed before requesting diagnostic tests. Assess a patient's risk of exposure to ticks rather than simply asking about tick bites, as many tick bites go unnoticed. Tests should not be used for 'screening' if there is little evidence that infection, either clinically or epidemiologically, has occurred, as the predictive value of a positive result is very low in this situation. False-positive results can occur with many other infections and inflammatory conditions (glandular fever, rheumatoid arthritis and syphilis), which leads to misdiagnosis and inappropriate treatments.

Usually, tests look for the presence of antibodies to *B. burgdorferi,* rather than the organism itself. Antibodies may not be present in the first few weeks after infection, but it is rare for tests to be negative in late-stage disease. Antibody tests on CSF are useful in suspected neuroborreliosis. If initial screening tests are positive, more detailed and specific tests, usually immunoblots (Western blots), should be performed by reference laboratories to establish whether these results are true positives or false positives.

Treatment

In the majority of individuals, symptoms usually resolve or improve within months, even without treatment. However, prompt treatment helps resolve symptoms more rapidly and patients with painful radiculopathy usually have markedly reduced symptoms and analgesia requirements shortly after starting antibiotics.

The most widely recommended treatment regimens are oral antibiotics, doxycycline 200 mg od, amoxicillin 500 mg tds or cefuroxime 500 mg bd for 2 weeks for erythema migrans and isolated facial palsy.

- Oral doxycycline 200 mg od or IV ceftriaxone 2 g od is recommended in acute neuroborreliosis for 14 days.
- IV treatment with ceftriaxone 2 g IV od for 28 days is recommended for late neurological presentations.

Prognosis

Clinical features of late neuroborreliosis may be slow to resolve. Retreatment may be indicated in occasional cases, but there is no evidence that prolonged or multiple courses of antibiotics are valuable.

A small minority of patients may continue to have prolonged subjective symptoms after appropriate treatment, similar to chronic fatigue syndrome or fibromyalgia. In such cases prolonged or multiple courses of antibiotics are not indicated. Referral to specialist clinics should be considered. Relief may be gained from intensive physiotherapy or cognitive behavioural therapy.

Malaria

The malaria parasite is transmitted by female *Anopheles* mosquitoes. Malaria is particularly endemic in the tropics. *Plasmodium falciparum* is the most common species, with *P. vivax* and *P. ovale* being relatively less common.

A complication of malaria is cerebral malaria. This is an encephalopathic illness and can present with delirium and/or seizures. Children, older adults and pregnant women are more at risk of developing this complication of malaria. Patients can also develop a retinopathy and cerebral oedema with increased intracranial pressure. Malaria diagnosis is made by visualizing blood smears on light microscopy to detect parasites. There is a high risk of death, and treatment is with prompt intravenous antimalarial treatment, such as with artesunate or quinine.

Prion diseases

Prion diseases are neurodegenerative diseases that have long incubation periods and progress relentlessly once clinical symptoms appear. Five human prion diseases are currently recognized:

- kuru
- sporadic Creutzfeldt–Jakob disease (sCJD)
- variant Creutzfeldt–Jakob disease (vCJD)
- Gerstmann–Sträussler–Scheinker syndrome
- fatal familial insomnia

These human prion diseases share common neuropathological features, including neuronal loss, proliferation of glial cells, absence of an inflammatory response and the presence of small vacuoles within neuropil, which produces a spongiform appearance. Bovine spongiform encephalopathy (BSE), one of a number of prion infections affecting animals, has focused public attention on these diseases with its possible link to variant CJD.

Prions are small infectious pathogens containing protein, but which lack a nucleic acid. They are characteristically resistant to a number of normal decontaminating procedures, and so disinfection and sterilization of prion-contaminated medical instruments require specific procedures.

Prion diseases are associated with the accumulation of an abnormal form of host protein, termed 'prion protein' (PrP). These changes are due to both variation in amino acid sequence and glycosylation of the PrP. Transport of the abnormal PrP to the nervous system, once it appears in the host, occurs via axons and appears to be neurotoxic, leading to apoptosis and cell death.

Creutzfeldt–Jakob disease

CJD is the most common of the human prion diseases. Sporadic, familial, iatrogenic and variant forms of CJD are all recognized.

Sporadic Creutzfeldt–Jakob disease

Sporadic CJD occurs with a frequency of 1 case per 1,000,000 population per year worldwide and accounts for 85% to 95% of all cases of CJD. Onset of disease is usually between 57 and 62 years of age. Rapidly progressive mental deterioration and myoclonus are the two cardinal features of sCJD. This usually progresses over a few months to akinetic mutism.

Variant Creutzfeldt–Jakob disease

vCJD was first described in 1996. As of 2012, there have been a total of 224 cases of probable vCJD reported worldwide. Available evidence suggests that vCJD represents bovine-to-human transmission of BSE, with most patients acquiring the disease through ingestion of infected meat products. Variant CJD presents with a progressive cognitive decline, with prominent neuropsychiatric features often accompanied by sensory symptoms. It presents at a younger age and has a more protracted course than sCJD (14 vs. 4–5 months).

Since 1989, when the specified bovine offal ban was first introduced, the use of all tissues most likely to contain the infective agent of BSE in products for human consumption, such as the brain, spinal cord, thymus, tonsils, spleen, intestines and, more recently, bones, are prohibited.

Iatrogenic Creutzfeldt–Jakob disease

Iatrogenic CJD has occurred following the use of cadaveric human pituitary hormones, dural graft transplants, corneal transplants, liver transplants and the use of contaminated neurosurgical instruments or stereotactic depth electrodes. Exact incubation periods for iatrogenic CJD are unknown but are estimated to be between 9 and 10 years.

Inherited prion diseases

These are caused by autosomal inherited mutations to the *PRNP* gene. Gerstmann–Sträussler–Scheinker syndrome and fatal familial insomnia form part of this group, the latter characterized by untreatable insomnia, dysautonomia and motor signs.

Diagnosis

The recent advent of very sensitive protein assays and our continued understanding of common genetic mutations in the diagnosis of CJD have rendered procedures such as brain biopsy unnecessary. This in combination with a compatible clinical presentation as supportive MRI, EEG and CSF analysis are sufficient to exclude other causes and establish CJD as the probable diagnosis:

- MRI can often demonstrate a high T2 and fluid-attenuated inversion recovery signal in the caudate and putamen in sCJD. In vCJD there may be high signal in the pulvinar and dorsomedial thalamus. In both forms of the disease, diffusion-weighted imaging may be more sensitive in showing cortical changes ('cortical ribboning').

- A characteristic EEG pattern of periodic synchronous biphasic or triphasic sharp wave complexes is observed in 67% to 95% of patients with sCJD, less so in vCJD.
- Detecting 14-3-3 protein in CSF is a specific test finding for sCJD but has low sensitivity. PrP conversion assays such as real-time, quaking-induced conversion in CSF have a reported sensitivity of around 90% in the diagnosis of CJD.

Treatment

There is no effective treatment for CJD, which is uniformly fatal. Death usually occurs within 1 year of symptom onset.

HINTS AND TIPS

A rapidly progressive dementia (over weeks or months), especially with myoclonus, should always be considered to be prion disease unless an alternative diagnosis can be made. This has implications for how all samples from the patient, including blood and cerebrospinal fluid, are handled by medical and laboratory staff.

Chapter Summary

- Bacterial meningitis is an essential diagnosis to consider in a patient presenting acutely with fever, headache, neck stiffness and photophobia, as mortality is high in untreated patients. Urgent management is with intravenous administration of a third-generation cephalosporin.
- In the early stages it can be hard to distinguish between viral encephalitis and bacterial meningitis. Cerebrospinal fluid (CSF) analysis is very helpful in aiding the diagnosis, as a lymphocytic CSF is likely due to viral encephalitis. Further CSF polymerase chain reaction study can then identify the particular pathogen.
- Neurological tuberculosis (TB) results from haematogenous spread of TB usually from the lungs and can present in multiple ways including tuberculous meningitis (affecting the brain), tuberculoma (affecting the brain and spine) and spinal TB (resulting in potential myelopathy).
- HIV can affect any part of the nervous system. Acute brain involvement is usually the result of opportunistic infections such as toxoplasmosis or *Cryptococcus* and related to a severely immunocompromised state.

UKMLA Conditions
Brain abscess
Encephalitis
Malaria
Meningitis
Raised intracranial pressure
Spinal cord compression
Stroke

UKMLA Presentations
Confusion
Decreased/loss of consciousness
Facial weakness
Fits/seizures
Headache
Neck pain/stiffness

Multiple sclerosis

EPIDEMIOLOGY

Multiple sclerosis (MS) occurs worldwide but is particularly common in North America, Australia and northern Europe. It has a prevalence of approximately 150 per 100,000 in the United Kingdom. The disease usually occurs in young White adults, with the peak age of onset for the relapsing–remitting form of the disease being between 20 and 30 years; this may convert to secondary-progressive MS at a mean age of 40 to 44 years. More females than males are affected in all forms of the disease.

PATHOGENESIS

The major mechanisms that cause MS are inflammation, demyelination and axonal degeneration in the later stages of the disease. The pathogenesis of MS is likely multifactorial, involving genetic factors (especially in the human lymphocyte antigen region), environmental factors and previous viral exposure (especially to Epstein–Barr virus).

PATHOLOGY

Areas of demyelination are found in the white matter of the brain and spinal cord. These areas are called 'plaques'. There is a particular predilection for certain sites within the central nervous system (CNS):

- periventricular region of the cerebral hemispheres
- corpus callosum
- brainstem (including medial longitudinal fasciculus), cerebellum and cerebellar peduncles
- cervical cord
- optic nerves

Histologically there is myelin destruction with relative preservation of axons. Plaques are a consequence of inflammatory infiltrates containing mononuclear cells and lymphocytes. Interstitial oedema occurs in acute lesions. Remyelination is rare and the mechanism of functional recovery is uncertain. It is postulated that chronic demyelination may eventually account for the loss of axons and subsequently the cell bodies. This may explain the clinical irreversibility of some of the relapses.

CLINICAL FEATURES

MS can present in a multitude of ways, the hallmark being that neurological symptoms are separated in location and time. MS is most commonly characterized by relapse, which is defined as the acute or subacute onset of clinical dysfunction that usually reaches its peak from days to several weeks, followed by a remission during which the symptoms and signs resolve to a variable extent. Three main patterns of disease progression are recognized:

- Relapsing and remitting: clearly defined relapses with full recovery or with some residual deficit upon recovery. Relapses are more common in early disease, and there is no disease progression during the periods between relapses. This makes up 85% to 90% of cases initially.
- Secondary progressive: when the disease starts with a relapsing–remitting picture, but eventually recovery from each successive relapse becomes less complete, and there is progression of disease between relapses causing the development of long-term disability. Approximately 40% of patients presenting with relapsing–remitting disease eventually develop secondary-progressive disease 10 years after disease onset. It is the progression of disease, rather than incomplete recovery from relapses, which causes disability.
- Primary progressive: disability worsens gradually from onset without true relapses or remissions, with a cumulative disability from the onset. Approximately 10% to 30% of patients may present with this form of disease.

There is a marked variability in the disease progression. Overall, studies have shown that the median time from disease onset to walking with a cane is 28 years. About 20% of patients with relapsing–remitting MS develop little or no disability after 10 years. Patients with primary-progressive disease, who tend to have a later age of onset and more even sex distribution, have a worse prognosis for ultimate disability compared with relapsing–remitting patients. Overall, the life expectancy of MS patients is reduced by 6 to 7 years compared with the general population, and severe disability is a major risk factor for premature death. Prognostic factors for MS are shown in Box 33.1. Pregnancy does not worsen the prognosis for those women with MS, and in fact there may be a reduction in relapse rates during pregnancy, which is probably compensated for by a higher relapse rate in the immediate period after delivery.

demyelination (i.e., MS). Up to 70% of cases fall into the latter category. In some patients, optic nerve demyelination may be asymptomatic and only discovered clinically by the presence of optic atrophy or by the use of visual evoked potentials (see Chapter 3).

COMMON PITFALLS

Papillitis can look similar to papilloedema through an ophthalmoscope. Papillitis causes early and profound loss in vision, with a central scotoma, impaired colour vision and pain on eye movement. In papilloedema, visual deterioration occurs only at a late stage, when there is enlargement of the blind spot and sometimes constriction of the fields.

The most common presentations of MS are discussed in the following subsections and shown in Table 33.1.

Optic and retrobulbar neuritis

Optic neuritis presents as subacute visual loss, usually unilateral, associated with a central scotoma and pain on ocular movement. Recovery is usual over a few weeks. The ophthalmological findings depend on whether the lesion is in the optic nerve head (papillitis) or in the optic nerve behind the eye (retrobulbar neuritis). In the former, a pink swollen disc is seen, whereas in the latter, the disc looks normal.

There are usually no residual symptoms following optic neuritis, although a relative afferent pupillary defect, small central scotomata and defects in colour vision may be demonstrated. Following an attack, optic atrophy (pale disc) often develops several weeks later.

Optic neuritis may be an isolated event (clinical isolated syndrome), or it may be a forerunner for further episodes of CNS

Brainstem/cerebellar presentation

Demyelination may initially affect the brainstem, including the cerebellar connections and medial longitudinal fasciculus (see Chapter 43) in the brainstem. Classical presentations include those described in Table 33.1.

Spinal cord lesion (myelopathy)

A spinal cord lesion (Fig. 33.1) is the most common presentation and results in a spastic paraparesis (thoracic cord) or tetraparesis (cervical cord), often with tonic spasms of the limbs. There is associated difficulty walking and sensory loss. Bladder symptoms are extremely common.

Lhermitte symptom, in which there is a brief, electric shock-like sensation down the limbs on flexion of the neck, may be present. It is indicative of lesions within the spinal cord, which can occur with processes other than demyelination (e.g., vitamin B_{12} deficiency before treatment).

Table 33.1 Common presenting symptoms in multiple sclerosis

Location	Frequency	Nature of symptoms
Spinal cord	50%	Motor – weakness, clumsiness, tonic spasms Sensory – numbness, tingling, burning, band-like sensation, Lhermitte phenomenon, altered temperature sensation Sphincter – urinary urgency/hesitancy/retention/incontinence, constipation, faecal incontinence, erectile dysfunction
Optic nerve (unilateral in 90%)	25%	Visual loss, blurred vision, reduced colour vision, pain on eye movement
Brainstem/cerebellum	20%	Dysarthria, dysphagia, diplopia, vertigo, facial numbness/weakness, trigeminal neuralgia, deafness, ataxia (trunk and limbs), nystagmus, pyramidal weakness due to corticospinal tract involvement, patchy sensory loss, tonic spasms
Cerebral hemispheres	5%	Hemiparesis, hemisensory loss, visual field deficit, dysphasia, seizures, cognitive impairment

Other symptoms

Patients with significant subcortical magnetic resonance imaging (MRI) lesion load can also present with subtle cognitive deficits. Seizures, fatigue and depression are also more common in patients with MS.

DIFFERENTIAL DIAGNOSIS

Differential diagnoses that should be considered include systemic lupus erythematosus, sarcoidosis, Behçet disease and hereditary disorders, such as the leucodystrophies, spinocerebellar ataxias and hereditary spastic paraparesis.

INVESTIGATIONS

Magnetic resonance imaging

Computed tomography scans do not accurately pick up areas of demyelination, whereas MRI is far more sensitive at showing the white matter disease. Hyperintense lesions are seen on T2-weighted images, typically in periventricular areas, the corpus callosum and juxtacortical white matter in the brain. Widespread MRI abnormalities are often seen at presentation,

despite the symptoms being isolated to one or two sites. Contrast enhancement of some lesions (suggesting active disease) and not of others on the same MRI suggests that the lesions are separated in time as well as space, and form an important criterion in making the diagnosis of MS.

Similar hyperintense lesions may be seen in cerebrovascular disease, neurosarcoidosis, vasculitis and lymphoma.

Cerebrospinal fluid examination

A mild lymphocyte pleocytosis may be present, especially during relapses. The protein may be slightly elevated. However, the presence of 'oligoclonal bands' (several intense bands of staining for immunoglobulin G on Western blotting) in the cerebrospinal fluid (CSF) but not in the serum is highly suggestive of MS. Oligoclonal bands in the CSF and often the serum (i.e., matched bands) may also be found in many chronic infective or inflammatory conditions involving the CNS.

Visual evoked potentials

If there has been demyelination at any time along the optic nerve (i.e., optic neuritis), whether symptomatic or asymptomatic, the conduction of visual images (usually a changing checkerboard) to the occipital cortex will be delayed. The normal response takes about 100 ms.

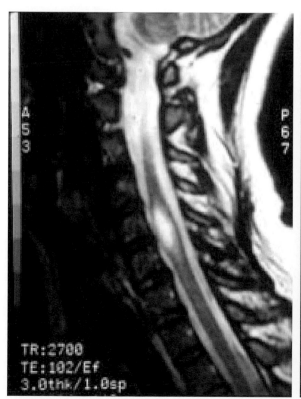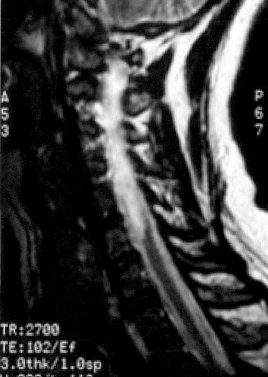

Fig. 33.1 Magnetic resonance imaging cord showing high signal cervical lesion. (From Walters RJ, Wills A, Smith P. *Specialist Training in Neurology*. Edinburgh: Mosby; 2007.)

DIAGNOSIS

The diagnosis of MS is based on the revised McDonald criteria. These are outlined in Table 33.2.

MANAGEMENT

Treatments for acute relapses

Corticosteroid therapy

Steroid therapy, given either intravenously or orally as methylprednisolone, is the mainstay treatment for severe acute relapses. This may shorten the duration of the relapse but does not affect eventual clinical outcome.

Disease-modifying treatment

β-Interferon and glatiramer acetate

Interferon-β1a and 1b and glatiramer acetate are drugs that suppress or modulate the immune system. The UK National Institute for Health and Care Excellence (NICE) and the Association of British Neurologists (ABN) guidelines suggest that they are used in ambulant patients with relapsing–remitting MS, where at least two relapses have occurred in the preceding 2 years, and in whom there is no progression between relapses. Patients with secondary-progressive MS may also be treated if their disability is primarily due to their relapses, which must occur at least annually. All three drugs are given as regular injections, and side effects can include flu-like symptoms, injection site reactions and the development of neutralizing antibodies. The effect of these drugs is to reduce relapse rates by about one-third over 2 years, and they may reduce the development of disability through prevention of those relapses, though the effect is modest. They do not modify progressively increasing disability that is unrelated to relapses. Furthermore, it is unknown whether these drugs reduce the accumulation of disability over the long term, and whether they prevent or slow entry into the secondary-progressive stage of the disease.

Other immunomodulatory agents

Consideration can be given to the use of other, more powerful immunomodulatory agents. Natalizumab is a monoclonal antibody that has been found to reduce the risk of sustained progression of disability by about 40% over 2 years and that of relapses by about 70% over 12 months. However, this drug is associated with an increased risk of opportunistic infections, including progressive multifocal leucoencephalopathy (PML), which can be fatal. Currently, the overall risk for this infection is 1.5 per 1000 patients, but the specific risk depends also on the duration of natalizumab

treatment, prior immunosuppressant treatment and previous infection with John Cunningham (JC) virus.

Fingolimod is an oral medication taken daily that prevents lymphocytes from crossing the blood–brain barrier and causing damage to nerve cells in the brain and spinal cord. NICE guidelines recommend its use in highly active relapsing–remitting MS: that is, patients who have an unchanged or increased relapse rate despite treatment with β-interferon. It reduces relapse rates by 52% compared with β-interferon, and disability progression by about 30% compared with placebo. The most common side effects associated with the drug include flu-like symptoms and elevated liver function tests. More rarely, cardiac arrhythmias and macular oedema can occur. Other disease-modifying agents include teriflunomide, dimethyl fumarate, alemtuzumab, cladribine, ocrelizumab and siponimod.

HINTS AND TIPS

Patients presenting with clinically isolated syndromes can be a therapeutic problem. In many countries disease-modifying treatment is offered to those patients with an initial demyelinating episode, and an abnormal MRI scan suggesting a high probability (about 60%) of conversion to MS. Although there is some evidence that disease-modifying treatment may delay conversion to clinically definite MS, it is unknown whether such treatments prevent or delay long-term disability. If the initial MRI is normal, the likelihood of developing MS is about 20%, and a repeat MRI should be obtained between 3 and 6 months.

Symptomatic treatment

An overview of the types of symptomatic treatment that are relevant in MS is shown in Table 33.3.

OTHER CENTRAL DEMYELINATING DISEASES

A number of other rarer diseases can cause demyelination within the CNS, but their presentation is very different from MS. These include:

- Acute disseminated encephalomyelitis: this monophasic syndrome presents following a viral illness or vaccination. It is fatal in as many as 30% of cases. The areas of white matter change can occur simultaneously in several parts of the CNS

Table 33.2 The 2017 McDonald criteria for diagnosis of multiple sclerosis in patients with an attack at onset or in patients with a disease course characterized by progression from onset (primary progressive multiple sclerosis).

		Number of lesions with objective clinical evidence	Additional data needed for a diagnosis of multiple sclerosis
Attack at onset	≥2 clinical attacks	≥2	None*
	≥2 clinical attacks	1 (as well as clear-cut historical evidence of a previous attack involving a lesion in a distinct anatomical location†)	None*
	≥2 clinical attacks	1	Dissemination in space demonstrated by an additional clinical attack implicating a different CNS site or by MRI‡
	1 clinical attack	≥2	Dissemination in time demonstrated by an additional clinical attack or by MRI§ OR demonstration of CSF-specific oligoclonal bands¶
	1 clinical attack	1	Dissemination in space demonstrated by an additional clinical attack implicating a different CNS site or by MRI‡ AND Dissemination in time demonstrated by an additional clinical attack or by MRI§ OR demonstration of CSF-specific oligoclonal bands¶
Progression from onset (primary progressive multiple sclerosis)	Primary progressive multiple sclerosis can be diagnosed in patients with: 1 year of disability progression (retrospectively or prospectively determined) independent of clinical relapse Plus two of the following criteria: • One or more T2-hyperintense lesions characteristic of multiple sclerosis in one or more of the following brain regions: periventricular, cortical or juxtacortical, or infratentorial. Unlike the 2010 McDonald criteria, no distinction between symptomatic and asymptomatic MRI lesions is required. • Two or more T2-hyperintense lesions in the spinal cord • Presence of CSF-specific oligoclonal bands		

If the 2017 McDonald Criteria are fulfilled and there is no better explanation for the clinical presentation, the diagnosis is multiple sclerosis. If multiple sclerosis is suspected by virtue of a clinically isolated syndrome but the 2017 McDonald Criteria are not completely met, the diagnosis is possible multiple sclerosis. If another diagnosis arises during the evaluation that better explains the clinical presentation, the diagnosis is not multiple sclerosis.
*No additional tests are required to demonstrate dissemination in space and time. However, unless MRI is not possible, brain MRI should be obtained in all patients in whom the diagnosis of multiple sclerosis is being considered. In addition, spinal cord MRI or CSF examination should be considered in patients with insufficient clinical and MRI evidence supporting multiple sclerosis, with a presentation other than a typical clinically isolated syndrome, or with atypical features. If imaging or other tests (e.g., CSF) are undertaken and are negative, caution needs to be taken before making a diagnosis of multiple sclerosis, and alternative diagnoses should be considered.
†Clinical diagnosis based on objective clinical findings for two attacks is most secure. Reasonable historical evidence for one past attack, in the absence of documented objective neurological findings, can include historical events with symptoms and evolution characteristic for a previous inflammatory demyelinating attack; at least one attack, however, must be supported by objective findings. In the absence of residual objective evidence, caution is needed.
‡The MRI criteria for dissemination in space: Dissemination in space can be demonstrated by one or more T2-hyperintense lesions that are characteristic of multiple sclerosis in two or more of four areas of the CNS: periventricular, cortical or juxtacortical, and infratentorial brain regions, and the spinal cord. Unlike the 2010 McDonald criteria, no distinction between symptomatic and asymptomatic MRI lesions is required. For some patients—e.g., individuals older than 50 years or those with vascular risk factors—it might be prudent for the clinician to seek a higher number of periventricular lesions.
§The MRI criteria for dissemination in time: Dissemination in time can be demonstrated by the simultaneous presence of gadolinium-enhancing and non-enhancing lesions at any time or by a new T2-hyperintense or gadolinium-enhancing lesion on follow-up MRI, with reference to a baseline scan, irrespective of the timing of the baseline MRI.
¶The presence of CSF-specific oligoclonal bands does not demonstrate dissemination in time per se but can substitute for the requirement for demonstration of this measure.
Taken from Thompson et al. Diagnosis of multiple sclerosis: 2017 revisions of the McDonald criteria, Lancet Neurology 2018 Feb;17(2):162-173.

and are often confluent and more symmetrical than in MS. Patients may also have other features that are unusual for MS, including fever, encephalopathy and seizures. Despite these features, this condition can be difficult to distinguish from an initial presentation of MS. Treatment is with steroids.

- PML: caused by JC papovavirus infection, especially in immunocompromised patients (e.g., 4% of patients with HIV).
- Neuromyelitis optica: a relapsing, autoimmune condition in which patients present with a demyelinating optic neuritis

Table 33.3 Symptomatic treatment in multiple sclerosis

Symptom	Treatment
Cognitive dysfunction	Disease-modifying treatment Cognitive rehabilitation techniques
Depression	Psychotherapy and/or pharmacotherapy
Pain	Mechanical pain – nonsteroidal antiinflammatory drugs, transcutaneous electrical stimulation (TENS), physiotherapy Neurogenic pain – anticonvulsants (e.g., gabapentin, pregabalin, carbamazepine, amitriptyline), antidepressants (e.g., amitriptyline), TENS
Ataxia and tremor	Physiotherapy and occupational therapy Medications – clonazepam, propranolol, isoniazid
Fatigue	Treatment of any underlying depression or nocturia Physiotherapy – graded exercise programmes Medications – amantadine or modafinil
Bladder dysfunction	Detrusor hyperreflexia causing urinary frequency and urgency – anticholinergics (e.g., oxybutynin, intravesical botulinum toxin) Detrusor-sphincter dyssynergia causing retention – intermittent self-catheterization Nocturia – antidiuretic hormone analogue DDAVP (desmopressin)
Spasticity	Physiotherapy Medications – baclofen, tizanidine, dantrolene (care must be taken not to reduce tone too far as it may exacerbate weakness)
Paroxysmal symptoms	Examples are muscle spasms, burning dysaesthetic pains, trigeminal neuralgia and other brief brainstem symptoms – best treated with sodium channel blockers such as carbamazepine

and myelitis either simultaneously or with an interval between them. Patients are typically positive for antibodies to aquaporin 4 or myelin oligodendrocyte glycoprotein (MOG). Treatment requires prolonged courses of steroids and immunomodulation (see Chapter 24).

- Leucodystrophies: metachromatic leucodystrophy (disorder of arylsulphatase A), adrenoleucodystrophy (accumulation of very-long-chain fatty acids).

- Vitamin B_{12} deficiency: can cause central demyelination.
- Central pontine myelinolysis: this is associated with too rapid a correction of sodium in patients who are hyponatraemic and often have a history of alcohol abuse. Demyelination occurs within the pons and the clinical presentation can vary from no symptoms to ataxia to a profound tetraplegia and pseudobulbar palsy.

● Chapter Summary

- Multiple sclerosis affects 150 per 100,000 people in the United Kingdom. The main mode of nerve damage in MS is demyelination and inflammation.
- The key CNS regions affected by MS are corpus callosum, periventricular, brainstem and spinal cord.
- Management of acute relapses (such as optic neuritis, pyramidal weakness) is with corticosteroids. Disease-modifying agents can be used if patients fulfil criteria and can reduce yearly relapses by up to 60%.

UKMLA Condition
Multiple sclerosis

UKMLA Presentations
Acute and chronic pain management
Acute change in or loss of vision
Facial weakness
Limb weakness
Speech and language problems
Urinary symptoms
Vertigo

The effects of vitamin deficiencies and toxins on the nervous system

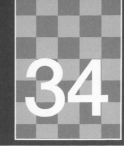

34

VITAMIN DEFICIENCIES

Nutritional deficiencies are particularly common in developing countries, but do occur in developed countries due to poor eating habits, alcoholism and malabsorption syndromes. The most common conditions are described in the following sections.

Vitamin B$_1$ (thiamine) deficiency

Deficiency of vitamin B$_1$ causes beriberi or Wernicke–Korsakoff syndrome.

Beriberi

Beriberi is caused by a staple diet of polished rice and results in either a polyneuropathy (dry beriberi) or marked generalized oedema with ascites and pleural effusions (wet beriberi).

Wernicke–Korsakoff syndrome

Wernicke–Korsakoff syndrome is more common in the Western world than beriberi and is caused primarily by chronic alcoholism with poor dietary intake of thiamine. The syndrome is composed of an acute phase (Wernicke encephalopathy) and a chronic phase (Korsakoff psychosis). The typical triad of Wernicke encephalopathy comprises:

- Ocular signs: with nystagmus and ophthalmoplegia.
- Ataxia: with a broad-based gait and cerebellar signs in the limbs, especially the legs.
- Confusion: with disorientation, apathy, agitation, amnesia, stupor and coma.

In over 80% of cases, there may also be signs of a peripheral neuropathy. In chronic cases, a slower amnestic syndrome develops, with selective impairment of short-term memory, which is made up for by confabulation (Korsakoff psychosis). The pathology of Wernicke–Korsakoff syndrome involves symmetrical damage to the mamillary bodies, thalamus, periaqueductal grey matter and cerebellum.

Treatment for Wernicke encephalopathy is intravenous thiamine followed by instigation of a normal diet and continued oral thiamine. Korsakoff psychosis is also treated with oral thiamine and a normal diet, but patients are often left with a severe cognitive deficit.

HINTS AND TIPS

In thiamine deficiency, glucose is inadequately metabolized and lactate and pyruvate accumulate. It is therefore essential to give thiamine immediately to any patient with suspected thiamine deficiency, before giving any sugar-containing substance, especially 5% dextrose or dextrose saline.

Vitamin B$_6$ (pyridoxine) deficiency

Vitamin B$_6$ deficiency causes a mainly sensory neuropathy and may be precipitated during isoniazid therapy for tuberculosis. Pyridoxine supplements should, therefore, be given when isoniazid is prescribed.

Vitamin B$_{12}$ deficiency

Deficiency of vitamin B$_{12}$ (cobalamin) can, rarely, result from nutritional deficiency (e.g., vegans) but is more often caused by malabsorption. The usual causes are pernicious anaemia, gastrectomy and diseases of the terminal ileum (e.g., Crohn disease, coeliac disease, Whipple disease, blind-loop syndrome). Up to 25% of patients with neurological damage caused by vitamin B$_{12}$ deficiency do not have haematological abnormalities (i.e., macrocytic megaloblastic anaemia). It can also be caused by inhalation of the recreational drug nitrous oxide.

Vitamin B$_{12}$ deficiency should be considered in any patient with a peripheral sensory neuropathy, myelopathy, optic neuropathy or dementia. The earliest symptom a patient may complain of is pins and needles in the feet, before signs of a myelopathy and impaired vibration and joint position sense due to dorsal column loss develop. The combination of a myelopathy and a peripheral sensory neuropathy is called 'subacute combined degeneration of the cord'.

Treatment with intramuscular vitamin B$_{12}$ must be started promptly. If treatment is initiated early, there can be complete recovery; if delayed, the progression may be halted, but there is little reversal. The condition can theoretically be made worse by giving folic acid without vitamin B_{12}.

Vitamin B_3 (nicotinic acid) deficiency

Nicotinic acid deficiency causes pellagra and is found in areas where the staple diet is maize. It is also found in chronic alcoholics who present with acute delirium. The classical clinical features comprise dermatitis, diarrhoea and dementia. More widespread neurological features include pyramidal and extrapyramidal signs and a peripheral neuropathy.

Vitamin D deficiency

This is associated with a proximal myopathy with wasting and weakness. It is most commonly seen in the elderly with poor diet and lack of sun exposure. It is also seen in immigrant populations, malabsorption syndromes, those treated with anticonvulsants and in chronic renal failure.

Vitamin E deficiency

Vitamin E is a fat-soluble vitamin that can become deficient in malabsorption syndromes, especially in cystic fibrosis, coeliac disease and diseases in which there is a reduced bile salt pool. There is a rare familial fat malabsorption syndrome with abetalipoproteinaemia associated with vitamin E deficiency.

Vitamin E deficiency primarily causes an ataxic syndrome, with areflexia and loss of vibration sense and proprioception, but with sparing of cutaneous sensation. It can mimic Friedreich ataxia. Treatment is with oral vitamin E.

TOXINS

There are numerous toxins capable of causing neurological symptoms, many of which are drugs prescribed for other medical conditions. The most common ones are listed in Table 34.1.

Table 34.1 Toxins and their neurological effects

Neurological complication	Toxin
Dementia	Alcohol, heroin use, carbon monoxide
Acute or subacute encephalopathy	Lead, mercury, manganese, thallium, solvent abuse, arsenic, tin
Drug-induced confusional state or psychosis	Antiparkinsonian drugs, steroids, isoniazid, alcohol withdrawal, lithium, amphetamines, cannabis, lysergic acid diethylamide
Lowered threshold of seizures	Alcohol, amphetamines, neuroleptics, tricyclics
Parkinsonism	Neuroleptics, antiemetics, reserpine, amiodarone
Chorea and/or dystonia	l-3,4-Dihydroxyphenylalanine, dopamine agonists, antiemetics, neuroleptics, trihexyphenidyl, manganese
Tremor	β2 agonists, lithium, sodium valproate, amiodarone, amphetamines, alcohol, levothyroxine
Cerebellar syndrome	Alcohol, phenytoin, mercury, carbamazepine
Ototoxicity	Aminoglycoside antibiotics, quinine, furosemide, overdose of aspirin
Optic neuropathy	Ethambutol, chloroquine, methyl alcohol, chloramphenicol, possibly pipe tobacco
Lens opacities	Steroids, chloroquine, amiodarone
Myelopathy	Nitrous oxide abuse, lathyrism (plant toxins)
Peripheral neuropathy	Gold, lead (motor), alcohol, organophosphates, medications including isoniazid, nitrofurantoin, vincristine, metronidazole, dapsone, sulphonamides, phenytoin, pyridoxine, cisplatin, amiodarone, tricyclics
Neuromuscular blockade	Botulinum toxin, organophosphate compounds, 'nerve gases', penicillamine, aminoglycosides (and other antibiotics) may exacerbate myasthenia
Myopathy	Alcohol, steroids, chloroquine, statins, zidovudine (azidothymidine)

Chapter Summary

- Thiamine (B_1) deficiency can cause neurological syndromes: beriberi that presents as a polyneuropathy and Wernicke–Korsakoff syndrome that presents as confusion, ophthalmoparesis and/or ataxia. B_{12} deficiency can present as both a myelopathy and a peripheral neuropathy.
- The full range of neurological symptoms can be caused by drugs, from antipsychotic medication associated with parkinsonism, alcohol with ataxia, nitrofurantoin with peripheral neuropathy and statins with myopathy.

UKMLA Conditions
Dementias
Wernicke encephalopathy

UKMLA Presentations
Abnormal involuntary movements
Altered sensation, numbness and tingling
Confusion
Diplopia
Fits/seizures
Tremor
Unsteadiness

Autoimmune conditions affecting the nervous system

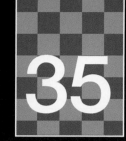

INTRODUCTION

Our understanding of neuroimmunology has increased dramatically in the last two decades and has resulted in the identification of a number of novel antibodies that target all parts of the nervous system. We will concentrate on conditions caused by centrally acting antibodies as they are the most commonly encountered in the clinical setting. The wide range of antibodies that are now known, and any associated malignancies, are given in Table 35.1.

ANTIBODY-MEDIATED ENCEPHALITIS

Limbic encephalitis

This condition caused by antibodies targeting the limbic system was first described in 1960. It usually occurs in later life and patients present with an encephalitis-like picture over weeks; features include loss of short-term memory, seizures and psychosis. Limbic encephalitis is commonly associated

Table 35.1 Paraneoplastic antibodies and associated tumours

Antibody	Syndrome	Most common associated cancer
Well-characterized paraneoplastic antibodies		
Anti-Hu (ANNA-1)	Encephalomyelitis (including cortical, limbic, brainstem encephalitis), cerebellar degeneration, myelitis, sensory neuronopathy and/or autonomic dysfunction	SCLC
Anti-Yo (PCA-1)	Cerebellar degeneration	Gynaecological, breast
Anti-Ri (ANNA-2)	Cerebellar degeneration, brainstem encephalitis, opsoclonus–myoclonus	Breast, gynaecological, SCLC
Anti-Tr	Cerebellar degeneration	Hodgkin lymphoma
Anti-CV2/CRMP5	Encephalomyelitis, cerebellar degeneration, chorea, peripheral neuropathy, sensory neuronopathy	SCLC, thymoma
Anti-Ma proteins	Limbic, hypothalamic, brainstem encephalitis, cerebellar degeneration	Germ cell tumours of the testis, lung cancer
Anti-amphiphysin	Stiff-person syndrome, encephalomyelitis	Breast, lung cancer
Anti-SOX1	Lambert–Eaton myasthenic syndrome, rapidly progressive cerebellar syndrome	SCLC
Anti PCA-2 (MAP1B)	Sensorimotor neuropathy, rapidly progressive cerebellar syndrome, encephalomyelitis	SCLC, NSCLC, breast cancer
Anti-KLHL11	Brainstem/cerebellar syndrome	Testicular
Antibodies that can occur with or without cancer		
Anti-AChR	Myasthenia gravis	Thymoma
Anti-VGCC	Lambert–Eaton myasthenic syndrome, cerebellar dysfunction	SCLC
Anti-NMDAR	Multistage syndrome with memory and behavioural disturbances, psychosis, seizures, dyskinesias and autonomic dysfunction	Teratoma
Anti-AMPAR	Limbic encephalitis, psychiatric disturbances	Miscellaneous solid tumours

Continued

Table 35.1 Paraneoplastic antibodies and associated tumours—cont'd

Antibody	Syndrome	Most common associated cancer
Anti-GABA	Seizures, limbic encephalitis	SCLC
Anti-VGKC	Limbic encephalitis and seizures (anti-LGI1), Morvan syndrome (anti-CASPR2)	Thymoma, SCLC, miscellaneous solid tumours
Anti-GlyR	Encephalomyelitis with muscle spasms, rigidity, myoclonus	Often no associated cancer
Anti-mGluR5	Encephalitis	Hodgkin lymphoma
Anti-GFAP	Meningoencephalitis	Gynaecological, adenocarcinomas
Anti-GAD65	Limbic encephalitis, stiff-person syndrome, cerebellar ataxia	SCLC, neuroendocrine tumors, thymoma
Anti-DPPX	Encephalitis with CNS hyperexcitability, progressive encephalomyelitis with rigidity and myoclonus	B cell neoplasms
Anti-AQP4	Neuromyelitis optica spectrum disorder	Adenocarcinomas
Anti-MOG	MOG antibody-associated disease	Gynaecological (rare)

AChR, *Acetylcholine receptor;* AMPAR, *α-amino-3-hydroxy-5-methyl-4-isoxazolepropionic acid receptor;* ANNA, *antineuronal-nuclear antibody;* AQP4, *aquaporin 4;* CASPR2, *contactin-associated protein-like 2;* CRMP5, *collapsing response-mediator protein;* DPPX, *dipeptidyl-peptidase-like protein;* GABA, *γ-aminobutyric acid;* GAD, *glutamic acid decarboxylase;* GFAP, *glial fibrillary acidic protein;* GlyR, *glycine receptor;* KLHL11, *Kelch-like protein 11;* LGI1, *leucine-rich glioma inactivated protein 1;* MAP1B, *microtubule-associated protein;* mGluR5, *metabotropic glutamate receptor 5;* MOG, *myelin oligodendrocyte glycoprotein 5;* NMDAR, *N-methyl D-aspartate receptor;* PCA, *Purkinje cell antibody;* SCLC, *small-cell lung cancer;* SOX1, *SRY-box transcription factor 1;* VGCC, *voltage-gated calcium channel antibody;* VGKC, *voltage-gated potassium channel antibody.*

with systemic malignancy (paraneoplastic) and often can predate the symptoms directly caused by the malignancy. Small-cell lung cancer is the most common associated tumour (Table 35.1).

Management ultimately involves treatment of the underlying malignancy, although immunosuppression such as intravenous immunoglobulin or plasma exchange can be offered to suppress the neurological symptoms.

Nonparaneoplastic limbic encephalitis

More recently cases have been identified with identical clinical features to paraneoplastic limbic encephalitis but without any underlying malignancy detected. In this group new associated antibodies have been identified in the serum such as voltage-gated potassium channel antibodies (VGKC), α-amino-3-hydroxy-5-methyl-4-isoxazolepropionic acid (AMPA) receptor antibodies (AMPAR) and γ-aminobutyric acid (GABA) receptor antibodies (GABAR). Immunosuppression as treatment in this context is more successful than in paraneoplastic limbic encephalitis.

Anti-NMDA receptor encephalitis

This condition is now increasingly recognized and the second most prevalent form of immune-mediated encephalitis after acute disseminated encephalitis and encephalomyelitis. It typically affects young women and has a characteristic clinical progression, starting with a fever prodrome, then psychiatric disturbance, then dyskinesias (usually face) and seizures and finally autonomic disturbance and encephalopathy, which usually requires intensive care support.

Anti-N-methyl D-aspartate (anti-NMDA) antibodies can be found in serum and cerebrospinal fluid. Importantly this condition is associated with malignancy, usually ovarian teratoma, which should be investigated for. Removal of the tumour dramatically improves rate of recovery in conjunction with immunosuppression such as plasma exchange. However, despite treatment, anti-NMDA receptor encephalitis is fatal in 5% of cases.

ANTIBODIES TARGETING THE PERIPHERAL NERVOUS SYSTEM

We have already discussed how neuronal-specific antibodies can affect normal function of the neuromuscular junction in conditions such as myasthenia gravis (see Chapter 28) and peripheral nerve in conditions such as acute motor axonal neuropathy, multifocal motor neuropathy (associated with anti-GM1 antibodies) and Miller–Fisher syndrome (associated with anti-GQ1B antibodies; see Chapter 27).

ANTIBODIES TARGETING MUSCLE

Idiopathic inflammatory myopathies can be associated with the presence of anti-Jo1 antibodies (found in about 20% patients with polymyositis and less commonly in dermatomyositis; see Chapter 29). Moreover, the likelihood of interstitial lung disease as part of the condition is increased with the presence of anti-Jo1. Immune-mediated necrotizing myopathy is a more severe form of idiopathic inflammatory myopathy that can be associated with the presence of anti-SRP (anti–signal recognition particle) antibodies and usually refractive to immunosuppressive therapy.

Myopathy may also be a feature of autoimmune connective tissue disorders such as Sjögren syndrome (associated with anti-Ro/La antibodies) and rheumatoid arthritis.

● Chapter Summary

- Limbic encephalitis is commonly associated with systemic malignancy (paraneoplastic) and often can directly predate the symptoms caused by the malignancy. Small-cell lung cancer is the most common associated tumour.
- Anti-NMDA (anti-N-methyl D-aspartate) receptor encephalitis has a characteristic clinical progression, starting with a fever, then psychiatric disturbance, then dyskinesias and seizures and finally autonomic disturbance and encephalopathy, which usually requires intensive care support.
- Idiopathic inflammatory myopathies (polymyositis and dermatomyositis) can be associated with the presence of anti-Jo1 antibodies.

UKMLA Conditions
Encephalitis
Myasthenia gravis

UKMLA Presentations
Behaviour/personality change
Confusion
Fits/seizures
Memory loss

Hereditary conditions affecting the nervous system 36

The genetic basis of neurological disease has been revolutionized by two methods of identifying disease genes. The first method is relevant in families where disease is inherited in a 'Mendelian' manner (such as autosomal dominant, autosomal recessive or X-linked). The second method, genome-wide association studies, uses hundreds and thousands of patients with the same disease to map the disease-causing mutation in human genes. As our understanding of the molecular pathophysiological consequences of these variants increases, genetic profiling will become readily available both as a diagnostic tool and in tailoring treatments for inherited conditions.

HINTS AND TIPS

The number of currently known inherited conditions affecting the nervous system has exponentially grown with advances in genetic techniques. Table 36.1 provides a nonexhaustive list of inherited diseases associated with topics covered in the book.

THE NEUROCUTANEOUS SYNDROMES

A number of inherited conditions involve disorders of organs derived from the ectoderm, causing tumours (benign and malignant), hamartomas (disorganized collections of blood vessels) and lesions in the skin and nervous system. Only the most common are outlined in the following subsections.

Neurofibromatosis

There are a number of different types of neurofibromatosis, but types 1 (peripheral predominance) and 2 (central predominance) are the most important.

Neurofibromatosis type 1 (von Recklinghausen disease)

Neurofibromatosis type 1 is an autosomal dominant condition caused by mutations in the neurofibromin gene (NF1) on chromosome 17. This gene encodes a protein called 'neurofibromin'.

Table 36.1 Rare mutations associated with common neurological presentations

Clinical feature	Condition	Genes associated
Headache	Familial hemiplegic migraine	FHM1 – voltage-gated calcium channel CACNA1A FHM2 – Na/K ATPase ATP1A2
Epilepsy	Benign familial neonatal convulsions Dravet syndrome	Voltage-gated potassium channel KCNQ2 Voltage-gated sodium channel SCN1A
Dementia	Alzheimer's disease	Presenilin 1 and 2 (PS1/PS2) Amyloid precursor protein (APP)
Movement disorders	Parkinson's disease	Parkin, LRRK2, PINK1
Motor system – myelopathy	Hereditary spastic paraparesis	SPG4 (spastin) SPG7 (paraplegin)
	Motor neuron disease	Superoxide dismutase (SOD), (C9orf72) associated with dementia
Peripheral nerve	Charcot–Marie–Tooth	Peripheral myelin protein 22 (PMP22) Myelin protein zero (MPZ)
	Distal hereditary motor neuropathy	Heat-shock protein (HSPB1I)
Neuromuscular junction	Congenital myasthenia gravis	(CHRNE) Postsynaptic Ach receptors (RAPSN) Rapsyn
Muscle	Duchenne/Becker muscular dystrophy	Dystrophin gene
Vascular diseases	Cerebral autosomal dominant arteriopathy with subcortical infarcts and leucoencephalopathy	Notch3 gene

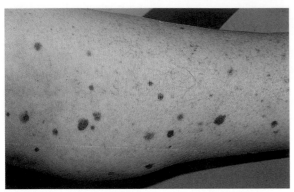

Fig. 36.1 Cutaneous manifestations of neurofibromatosis type 1. (From Gawkrodger DJ, Ardern-Jones MR. Neurocutaneous disorders and other syndromes. In: *Dermatology: An Illustrated Colour Text*. 6th ed. Amsterdam: Elsevier; 2017.)

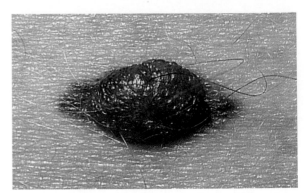

Fig. 36.2 Adenoma sebaceum: classic raised reddish nodules found over the nose and cheeks in tuberous sclerosis. (From Gawkrodger DJ, Ardern-Jones MR. Neurocutaneous disorders and other syndromes. In: *Dermatology: An Illustrated Colour Text*. 6th ed. Amsterdam: Elsevier; 2017.)

The mutation has an incidence of 1 in 4000. Clinically, it is characterized (Fig. 36.1) by:

- Neurofibromata: lying along peripheral nerves.
- Café-au-lait spots: multiple pale-brown macules, especially on the trunk – they are found in the normal population, but more than five lesions of over 1.5 cm in an adult is abnormal.
- Cutaneous fibromata (molluscum fibrosum): subcutaneous, soft, often pedunculated and usually multiple.
- Axillary freckling.
- Lisch nodules: small hamartomas of the iris.
- Other associated features include:
  - Neural tumours: there is a higher incidence of neural tumours than in the general population (e.g., meningioma, vestibular schwannomas on the eighth nerve, gliomas and spinal root neurofibroma).
  - Skeletal abnormalities: 50% of patients have a scoliosis.
  - Endocrine abnormalities: associated phaeochromocytoma, medullary carcinoma of the thyroid.
  - Learning difficulty and epilepsy: in 10% to 15% of patients.
  - Renal artery stenosis.
  - Obstructive cardiomyopathy.
  - Pulmonary fibrosis.

Neurofibromatosis type 2

Neurofibromatosis type 2 is an autosomal dominant condition caused by mutations in the *NF2* gene on chromosome 22. This gene encodes a protein called 'merlin'. The mutation has an incidence of 1 in 50,000. Clinically, it is characterized by few skin and skeletal manifestations and the presence of bilateral eighth nerve vestibular schwannomas (previously referred to as 'acoustic neuromas'). Other intracranial and intraspinal tumours may be present and include brain and spine meningiomas, ependymomas and astrocytomas.

Treatment

Intracranial tumours require excision and, if necessary, radiotherapy. Cosmetic surgery may be required for the cutaneous manifestations. Genetic counselling is important.

> **HINTS AND TIPS**
>
> Genetic diagnoses have major implications for patients and their families. Genetic counselling is therefore a critical part of any consultation. This should include a discussion of the clinical features of the disease, prognosis, treatment options, mode of inheritance and consequences for other family members. Further pretest counselling may also be needed to assess a patient's understanding of the impact of a diagnosis on themselves, their employment, insurance policies and relationships and assess their support structures. Informed consent is mandatory for all genetic testing.

Tuberous sclerosis

Tuberous sclerosis is an autosomal dominant condition with an incidence of 1 in 10,000. It is caused by either the *TSC1* or *TSC2* genes, which encode for the proteins hamartin and tuberin, respectively.

The condition is characterized by:

- Skin lesions including facial angiofibromata (previously called 'adenoma sebaceum'; Fig. 36.2), depigmented patches

If epilepsy is sufficiently intractable, lobectomy or even hemispherectomy may be required.

HEREDITARY ATAXIAS

There are a large number of inherited conditions accompanied by varying clinical features of cerebellar degeneration, either alone or in combination with spinal degeneration, and these are referred to as the 'hereditary ataxias'. Three of the more common conditions are outlined in the following subsections, but they are all rare.

Friedreich ataxia

Friedreich ataxia is an autosomal recessive condition caused by an expanded trinucleotide repeat (GAA) in the frataxin gene on chromosome 9. The severity of the disease phenotype depends on the number of trinucleotide repeats. Frataxin is especially found in the spinal cord, heart and pancreas and not in the cerebellum or cerebrum.

Within the spinal cord there is progressive degeneration of the posterior columns, corticospinal tracts and dorsal and ventral spinocerebellar tracts. Clinical features include:

- Ataxia: spreading from distal legs.
- Dysarthria.
- Sensory neuropathy: absent ankle jerks, absent joint position and vibration sense.
- Pyramidal signs: upgoing plantar responses (despite absent ankle jerks).
- Optic atrophy.
- Skeletal abnormalities: pes cavus and scoliosis.
- Cardiomyopathy and associated arrhythmias.
- Diabetes.

Patients often die from the cardiac complications (heart failure and arrhythmias) rather than from the neurological complications.

Ataxia telangiectasia

Ataxia telangiectasia is an autosomal recessive disorder causing progressive cerebellar ataxia, ocular and cutaneous telangiectasia and immunoglobulin A (IgA) immunodeficiency. Death is often by the third decade from infection or lymphoreticular malignancy.

Spinocerebellar ataxias

The predominant symptom of the spinocerebellar ataxias (SCAs) is one of progressive cerebellar ataxia inherited often in an autosomal dominant manner. The SCAs may present as a

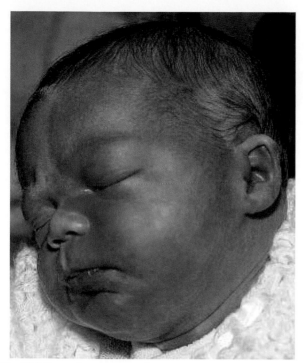

Fig. 36.3 Port-wine naevus in Sturge–Weber syndrome. (From Baselga E. Vascular malformations. In: Bolognia J, Jorizzo J, Schaffer J, eds. *Dermatology*. 4th ed. Elsevier; 2018.)

(ash-leaf macule), 'shagreen' patches and subungual fibromata around the finger and toe nails.
- Epilepsy and varying degrees of learning disability. Slowly expanding cerebral tumours, such as hamartomatous 'tubers' and astrocytomas, can also occur and provoke seizures.
- Tuberous sclerosis also increases the susceptibility to systemic tumours that may affect the kidney, lung or muscle.

Treatment

The epilepsy is often resistant to treatment. Surgery may be required for large cerebral tumours, especially if hydrocephalus develops. Careful regular evaluation and follow-up of these patients must be made to provide a possibility of early treatment for the neoplastic complications.

Sturge–Weber syndrome

Sturge–Weber syndrome has no clear inheritance pattern. It is characterized by an extensive port-wine naevus or 'stain' on one side of the face (Fig. 36.3), usually within the first and second divisions of the trigeminal nerve, and an underlying leptomeningeal angioma. There may be atrophy of the affected hemisphere, epilepsy and congenital glaucoma.

pure ataxia (such as SCA6) or be associated with a wide range of signs, including a degenerative retinopathy (SCA7), spasticity, parkinsonism (SCA3) and a peripheral neuropathy.

INBORN ERRORS OF METABOLISM

Numerous rare metabolic conditions can cause abnormalities of both the central and peripheral nervous system. Two of the more common examples of these will be discussed briefly.

Acute intermittent porphyria

The porphyrias comprise a heterogeneous group of disorders of haem synthesis, causing an overproduction of porphyrins. Acute intermittent porphyria, an autosomal dominant disorder occurring in adult life, is often associated with neurological complications. It can be precipitated by medications, sepsis or alcohol.

Clinical features and their frequency are as follows:

- Abdominal pain: 90%; these patients are often admitted with unexplained abdominal pain.
- Peripheral neuropathy: 70%; usually an acute motor neuropathy that can present like Guillain–Barré syndrome.
- Hypertension and a sinus tachycardia: 70%.
- Psychiatric disturbance such as mania and depression: 50%.
- Seizures: 15%.

To secure the diagnosis, the urine is screened for porphobilinogen levels. However, testing the blood for reduced erythrocyte porphobilinogen deaminase and raised aminolaevulinic acid synthetase is most sensitive.

Management is largely supportive, with a high carbohydrate intake and a haematin infusion. Any medication that precipitates this condition should be avoided.

Wilson disease (hepatolenticular degeneration)

Wilson disease is a rare autosomal recessive disorder of copper metabolism. There is a deficiency of caeruloplasmin protein, which binds copper, resulting in copper deposition in various organs, especially in the liver and the basal ganglia in the brain. It is caused by mutations in the *ATP7B* gene, and clinical features comprise:

- Movement disorders: a wide range of movements can occur, including tremor, early dysarthria and dysphagia, dystonia, parkinsonism and chorea.
- Cirrhosis of the liver.
- Kayser–Fleischer ring: a fine brown deposition of copper in Descemet membrane of the cornea, which may ultimately form a ring. This may be visible to the naked eye, but slit-lamp examination is usually necessary.
- Neuropsychiatric features such as depression, mania and psychosis.

Diagnosis is by measurement of a low serum caeruloplasmin and total serum copper, with elevated unbound or 'free' copper. There is high urinary copper excretion and liver biopsy may show massive copper deposition. Treatment involves a lifelong low-copper diet and a chelating agent such as penicillamine. Liver transplantation is sometimes performed.

● Chapter Summary

- Neurofibromatosis types 1 and 2 and tuberous sclerosis fall into a group called 'inherited neurocutaneous disorders'. All three have distinct presentations; *NF1* is associated with cutaneous fibromata and café-au-lait spots, *NF2* is associated with bilateral vestibular schwannomas and *TS* is associated with facial angiofibromata and hamartomatous 'tubers' in the brain.
- Friedrich ataxia is an autosomal recessive inherited condition that affects corticospinal and dorsal column tracts, resulting in pyramidal weakness and sensory neuropathy in addition to the ataxia.
- The porphyrias comprise a heterogeneous group of disorders that cause an overproduction of porphyrins. Clinical features include a peripheral neuropathy, abdominal pain and organic psychosis.

UKMLA Conditions
Dementias
Epilepsy
Motor neurone disease
Parkinson's disease

UKMLA Presentations
Abnormal involuntary movements
Fits/seizures
Unsteadiness

Functional neurological disorders

Functional disorders are common in neurology. There are different terms that are used to describe functional disorders, and whichever term the patient and/or doctor feel comfortable with can be used. Functional suggests a change in the function of, rather than the structure of the nervous system. Dissociation refers to the feeling of disconnect from one's own body (depersonalization) and disconnect from one's environment (derealization) that some patients experience. Non-organic refers to the symptom not being caused by an organic neurological pathology, such as a stroke or multiple sclerosis. Other terms such as psychosomatic, psychogenic, conversion disorder and medically unexplained tend to not be used as frequently. It is important to note that organic and functional disorders can coexist in a patient, and functional overlay is also common, where an organic neurological pathology is exacerbated by a functional neurological disorder.

Other conditions which do not fall under the umbrella of functional disorders are hypochondriasis which is excessive and intrusive health anxiety, factitious disorder which is the fabrication of symptoms to obtain medical care, Munchausen syndrome, where a patient with factitious disorder visits different healthcare providers changing their story, and malingering, which is the fabrication of symptoms to obtain a material gain.

This chapter will focus on the more frequent types of functional disorders seen in neurology.

DISSOCIATIVE/NONEPILEPTIC ATTACKS/SEIZURES

These are common and can also be referred to as pseudoseizures. They can happen in patients with epilepsy, with organic seizures and dissociative seizures happening on different occasions in the same patient. In young patients with dissociative seizures, these are more common in women than men. In middle-aged and older patients, men and women are affected more equally. In comparison to organic seizures, dissociative seizures are longer (>5 minutes), have a gradual rather than a sudden onset, and a fluctuating course. A patient having a dissociative seizure may resist eye opening and have more asynchronous, thrashing movements. Observations during the dissociative seizure including oxygen saturations, blood pressure and heart rate may be unchanged, but breath holding during a dissociative event can lead to a reduction in oxygen saturations. Useful investigations are a video electroencephalography (EEG) during a typical dissociative seizure, which does not show epileptiform activity or the semiology of an organic seizure. It is helpful to ask if the patient is happy for a friend or relative to video any events which happen outside of the hospital setting, so that these can be reviewed in clinic for the aforementioned clinical features.

FUNCTIONAL WEAKNESS

This is a common symptom and can come on suddenly after an injury, or more gradually after pain or fatigue. To help diagnose functional weakness, observe the patient for any inconsistencies, such as weakness while performing the formal neurological examination, but then improving when distracted or performing a different task. There can be a give-way quality to the weakness, and encouraging the patient leads to improvement of the weakness. A further test is Hoover's sign (Fig. 37.1). When the patient is asked to extend the right hip, this appears weak, but upon flexing the left hip, the right hip extends, which is a normal physiological response. It can be useful to demonstrate this sign to the patient, to show that the weakness improves when they are distracted. This establishes that there is no structural issue with the nervous system causing the leg to be weak, and can be an encouraging sign for the patient. Hoover's sign can be falsely positive in patients with significant limb pain or neglect. With functional facial weakness, the patient may have overcontraction of orbicularis oculi and platysma.

FUNCTIONAL TREMOR

Functional tremors can have a rapid onset and tend to have a variable frequency. They can vary from day to day and can improve when a patient is distracted and asked to perform a different task. They can worsen if the examiner tries to hold the limb still. There is also the phenomenon of entrainment, where if the patient is asked to copy a rhythmic movement with the unaffected side, the tremor entrains to the same frequency as the rhythmic movement being made with the unaffected side.

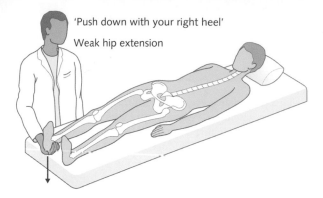

'Push down with your right heel'

Weak hip extension

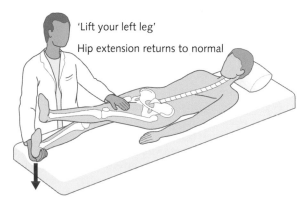

'Lift your left leg'

Hip extension returns to normal

Fig. 37.1 Hoover's sign. (From Innes JA, et al. *Macleod's Clinical Examination.* 14th ed. Elsevier; 2018.)

ASSESSMENT AND MANAGEMENT OF FUNCTIONAL NEUROLOGICAL DISORDERS

It is helpful to ensure the patient feels that they are being listened to and often an explanation of their condition can help greatly with the symptoms. Listing all the symptoms they are experiencing is important. Find out if there are any triggers for their symptoms. It is also important to ask about dissociation, which is feeling disconnected from the world around them and feeling disconnected from their own body. Asking about previous functional conditions is also important. Sensitively ask about symptoms of panic attacks, anxiety and depression. Asking about previous life events or trauma is not useful early in the assessment and can be counterproductive, but this could be discussed further down the line.

Investigations may be needed if it is unclear from the first assessment whether these are functional or organic symptoms; therefore tests such as neuroimaging and EEG can be obtained as necessary. It is important to note that neuroimaging can reveal incidental and unrelated findings to the symptoms reported, and this should be discussed in advance of the imaging with the patient. Video EEG is a very important and useful test for dissociative seizures.

It is vital to note that patients are not making up their symptoms. Being clear with patients regarding this allows them to understand that they are being taken seriously. It is important to explain that they have a functional neurological disorder, which means that the nervous system is structurally normal but is not functioning properly. Explaining that they do not have an organic neurological disorder, and the impact of dissociation on their symptoms can also help. A good explanation of the condition can help greatly with management and recovery. Demonstrating their functional signs to them can also be helpful, such as by showing the patient their positive Hoover's sign to establish that their hip extension improves upon distraction (Fig. 37.1). This also establishes how the diagnosis has been made. Furthermore, discussing that this is a common condition can be helpful. Explaining that there is a good chance of improving as there are no structural issues with the nervous system is also helpful for their recovery. The websites neurosymptoms.org and fndhope.org give further explanations about functional neurological conditions for patients. These website addresses can be given to patients to allow them to read about their condition and learn more about management strategies.

Discussing sensitively if appropriate that depression and anxiety can exacerbate the condition can also help. If the patient is in agreement, referral for specialist psychiatry/psychology input can also be very helpful. Referral should be made to a psychiatry/psychology team with experience in functional disorders. They may offer cognitive behavioural therapy to help to change the patient's pattern of thinking and behaviours. Antidepressants, such as tricyclic antidepressants or selective serotonin reuptake inhibitors, or beta-blockers as an anxiolytic for somatic anxiety symptoms can also be helpful. Physiotherapy can be very helpful, therefore patients can be referred for this. There are also specialist functional neurological disorder services, which offer a multidisciplinary approach with psychiatry, psychology, physiotherapy, occupational therapy and mental health nurse teams all involved in assessing and managing the patient. This offers a holistic approach to the management of these conditions, and in some cases patients can be referred to these services.

● Chapter Summary

- Functional neurological disorders are common and can coexist in patients with organic neurological diseases.
- Management is centred around a good explanation of the condition to patients, and psychiatry/psychology and physiotherapy input can be helpful in some cases.

UKMLA Presentations
Facial weakness
Fits/seizures
Limb weakness
Tremor

Adnexal (eyelids, lacrimal system and orbit) 38

EYELID

Disorders of the eyelid are common and affect both adults and children, they frequently present to the general practitioner and is commonly associated with a conjunctivitis.

The anatomy of the eyelid is shown in Fig. 38.1.

Disorders of eyelids can be divided into:

- allergic disorders
- infections
- benign tumours
- malignant tumours

Allergic disorders

These are summarised in Table 38.1.

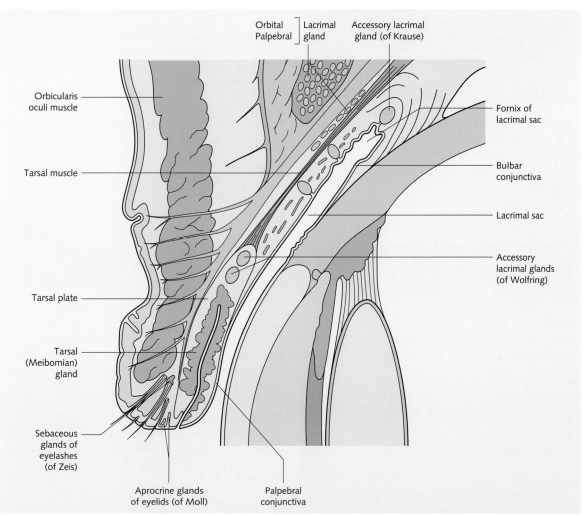

Fig. 38.1 The anatomy of the eyelid. Note how the conjunctiva starts (palpebral) on the posterior aspect of eyelid and reflects (fornix) on to the sclera towards the corneal limbus (bulbar). (From *Crash Course: Ophthalmology, Dermatology, and ENT*. 3rd ed. Elsevier.)

Table 38.1 Summary of allergic disorders of the eyelid

	Symptoms	Signs	Treatment
Acute allergic oedema	Sudden onset, itching	Pitting eyelid oedema	Systemic antihistamines
Contact dermatitis	Itching, tearing	Eyelid swelling, erythema, crusty skin	Removal of cause, mild topical hydrocortisone
Atopic dermatitis (eczema)	Itching	Eyelid crusting, erythema, discharge from secondary infection	Emollients, topical hydrocortisone cream, antibiotics

(From *Crash Course: Ophthalmology, Dermatology, and ENT*. 3rd ed. Elsevier.)

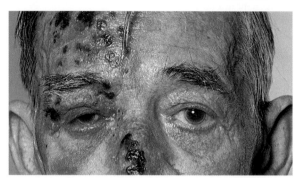

Fig. 38.2 Herpes zoster ophthalmicus – involvement of nose indicating eye involvement (Hutchinson sign). (From Spalton D, Hitchings R, Hunter P. *Atlas of Clinical Ophthalmology*. 3rd ed. St Louis: Mosby; 2004, with permission.)

Infections

These may be acute or chronic.

Acute herpes zoster ophthalmicus

Common, unilateral condition caused by the varicella zoster virus (shingles). It affects the elderly, and it is important to consider systemic immunocompromise in the young (see Fig. 38.2).

Symptoms

Acute pain and headache in the distribution of the first division of the trigeminal nerve. A vesicular rash follows this.

Signs

Maculopapular rash, which progresses to crusty vesicles, oedema and swelling. There may be an associated keratopathy and uveitis.

> **HINTS AND TIPS**
>
> Look out for Hutchinson sign: rash on the tip/side of the nose. This indicates nasocilliary involvement and strong risk factor for ocular involvement.

Treatment

Oral aciclovir treatment is usually given within 72 hours. IV antivirals may be considered if there is a very severe infection, or if the patient is immunocompromised. Ocular involvement requires an urgent ophthalmology review.

Primary herpes simplex

Uncommon, unilateral, typically affecting children, patients with atopic dermatitis who may be using steroids and the immunocompromised.

Signs

Crops of vesicles which are creamy-yellow and may rupture leading to a conjunctivitis.

Treatment

Topical aciclovir.

Other acute conditions

Acute rare conditions which may also affect the eyelids include:

- impetigo
- erysipelas
- necrotizing fasciitis

Chronic infections

This is most commonly due to chronic blepharitis secondary to *Staphylococcus aureus* and can affect both the anterior and posterior lid margins.

Chronic blepharitis

Chronic blepharitis is a common condition and tends to be controlled in susceptible individuals rather than cured. It is commonly seen in patients with acne rosacea and atopic eczema (Fig. 38.3).

Symptoms

Irritated crusty eyes, excess 'sleep' in the mornings, lacrimation.

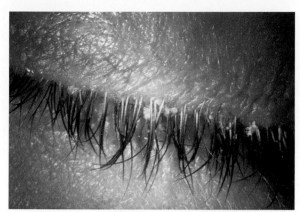

Fig. 38.3 Chronic blepharitis associated with chronic staphylococcal infection. (Photograph courtesy of Dr Robert Kersten, University of Utah, Moran Eye Center.)

Signs
Lid margin crusting and scaling, debris around the lash roots, loss of lashes and greasy plugs in the meibomian glands, lid margin erythema, greasy tear film.

Associated ocular signs: these include secondary conjunctivitis and marginal keratitis.

Treatment
- Lid hygiene (warm cotton buds dipped in bicarbonate solution or baby shampoo).
- Topical tear film supplements.
- Topical fusidic acid.
- Systemic tetracyclines.

BENIGN TUMOURS

Chalazion

A chalazion is the most common type of benign eyelid lump. It occurs when a meibomian gland becomes obstructed leading to a granuloma within the tarsal plate.

Symptoms and signs
Painless swelling in the posterior lamella, which may discharge either anteriorly or posteriorly.

Treatment
Hot compresses encourage discharge, and most are self-limiting. It is important to treat any associated blepharitis or cellulitis. Incision and curettage may be required in recalcitrant cases.

Molluscum contagiosum

Molluscum contagiosum is an umbilicated, pearly-looking lid margin cyst caused by the pox virus.

Symptoms and signs
Irritated red eyes caused by viral discharge from the cysts with a secondary follicular conjunctivitis.

Treatment
Excision of the lesion with cautery to the base.

Other cysts

These are the result of obstruction of the other glandular structures within the eyelid. They are usually asymptomatic and are excised for cosmetic reasons. They include:

- Cyst of Moll (obstruction of a sweat gland)
- Cyst of Zeiss (obstruction of accessory sebaceous gland)

MALIGNANT TUMOURS

Basal cell carcinoma

This is the most common malignant eyelid tumour and accounts for 90% of all eyelid malignancies. Ten percent of all basal cell carcinomas (BCCs) occur on the eyelids (see Fig. 38.4).

Symptoms and signs
Painless lesion which may be nodular, sclerosing or ulcerative ('rodent ulcer'). It is associated with lash loss and a pearly margin. It is slow-growing, locally invasive, and non-metastasizing.

Treatment
Excision biopsy with margin control with either cryotherapy or radiotherapy.

Squamous cell carcinoma

This is much less common than BCC; however, it is potentially more aggressive with regional lymph node metastasis or perineural spread. It accounts for 5% to 10% of eyelid malignancies. Clinically, it may be indistinguishable from BCC (see Fig. 38.5).

Treatment
Excision with margin control.

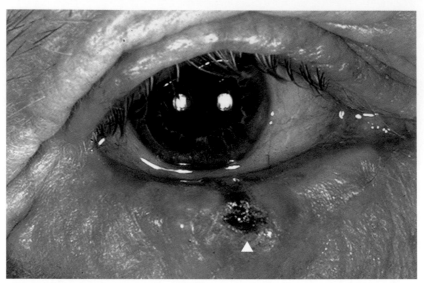

Fig. 38.4 Basal cell carcinoma. There is an ulcerated wound in the lower eyelid. Two labels pointing to the wound read, central ulceration and basal cell carcinoma. (From Klatt E. *Robbins and Cotran Atlas of Pathology*. 4th ed. Elsevier; 2020.)

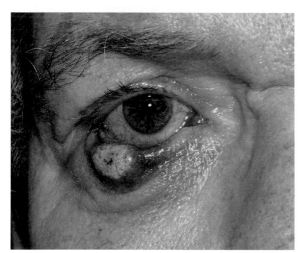

Fig. 38.5 Squamous cell carcinoma. Mechanical ectropion resulting from a large lower-eyelid mass. (From Yanoff M, Duker J. *Ophthalmology*. 6th ed. Elsevier; 2023.)

EYELID MALPOSITIONS

Entropion

This is an in-turning of the lower and, more rarely, the upper lid.

Ectropion

This is an out-turning of the lower lid. See Tables 38.2 and 38.3.

Ptosis

There are many causes of ptosis and each case requires careful history and examination.

History and symptoms

Important points are age of onset, duration and associated symptoms such as fatiguability, diplopia, and variability.

Signs

Important measurements are vertical fissure height and levator function. It is important to measure fatiguability and ocular motility, look for jaw winking and check the Bell phenomenon.

Treatment

Treatment is related to the cause. Medical conditions such as myasthenia, which causes myogenic ptosis, require a neurological referral. There are various surgical options, depending on the age of the patient and the clinical diagnosis.

LACRIMAL SYSTEM

Tears are trilayered and are predominantly formed by the lacrimal gland. Tears cling and stick to the surface of the eye from conjunctival mucus-secreting glands and do not evaporate from the surface of the eye due to a coating of oil, which is secreted by the meibomian glands. The anatomy of the lacrimal system is shown in Fig. 38.6. It is important to exclude and

Table 38.2 Summary of entropion eyelid malpositions

Cause	Pathogenesis	Treatment
Involutional	Age-related regeneration of the elastic tissues within the eyelid leads to horizontal laxity	Temporary treatment in casualty – lubricants and eyelid taping to reduce irritation from lashes Permanent treatment is with surgical correction
Cicatricial	Severe scarring of the palpebral conjunctiva pulls the lid inwards towards the globe (chemical injuries, trauma and inflammation)	Bandage contact lens prevents eyelash rubbing against the cornea Permanent treatment is with anterior lamellar rotation +/– composite grafts
Congenital	Improper development of the inferior retractor aponeurosis	Often self-limiting. In symptomatic cases, surgical correction

(From *Crash Course: Ophthalmology, Dermatology, and ENT*. 3rd ed. Elsevier.)

Table 38.3 Summary of ectropion eyelid malpositions

Classification	Pathogenesis	Treatment
Involutional	Ageing changes in the elastic tissues within the eyelid leading to lower lid laxity	Surgical correction of the lid laxity
Cicatricial	Scarring and contracture of the skin pulling the eyelid away from the globe	Eliminate any chemical cause, for example, preserved eye drops. Surgical correction
Paralytic	Ipsilateral facial nerve palsy	Lubrication, surgical correction including a temporary tarsorrhaphy to reduce corneal exposure
Mechanical	Tumours on or at the lid margin leading to eversion	Removal of the cause

(From *Crash Course: Ophthalmology, Dermatology, and ENT*. 3rd ed. Elsevier.)

Table 38.4 Summary of categories of ptosis

Classification	Mechanism	Cause
Mechanical	The lid is pulled down due to the gravitational effect of a mass or scarring	Large lid lesions pulling down lid Scarring Dermatochalasis (pseudo-ptosis) Oedema
Aponeurotic	A defect in the levator aponeurosis	Involutional (senile) Postoperative (perhaps due to stretching from the eyelid speculum)
Myogenic	Myopathy of the levator muscle or neuromuscular junction disease	Myasthenia gravis Myotonic dystrophy Congenital ptosis Blepharophimosis syndrome
Neurogenic	Innervational defect	III nerve palsy Horner syndrome Marcus Gunn jaw winking

(From *Crash Course: Ophthalmology, Dermatology, and ENT*. 3rd ed. Elsevier.)

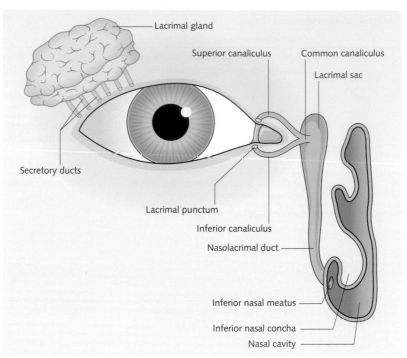

Fig. 38.6 Lacrimal system. Tears from the lacrimal gland traverse the cornea, enter the puncta, travel along the canaliculi to the lacrimal sac, thence to the nasolacrimal duct, and then pass into the inferior nasal meatus. (From *Crash Course: Ophthalmology, Dermatology, and ENT*. 3rd ed. Elsevier.)

treat any cause of reflex lacrimation such as trichiasis, blepharitis or dry eyes.

Symptoms and disorders of the lacrimal system

The main symptom related to the lacrimal system is excess tearing, known as 'watery eye'. This can be caused by two conditions:

- hyperlacrimation
- epiphora

Hyperlacrimation

Hyperlacrimation is where there is reflex lacrimal hypersecretion secondary to ocular surface abnormality. Treatment in these cases is to treat the underlying cause.

Epiphora

Epiphora is the compromise of lacrimal drainage due to:

- Congenital obstruction.

- Eyelid malposition displacing the lacrimal punctum out of the tear lake.
- Lacrimal obstruction along the drainage system which may be partial or complete.
- Lacrimal pump failure due to weakness of the orbicularis oculi, for example, secondary to facial nerve palsy.

Adult nasolacrimal duct obstruction

Symptoms
Sticky, watery eye where the conjunctiva is white. Symptoms worsen in wind or the cold weather.

Signs
Include punctual stenosis, blocked system on syringing via the canaliculus with saline. A dacryocystogram may be used to identify the location of the blockage.

Treatment
Dacryocystorhinostomy (DCR) connects the mucosal surface of the lacrimal sac to the nasal mucosa by removing the intervening bone.

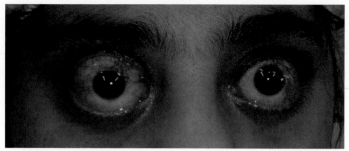

Fig. 38.7 Active thyroid eye disease in a 32-year-old woman. There is proptosis, upper and lower eyelid retraction, conjunctival injection on both sides. (From Rezaei N. *Translational Autoimmunity, Volume 4*. Academic Press; 2022.)

ORBITAL DISEASE

The orbit is composed of the bony and soft tissue structures that surround the globe. It has several important functions including protection of the globe, attachments to stabilize ocular movement and connective tissue structures which transmit nerves and blood vessels. The expression of diseases in terms of clinical signs is often similar despite the large variety of diseases which can affect the orbit. A detailed history and examination is vital.

Differential diagnosis of orbital disease

Dysthyroid eye disease

Dysthyroid or thyroid eye disease (TED) is the most common cause of both bilateral and unilateral axial proptosis in adults and is permanent in 70% of cases. Although associated with thyrotoxicosis, it is uninfluenced by the treatment of hyperthyroidism because patients can be clinically and biochemically euthyroid. TED is an organ-specific autoimmune IgG-mediated disease leading to infiltration of muscles and fat surrounding eye (see Fig. 38.7).

There are two stages:

1. Acute inflammatory (risk of sight loss): lasts approximately 12 to 18 months, causing proptosis, and may cause compressive optic neuropathy.
2. Chronic fibrotic: leading to a restrictive myopathy and diplopia. Aqueous humour outflow obstruction from the eye may occur, leading to increased intraocular pressure and thus secondary glaucoma.

Risk factors include smoking and female gender. Graves disease affects 2% of females in the United Kingdom. Therefore, male smokers with TED have the worst prognosis. The symptoms and signs of TED are listed in Table 38.5. An alternative method of remembering symptoms and examination pointers is to use the acronym of the American Thyroid Association, NO SPECS (see Hints and Tips).

Table 38.5 Features of thyroid eye disease

Symptoms:
- Nil
- Grittiness (e.g., superior limbic keratoconjunctivitis)
- Redness
- Eyelid swelling
- Diplopia
- Cosmetic appearance, 'bulgy'/'staring' eyes (Kocher sign)
- Visual loss

Signs:
- Lid retraction (Dalrymple sign) – primary due to fibrotic contracture of the levator, secondary due to overaction of the levator/superior rectus complex if there is hyperphoria produced by fibrosis of the inferior rectus
- Lid lag on down gaze (von Graefe sign)

(From *Crash Course: Ophthalmology, Dermatology, and ENT*. 3rd ed. Elsevier.)

Investigation
- CT orbit.
- Proptosis (2/3 of globe should lie within the orbital rim).
- EOM (extraocular muscle) infiltration and enlargement (inferior rectus (IR) and medial rectus (MR) most commonly involved).
- Thyroid function tests (TSH, T3 and T4).

Treatment
- Manage thyroid dysfunction.
- Ocular lubricants alone (in mild cases for corneal exposure).
- Glaucoma topical medications (for secondary or posttrabecular glaucoma).
- Acute optic nerve compression (5% of patients).
- Systemic corticosteroids.
- Orbital radiotherapy.
- Surgical orbital decompression.

Chronic phase:

- Diplopia: squint surgery, prisms, botulinum toxin.
- Cosmetic: orbital decompression; lid surgery, e.g., blepharoplasty, lid lowering, etc.

Infective disorders

Orbital cellulitis is an important, potentially visually threatening disorder. The most serious complications are blindness and secondary central nervous system infection leading to a brain abscess.

Symptoms and signs

Swelling of the eyelid tissues. Preseptal cellulitis is a superficial skin infection, which is anterior to the orbital septum.

Signs of orbital cellulitis, a sight-threatening condition, are pain on movement, conjunctival injection, restriction of eye movements with diplopia, proptosis, reduced vision, relative afferent papillary defect, and feeling systemically unwell with an associated pyrexia.

Examination

Full ocular and orbital examination must be carried out.

Treatment

Admit and give intravenous broad-spectrum antibiotics until pyrexia resolves and vision returns to normal.

● Chapter Summary

- Disorders of the eyelid can be divided into allergic disorders, infections, benign, and malignant tumours.
- Allergic disorders of the eyelid include acute allergic oedema, contact dermatitis, and atopic dermatitis. It is important to consider the timing of symptoms in order to differentiate between them.
- Main infectious disorders that affect the eyelid include herpes zoster ophthalmicus and herpes simplex virus – both require aciclovir as management.
- Most common benign tumour is a chalazion – treatment is conservative and hygiene advice. Malignant tumours include basal cell carcinoma and squamous cell carcinoma.
- Hyperlacrimation is where there is reflex lacrimal hypersecretion secondary to ocular surface abnormality.
- TED symptoms and examination can be remembered through acronym NO SPECS.
- Orbital cellulitis is a vision-threatening disorder and knowing how to differentiate between preseptal cellulitis is key. Pain on eye movement is a core feature of orbital cellulitis.

UKMLA Conditions
Benign eyelid disorders
Blepharitis
Periorbital and orbital cellulitis
Thyroid eye disease

UKMLA Presentations
Allergies
Eye pain/discomfort
Facial/periorbital swelling
Ptosis

Anterior segment (cornea and cataract)

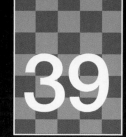

39

CORNEA

Introduction

The cornea is avascular and is the major refractive interface in the eye accounting for two-thirds of the refractive power, with the lens providing a third. It has clarity owing to the regular alignment of collagen fibrils, such that parallel light rays can pass through unobstructed. Any compromise from corneal disease leads to corneal opacity, reduced vision and the need for a corneal graft. Therefore, adequate medical treatment will avoid the progression of the disease process.

The cornea, particularly involving the stromal layer (see Table 39.1), is the part of the eye that is operated on during laser refractive surgery such as photorefractive keratectomy (PRK) and laser in situ keratomileusis (LASIK).

Table 39.1 Description of the five anatomical layers of the cornea

Corneal layer	Description
Epithelium	A multicellular layer providing the main external defense to disease (e.g., bacteria).
Bowen's membrane	The basement membrane to epithelium.
Stroma	Approximately 90% of the corneal mass. It is essentially acellular, except for a few keratocytes. A relatively dehydrated state must be maintained to preserve clarity.
Descemet's membrane	An acellular structure. It provides support for the endothelium.
Endothelium	A monolayer of nonrenewing cells. These very important cells are responsible for maintaining the dehydrated state. They pump fluid actively out of the stroma. Any compromise of the endothelium leads to stromal oedema and clouding, e.g., in Fuchs endothelial dystrophy.

From *Crash Course: Ophthalmology, Dermatology, and ENT.* 3rd ed. Elsevier.

Infection

Corneal infection can be a major cause of sight-threatening disease. Patients may have bacterial, protozoan or viral disease. See Table 39.2.

Bacterial

These infections are rare in the absence of a corneal epithelial defect. They are therefore seen in the context of contact lens wearers and/or ocular surface compromise such as entropion, dry eye, corneal anaesthesia (congenital, diabetes mellitus or acoustic neuroma) or immunocompromised.

Management

A corneal scrape is taken and treatment is started. This is usually a quinolone (good broad-spectrum cover) such as guttae ofloxacin. Intensive treatment (hourly drops) continues over 48 hours and clinical response is assessed. Steroids may then be required to reduce stromal scarring.

Rapid identification of the organism can prevent endophthalmitis and loss of vision.

Protozoan

Corneal acanthamoeba infection is associated with soft contact lens wear and poor lens hygiene, particularly the use of tap water. Infection is characterized by a red eye with intense pain which is out of proportion to the other clinical signs.

Classic signs include a ring ulcer with stromal immune ring (Wessely ring), perineural infiltrate and anterior segment inflammation.

Diagnosis is obtained with deep corneal scrapes, biopsy or confocal microscopy. Treatment includes Brolene, polyhexamethylene biguanide (PHMB) and ketoconazole.

Chronic infection from stromal acanthamoeba cysts can lead to scarring and may require corneal transplantation.

Viral keratitis

Many viruses may affect the cornea including herpes simplex and zoster. Herpes simplex virus (HSV) can affect the epithelium, stroma or endothelium (Fig. 39.1).

Table 39.2 Key differentiating features of the different types of infective keratitis

	Bacteria	Viral	Fungal	Protozoan
Presentation	Pain and discharge	Discomfort and gritty feeling	Less pain	Disproportionate pain to clinical signs
	Blurry vision	Corneal anaesthesia/ reduced sensation	More blurred vision + redness	
Signs	Hypopyon	Dendric ulcer Hypopyon less likely Raised IOP*	Fluffy edges Satellite lesions	Pseudodendrites
Risk factors	Contact lens Entropion Dry eye Immunocompromised		Immunocompromised Steroid use, vegetative trauma, previous surgery	Contact lens, poor hygiene
Common organism	*Staphylococcus aureus Staphylococcus epidermidis Streptococcus pneumoniae Enterobacter (Coliforms, Proteus, Klebsiella)*	Herpes simplex virus Varicella zoster virus Adenovirus		Acanthamoeba
Management	Urgent ophthalmology referral Corneal scrape Contact lens advice Topical antibiotics (chloramphenicol)	Topical acyclovir Cycloplegic, e.g., atropine		Deep corneal scrapes and/or biopsy Brolene, polyhexamethylene biguanide (PHMB) and ketoconazole

Epithelial disease

This is characterized by the classic dendritic or geographic (more advanced) forms. The central defect stains with fluorescein and the edges stain with Rose Bengal (stains dead cells). Treatment is with topical antiviral and a cycloplegic (Fig. 39.1).

A neurotrophic ulcer is another form of epithelial disease, which looks like a nonhealing corneal abrasion and requires additional treatment such as lubricants, patching, botulinum ptosis or a conjunctival flap.

HINTS AND TIPS

Reduced corneal sensation (particularly in unilateral disease) is suggestive of a previous HSV infection.

Stromal disease

The classic form is referred to as a disciform keratitis. This may or may not be associated with epithelial or endothelial disease.

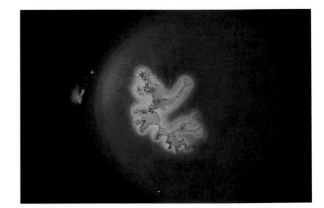

Fig. 39.1 A dendrite typical of herpes simplex keratitis with epithelial ulceration, raised edges and terminal bulbs. (From Salmon J. *Kanski's Clinical Ophthalmology: A Systematic Approach*. 9th ed. Elsevier; 2020.)

There is a central ring opacity with corneal oedema and fine keratic precipitates (KPs).

This immune process may progress to scarring with vascularization. Careful treatment with topical steroid and cycloplegic is required.

Herpes zoster

The multiple epithelial pseudodendrites and anterior stromal infiltrates are responsive to topical steroids.

The main treatment is with systemic antivirals (see section on uveitis, Chapter 43).

Inflammation

The cornea may suffer from nonmicrobial keratitis which may be due to either local or systemic disease. These conditions classically lead to inflammation, corncal infiltrate and corneal thinning/melting.

The mainstay of treatment, in all scenarios, is topical steroid drops (except with extreme thinning) and topical antibiotic, though occasionally systemic steroids are required.

Ocular disease

There are numerous ocular conditions that may lead to a nonmicrobial keratitis. Two of these include marginal keratitis and vernal keratoconjunctivitis.

Marginal keratitis

This relatively common condition is associated with blepharitis, specifically anterior blepharitis secondary to a staphylococcus infection. Staphylococcal hypersensitivity leads to peripheral infiltrate and thinning.

Treatment is topical steroid and lid hygiene (to treat blepharitis).

Vernal keratoconjunctivitis

This is a superiorly located ulcer found in patients with marked allergic eye disease. It is due to giant papillae under upper lid.

Treatment is with topical steroid and anti allergic eye drops (e.g., opatanol and olopatadine).

Keratoconus

This ectatic dystrophy is characterized by a gradual deterioration in vision (due to worsening astigmatism) in adolescence. It rarely presents in its acute form, corneal hydrops, which is due to a split in Descemet membrane (Fig. 39.2).

Characteristic clinical signs include:

- Conical cornea (apex usually inferiorly placed).
- Corneal thinning and scarring.
- Vogt striae (fine lines on posterior corneal surface).
- Fleischer ring (iron line on corneal epithelium, at the base of the cone).
- Munson sign (bulging of lower lid on down gaze).

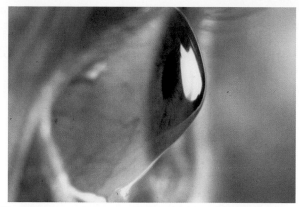

Fig. 39.2 Keratoconus cornea showing cone-like protrusion. (From Levin L, Albert D. *Ocular Disease: Mechanisms and Management.* Philadelphia: Saunders/Elsevier; 2010.)

- 'Scissor reflex' on retinoscopy.
- Corneal topography (steep and thin apex).

Treatment of keratoconus is initially refractive (glasses and/or contact lenses: patients need to use rigid lenses to treat astigmatism). If patients become intolerant of contact lenses, a corneal graft is offered. Treatment of acute corneal hydrops (which is very painful) is with topical steroid and topical cycloplegic.

TRAUMA

Epithelial abrasion and recurrent erosion

Epithelial abrasion

Epithelial abrasions are very common and usually easily treated as the epithelium usually heals very quickly.

A green epithelial defect is visible under blue light following instillation of fluorescein stain (Fig. 39.3).

Small abrasions are treated with a short (5–7 days) course of topical antibiotic drops, larger abrasions with ointment (usually chloramphenicol or Fucithalmic (fusidic acid)). Cycloplegics (e.g., cyclopentolate) and/or patching (for 24 hours; not in children) may be added.

Recurrent erosion syndrome

A few patients with previous traumatic abrasions (classically those following fingernail injury or paper cuts) get spontaneous recurrent abrasions recurrent erosion syndrome (RES).

Patients describe pain on waking and opening eyes; if mild it settles over a few hours. It can be tremendously debilitating. Bilateral RES may indicate a corneal dystrophy.

Treatment is aimed at the acute phase and prevention of recurrences:

- Acute treatment as for abrasion.
- Long-term treatment includes bland eye cream (e.g., lacrilube ointment) at night time, with or without lid taping/patching.

If it is still problematic, consider the following, in this order:

- debridement
- bandage contact lens
- anterior stromal puncture
- phototherapeutic keratoplasty (PTK)

Perforation

Corneal perforation is a very serious condition and may lead to long-term sight loss. It can be due to acute injury (laceration) or to intrinsic corneal disease, thinning and perforation (e.g., corneal melt secondary to rheumatoid arthritis). This distinction is important as the treatment of the two is quite different.

Corneal laceration

Lacerations may be partial - or full-thickness lacerations.

Partial-thickness laceration

Be sure of the diagnosis first! Ensure that the wound is Seidel negative (i.e., no wound leak).

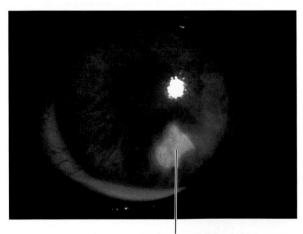

Corneal abrasion

Fig. 39.3 Corneal abrasion demonstrating fluorescein pooling of a small inferior epithelial defect. (From Kaiser P, et al. *The Massachusetts Eye and Ear Infirmary Illustrated Manual of Ophthalmology*. 4th ed. Saunders; 2014.)

Treat as for a corneal abrasion unless there is wound gape, in which case a corneal suture should be placed.

Full-thickness laceration

This is an emergency. The globe should be closed within 24 hours if possible.

The key signs are:

- Sudden reduced vision, often following a hammering/drilling injury.
- Low intraocular pressure.
- Shallow anterior chamber.
- Cataract (lens often damaged as well).

Once diagnosed the following treatment should commence:

- Shield or cartella (i.e., NO PAD).
- Patient should be starved ready for a general anaesthetic (avoid local anaesthetic if possible).
- Systemic broad-spectrum antibiotics (e.g., oral ciprofloxacin has good vitreous/ocular penetration).
- Check tetanus status and administer as necessary.
- CT scan.
- Corneal repair with 10/0 nylon sutures.

Long-term management may include contact lens for astigmatism or cataract extraction.

Alkali burn

Corneal alkali burns are potentially very serious; this is because of the rapid absorption and intraocular penetration of the alkali, leading to both superficial and intraocular complications.

The key external features are limbal ischaemia and limbal stem cell damage; this will largely account for the longer-term prognosis (Fig. 39.4).

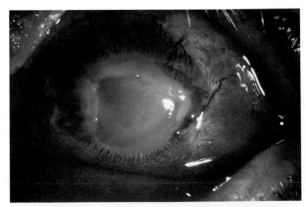

Fig. 39.4 Chronic nonhealing corneal ulcer after a severe alkali burn. (From Krachmer J, Palay D. *Cornea Atlas*. 3rd ed. Saunders; 2014.)

Treatment

- After irrigation, the fornices should be swept with cotton swab or glass rod.
- Topical antibiotic and cycloplegic.
- Analgesia (oral).
- Topical steroid if intraocular inflammation.
- Sodium citrate (reduce risk of corneal melt). If melting occurs, use collagenase inhibitor (acetylcysteine 10%–20%).
- Always check intraocular pressure and treat as appropriate.
- Bandage contact lens.

UV keratitis

UV keratitis is also known as 'arc eye'. Most commonly seen in welders who do not wear a protective mask and also seen in UV sunbed users.

Patients present in great pain and clinically there are multiple small epithelial defects (punctate epitheliopathy).

Treatment is with a short course of topical antibiotic ointment and cycloplegic.

CATARACT

A cataract is an opacity of the crystalline lens in the eye. The most common operation performed worldwide is cataract surgery. It is also one of the commonest causes of blindness worldwide. The commonest symptoms are blurring of vision and glare (Fig. 39.5).

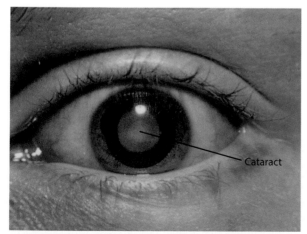

Fig. 39.5 The lens appears cloudy due to cataract. (From Leonard P. *Building a Medical Vocabulary*. 11th ed. Saunders; 2022.)

Symptoms

Blurred vision

Initially, the patient will be able to alleviate their blurred vision by attending their optician frequently. This will allow patients to update their prescription, as an increasing cataract causes a myopic shift. The patient may be able to read unaided, due to being more short sighted, but eventually glasses will not help either for reading or for distance.

Glare

The patient will notice streaking or dazzling rays of light, particularly when looking at oncoming car headlights at night. It is worse when in dark surroundings when pupils dilate. The patient may have only a slight reduction in visual acuity, but relatively much poorer contrast sensitivity. Updating the spectacles will not have any effect on this symptom.

Risk factors

Risk factors for developing cataracts include:

- age (more exposure to UV light)
- diabetes
- uveitis
- trauma

UV light is more of a problem in causing cataract in Asia or Africa at younger age than in the cloudy United Kingdom.

> **HINTS AND TIPS**
>
> Snellen acuity may overestimate visual function in patients with posterior subcapsular cataract.

Anatomy of the lens

The crystalline lens is situated in the eye between the anterior and posterior segments of the eye. It is suspended in place by zonules, which are fibres that run from the ciliary body to the equator of the lens. The shape, and thus power, of the lens is varied by ciliary muscle contraction or relaxation. Relaxation of the muscle leads to tightening of the zonules with a reduction in the lens curvature and focusing power (for distant vision). During the near reflex, the ciliary muscle contracts, allowing relaxation of the zonules to allow increased lens curvature, and thus increase in focusing power. The lens gets larger or fatter as we get older with the anterior lens epithelial cells laying down new fibres.

Common types of cataract

- Nuclear sclerosis (clouding of the central lens, associated with gradual reduction in vision and myopic shift 'index myopia'). This is the commonest form of cataract.
- Posterior subcapsular (opacity, often focal of the posterior lens, which can be quite debilitating and perceived to deteriorate quickly, even over weeks). This rapid deterioration reflects the site of opacity near the visual axis. They also complain of glare (poor vision in bright light).
- Cortical (radial spoke-like opacity in the anterior lens). These rarely affect vision unless they involve the centre directly.

Traumatic cataract

Cataracts may form following:

Blunt trauma
Blunt trauma may lead to a classical anterior subcapsular cataract (Vossius ring cataract) which happens spontaneously or soon after the trauma. A nuclear sclerotic cataract may develop over a longer period.

Penetrating trauma
A cataract will follow penetrating trauma if the capsule has been breached; this is due to lens hydration.

Ionizing radiation
Radiation to the head may lead to cataract formation over time.

Postoperative
It is well described that patients will often experience worsening or development of cataract following ocular surgery, such as vitrectomy or trabeculectomy. It is hypothesized that this may be due to postoperative intraocular inflammation. It may also develop following direct trauma to the lens, such as from vitrectomy instruments.

SYSTEMIC DISEASE

Diabetes

Diabetic patients develop cataracts younger in life than nondiabetic patients and they classically are like senile cataract phenotypically.

Senile (nuclear sclerosis, posterior subcapsular and cortical cataract).

Hypocalcaemia: small white flecks, seen in severe deficiency.
Galactosaemia: galactose-1-phosphate uridyl transferase (GPUT) deficiency; auto recessive.
Wilson disease: cortical, anterior 'sunflower cataract'.
Myotonic dystrophy: cataracts are specular and polychromatic in nature.

Toxic cataract

Certain medications can lead to cataract formation. They include:

- Systemic steroids (they classically cause posterior subcapsular cataract)
- Anticholinesterases
- Antipsychotics
- Amiodarone (cataract and corneal deposits)

Associated with ocular disease

There are certain ocular conditions that are associated with increased frequency and earlier onset of cataract.

Intraocular inflammation

Patients with chronic uveitis can develop cataract. Topical or systemic steroids, used for uveitis, can themselves induce cataracts.

Other ocular conditions

Other ocular conditions that lead to cataract include:

- High myopia.
- Angle closure glaucoma (classically leads to anterior capsule opacities, 'glaucomflecken').
- Pseudo-exfoliation syndrome.
- Retinitis pigmentosa (posterior subcapsular cataract).
- Stickler syndrome.

Symptoms
Loss of vision
Patients often complain of gradual loss of vision over 6 to 12 months. This loss of vision may be absolute (uncorrectable with lenses) or refractive (myopic shift) (Fig. 39.6). Occasionally patients will describe a rapid loss of vision with cataract that occurs in the following scenarios:

- Posterior subcapsular cataract.
- Post-traumatic.

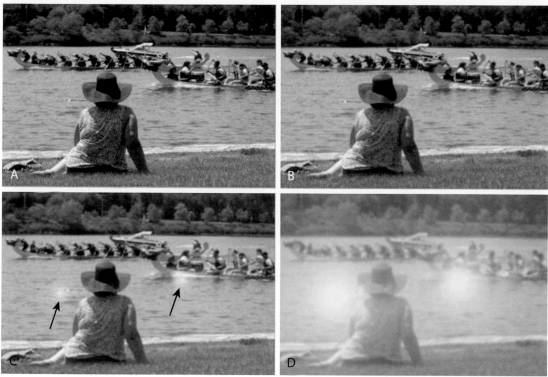

Fig 39.6 Eye disease simulations: cataract. (A) Vision with a clear lens. (B) Mild cataract. There is a generalized mild blurriness, often described as seeing through a film. (C) Moderate cataract. Details on faces are no longer visible and there is the beginning of glare with reflected sunlight (*arrows*). At night, halos around light may develop. (D) Severe cataract. Diffuse blurred vision with glare obscuring people and objects. (From Schmidt CH, et al. Eye Disease in Medical Practice: What You Should Know and Why You Should Know It. *Medical Clinics of North America.* 2021:105(3); 397-407.)

- Incidental identification upon covering the better eye (e.g., following ocular examination).

Glare/reduced contrast sensitivity

Patients may complain of poor vision in bright light, usually associated with posterior subcapsular cataract. Snellen acuity may underestimate real visual handicap.

Monocular diplopia

This rare symptom of double vision from one eye, while the other is closed, is occasionally reported.

Signs

Patients are noted to have lens opacity. There may be other signs associated with the cataract such as:

- inflammation
- pseudo-exfoliation syndrome
- anterior segment dysgenesis

Management of cataract

The definitive management of cataract is surgical removal with an intraocular lens implant. Cataract extraction is the commonest surgical procedure performed worldwide.

Conservative measures

Occasionally patients decline surgery, or it may not be indicated. The measures employed to maximize vision are glasses, improved light and/or magnifying glasses.

Surgical removal

The emergence of phacoemulsification has revolutionized the management of cataract. The best time to operate is when the patient is having problems with their level of vision, which is disabling and interfering with their daily activities (e.g., reading, driving, television, crossing the road) despite correct and up-to-date spectacles.

The aim of the microscope-assisted surgery is to remove the cloudy natural lens from the eye and replace it with a plastic intraocular lens (IOL).

Postoperative follow-up

Patients are usually seen:

- Week 3 postop- where they should then have a postoperative refraction when they finish their course of drops.
- If there has been an intraoperative complication patients are seen at day 1 postop.

Patients take antiinflammatory (steroid) and antibiotic drops, either combined or separate.

Postoperative complications

Endophthalmitis

- Early (onset of a very painful red eye in the first few days postoperatively with a hypopyon).
- Late (chronic inflammation with or without hypopyon).

This devastating complication affects about 0.1% of intraocular surgeries.

The management is outlined in Chapter 42.

Raised intraocular pressure

Most problems with pressure rise relate to retained viscoelastic in the immediate postoperative period.

Other causes of raised pressure include:

- inflammation
- steroid response glaucoma

Inflammation

Some patients experience prolonged or recurrent bouts of inflammation. They can usually be controlled with topical medications; some require oral or peribulbar steroids.

Retinal detachment

- About 1.150 patients experience a retinal detachment postoperatively. This rate increases dramatically if there is a posterior capsular rupture with vitreous loss.
- High myopia and pre-existing lattice degeneration also increase the risk.

Posterior capsular opacification

- This is a common complication of cataract surgery but seen less often with the application of newer lens design and materials.
- Patients describe a gradual reduction in vision.
- There is obvious thickening of the posterior lens capsule on slit lamp examination.
- Treatment is with YAG laser capsulotomy, which punches a hole in the posterior capsule.

● Chapter Summary

- Bacterial keratitis is usually caused by a disruption in the corneal epithelium. Risk factors include contact lens wearers and anything that could cause ocular surface compromise.
- Remember to test for corneal sensation when suspecting viral keratitis, as absent/reduced sensation makes it more likely.
- Protozoan keratitis usually causes disproportional pain to clinical signs.
- An epithelial defect can be detected using fluorescein stain under a blue light.
- Full-thickness laceration is an ophthalmic emergency. Key symptoms sudden reduced vision, low IOP, shallow anterior chamber. The globe should be closed within 24 hours.
- A cataract is an opacity of the crystalline lens in the eye, and it is one of the most common causes of blindness worldwide. Most prominent symptoms are blurring of vision and glare.
- Management of cataract usually is surgical removal and placement of a plastic intraocular lens. Postoperative complications to be aware of are endophthalmitis, raised IOP, inflammation, retinal detachment and posterior capsular opacification.

UKMLA Conditions
Blepharitis
Cataracts
Infective keratitis

UKMLA Presentations
Diplopia
Eye pain/discomfort
Eye trauma
Foreign body in eye
Gradual change in vision
Red eye

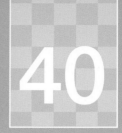
INTRODUCTION

Glaucoma is a group of diseases defined by a characteristic pattern of progressive optic neuropathy. There is associated irreversible damage to the visual field with the progressive reduction in light sensitivity of peripheral and, later, central vision.

Glaucoma is the second most common cause of blindness worldwide and the most common cause of irreversible blindness. The only proven treatments are aimed at reduction of intraocular pressure (IOP).

PATHOPHYSIOLOGY

Progressive loss of retinal ganglion cells with a pathognomonic excavation of the optic nerve head leads to a 'cupped' disc. Damage is usually related to the level of IOP. The balance between inflow of fluid produced by the ciliary body and outflow through the trabecular meshwork determines the IOP. In most glaucomas the rate of fluid outflow is reduced, e.g., by trabecular meshwork changes or abnormal trabecular meshwork contact with the iris.

Visual field testing can usually detect damage only when 30% to 50% of ganglion cells have already been lost. Either optic disc or visual field may show detectable change first. Techniques such as three-dimensional laser tomography of the optic nerve or nerve fibre layer thickness measurement by polarized light can also detect early changes. All these technologies can also be used to detect change.

> ### ETHICS
>
> Patients are often unaware of even functionally significant visual loss due to cortical 'filling in' of scotoma. It is crucial to explain that we aim to save vision for the future, but cannot repair what is lost, to help patients understand the objectives and limitations of treatment while the disease is still in this asymptomatic stage.

GLAUCOMA EXAMINATION

Glaucoma examination may detect:

1. Raised IOP
2. Optic disc cupping
3. Visual field defects
4. Open or closed angle on gonioscopy

Aqueous pathway

The aqueous humour is produced by the ciliary body, passes in front of the lens and behind the iris, then through the pupil and over the iris to the periphery towards the angle where it then passes through the trabecular meshwork, the canal of Schlemm, then outwards to the episcleral vessels.

The adult eyeball is a rigid box, since the cornea and sclera cannot stretch. If raised IOP occurs, then the pressure is transmitted posteriorly towards the optic disc. The optic disc surface looks like a flat saucer/plate (i.e., plan view), but can be squashed and deformed to become more of a teacup shape in three dimensions, hence the term optic disc 'cupping' or 'cupped' (see Fig. 40.1).

> ### HINTS AND TIPS
>
> #### PATHWAY OF AQUEOUS HUMOUR DRAINAGE
>
> Ciliary body produces aqueous humour → through pupil → iris → peripheral drainage 'angle' → trabecular meshwork → canal of Schlemm → episcleral vessels

PRIMARY GLAUCOMAS

Primary open angle glaucoma

Primary open angle glaucoma (POAG) is the most common form of glaucoma in most races. In most patients, idiopathic age-related changes to the trabecular meshwork increase resistance to fluid outflow and the IOP rises. However, in up to a

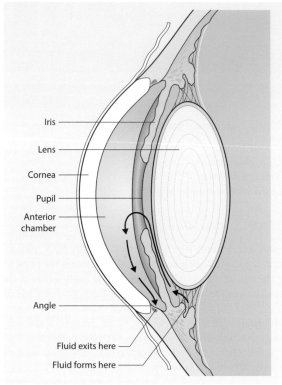

Fig. 40.1 Cross-sectional diagram indicating the drainage 'angle'. (From *Crash Course: Ophthalmology, Dermatology, and ENT*. 3rd ed. Elsevier.)

Table 40.1 Risk factors for primary open angle glaucoma	
Greater age	Exponential increase after age 40, to 10%–20% over 80 years old
Raised IOP	Also increases *rate* of damage
Affected first-degree relative	10%–30% increased risk
Race	Risk in those of African origin is 5× that of Caucasians
Myopia	Higher risk with greater myopia
Thin corneas	Higher risk
Larger optic discs	Higher risk

From *Crash Course: Ophthalmology, Dermatology, and ENT*. 3rd ed. Elsevier.

HINTS AND TIPS

Primary open angle glaucoma (POAG) is a diagnosis of exclusion that can be made only when other causes, perhaps needing different treatment, have been ruled out (e.g., angle closure, previous trauma). A normal open angle (i.e., where iris and cornea meet) on gonioscopy is a requirement for a diagnosis of POAG.

RED FLAG

Consider acute angle closure in any patient with an acute red eye who is systemically unwell.
Look out for:
-Severe pain (ocular/headache)
-Visual symptoms – ↓ visual acuity, haloes
-Semi-dilated, poorly reactive pupil
-Hazy cornea

third the IOP is within statistically normal limits for that population. Non-pressure-related mechanisms are likely to be more important in these cases.

Slowly progressive damage remains asymptomatic until the late stages, this is often detected during routine optometry appointments. However, objective measures of visual function and performance are affected before patients notice loss of vision and even asymptomatic patients are more likely to suffer falls and car crashes.

Ocular hypertension is raised IOP without optic nerve damage – approximately 1 in 20 people over the age of 40 have IOP higher than a population defined normal. Patients may be treated or monitored for signs of change, depending on other risk factors (Table 40.1).

Features may include:

- Peripheral visual field loss – nasal scotomas progressing to 'tunnel vision'.
- Decreased visual acuity.
- Optic disc cupping.

Primary angle closure glaucoma or acute angle closure glaucoma

Primary angle closure is defined by abnormal contact between peripheral iris and trabecular meshwork without other

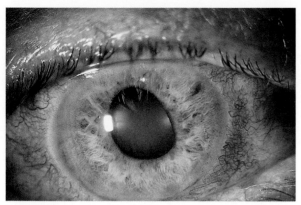

Fig. 40.2 Acute angle - closure glaucoma: the eye is red; the pupil is oval. Part of the cornea is hazy. (From Curtis K, et al. *Emergency and Trauma Care for Nurses and Paramedics.* 3rd ed. Elsevier; 2019.)

additional cause (e.g., vitreous cavity blood pushing the lens forwards).

This is a condition where the pressure in the eye rises acutely to very high levels (typically >60 mmHg). A Goldmann tonometer is used to measure IOP.

Symptoms

- Headache.
- Severe pain in the eye or over the brow.
- Photophobia
- Loss of vision.
- Nausea and vomiting.
- There may be a history of seeing 'halos' around lights which signify sub acute attacks of angle closure glaucoma.

Do not always assume nausea and vomiting is from abdominal aetiology.

Signs

- Visual acuity is severely reduced (typically worse than 6/60 or even counting fingers).
- Redness and hazy cornea due to oedema is noticeable, particularly when compared to the other side.
- The pupil is oval, semidilated and reacts poorly to light.

Risk factors

- Elderly (get cataract which may be thicker/swollen not just cloudy/opaque).
- Hypermetrope (may account for young Mongolian/ Singaporean age group).

What to do

The symptoms and signs of acute glaucoma are so obvious that the diagnosis is easy. Beware of the patient who may not have ALL of the signs and symptoms mentioned, so have a high index of suspicion.

Acute glaucoma is an emergency and should prompt urgent referral to an ophthalmologist. Ring the on-call ophthalmologist and discuss whether any treatment is required before the patient is transferred (see Fig. 40.2).

Background/principle

There is not much space between the iris and lens capsule so that aqueous fluid is sequestered/trapped behind the iris and pushes the iris forwards. The space/angle between the iris and cornea becomes smaller and ultimately closes. A vicious cycle is set up and the pressure in the eye shoots up towards 60 mmHg. The retina, iris and cornea become very ischaemic. Hence the drop in vision, poorly reactive pupil and corneal oedema.

The cycle of events is broken by decreasing the eye pressure, improving the view through the cornea to the iris and performing laser iridotomy so that the aqueous can gush forwards through the lasered mini-pupil and allow the iris to flop back posteriorly and reopen the angle.

There is about a 4-hour window from the time of extremely elevated IOP until the retina becomes so ischaemic that it dies. Blood is finding it extremely difficult to enter the eye posteriorly to the retina and anteriorly to the iris. This leads to retinal ganglion cell loss and nerve fibre layer loss at the optic disc, which leads to irreversible glaucomatous (optic disc cupping) damage.

Treatment

1. Carbonic anhydrase inhibitor – intravenous acetazolamide.
2. Combination of topical medications (also see POAG section). May include:
   I. Cholinergic (miotic) (e.g., pilocarpine)

II. Beta-blockers (e.g., timolol, Betagan)

III. Alpha-2 adrenergic agonists (e.g., apraclonidine)

Definitive management option would be lens extraction to make space within the eye, or bilateral peripheral laser iridotomy to remove pupil block. Laser iridotomy in the unaffected eye is to prevent acute angle closure from developing due to the high risk.

TREATMENT

The only proven treatments are all aimed at reduction of IOP.

The principles of treatment are:

- Define the lowest IOP needed to halt or slow progression of visual field loss sufficiently to prevent functionally significant blindness within a patient's lifetime. Pressures in the low teens may be required.
- Treat underlying causes and any angle closure if present.
- Treat in a stepwise fashion with more effective, simpler dosing schedule drugs first.

- Consider surgery, occasionally laser, if maximally tolerated treatment is insufficient.

Medical

A number of different classes of drugs are widely used.

Concordance with treatment is the biggest barrier to effectiveness. Simpler dosing regimes and combined drug preparations help. Allergy to drugs or the preservatives used in them also limits usage (see Table 40.2).

Laser

Several glaucoma laser treatments can be used depending on the type of glaucoma (see Fig. 40.3 and Table 40.3).

Surgical

Trabeculectomy

A flap of sclera is lifted beneath the conjunctiva and a hole is made into the anterior chamber.

Table 40.2 Medical treatment of glaucoma

Class of drug and examples	Mechanism of action	Contraindications and side effects
Beta-blockers Timolol Levobunolol Betaxolol Carteolol	Reduce production of aqueous by the ciliary body	Reversible airways obstruction (asthma or COPD) Can cause heart block and bradycardia Reduced exercise tolerance
Alpha-2 adrenergic sympathomimetic agonists Brimonidine Apraclonidine	Reduce production of aqueous by the ciliary body and small increase in outflow	Contraindicated in severe cardiovascular disease. Apraclonidine crosses the blood–brain barrier – causes drowsiness and lethargy in elderly. Allergy and skin/conjunctival hypersensitivity
Parasympathomimetic agents – pilocarpine	Increases outflow: ciliary muscle contraction opens trabecular meshwork	Pupillary constriction, induced myopia, iris–lens adhesions, brow ache and risk of retinal detachment
Carbonic anhydrase inhibitors Systemic: acetazolamide Topical dorzolamide or brinzolamide	Reduce production of aqueous by the ciliary body	Allergy and skin/conjunctival hypersensitivity: these are sulphonamide derivatives with risk of Stevens–Johnson syndrome. Systemic – nausea, lassitude, depression, paraesthesiae, renal stones, electrolyte imbalance
Prostaglandin analogues Bimatoprost Latanoprost Travoprost	Increase uveoscleral outflow of aqueous	Excess lash growth Periocular and iris pigmentation change
ALL DROPS	Preservatives	Risks of preservative allergy and lower subsequent surgical success

From *Crash Course: Ophthalmology, Dermatology, and ENT*. 3rd ed. Elsevier.

Table 40.3 Glaucoma laser treatments

Types of laser treatments	Description
Selective laser trabeculoplasty (SLT)	Directly treats the trabecular meshwork and aims to stimulate remodelling of tissues and reduce outflow obstruction. It is useful in reducing eye pressure and can be offered first line instead of eye drops for open angle glaucoma.
Laser peripheral iridotomy	Used in angle closure glaucoma to prevent forward bowing of the iris and so increase access of aqueous to the trabecular meshwork.
Argon laser iridoplasty	A ring of peripheral iris is thinned to improve aqueous access to the trabecular meshwork in some angle closure patients where laser iridotomy is insufficient.
Trans-scleral diode laser	Used for ciliary body ablation which reduces aqueous production through destruction of the ciliary body tissues. It is hard to predict the response and so is used mainly in patients who cannot undergo surgery.

Releasable sutures close the scleral flap and allow postoperative adjustment to the rate of flow. Drainage is into the 'bleb' – a cyst-like structure protected by the upper lid. This may be considered in refractory cases.

Glaucoma drainage devices – 'tubes'

In some conditions, or after failed trabeculectomy surgery, insertion of a drainage tube may be more successful than a trabeculectomy. A plastic tube drains fluid behind the equator of the globe.

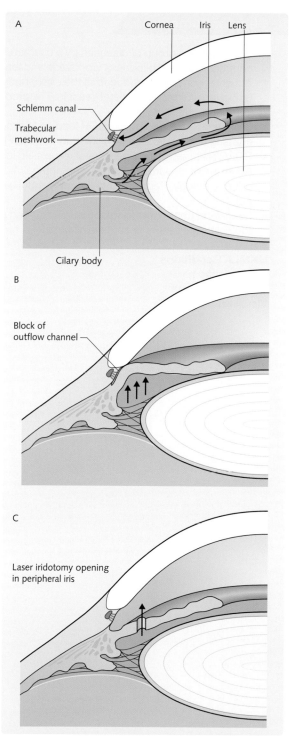

Fig. 40.3 Laser iridotomy. (A) Normal open angle, (B) closed angle, (C) reopened angle following iridotomy. (From *Crash Course: Ophthalmology, Dermatology, and ENT*. 3rd ed. Elsevier.)

● Chapter Summary

- Glaucoma is a group of diseases by a characteristic pattern of progressive optic neuropathy – second most common cause of blindness worldwide and leading cause of irreversible blindness worldwide.
- Aqueous humour is produced in the ciliary body and drained via trabecular meshwork into the canal of Schlemm and then episcleral vessels. The production of aqueous humour and outflow determines the intraocular pressure (IOP).
- Glaucoma is caused by high IOP leading to progressive loss of ganglion cells which leads to optic disc cupping and visual field defects ('tunnel vision').
- POAG features include peripheral visual field loss, decreased visual acuity and optic disc cupping.
- Acute angle closure glaucoma is an ophthalmic emergency and requires an urgent referral to ophthalmology. Red flags include red painful eye, loss of visual acuity, hazy cornea and fixed mid-dilated pupil.
- Long-term treatments for glaucoma are aimed at reduction of IOP which can include use of IOP lower topical drugs, lasers or surgical options.

UKMLA Conditions
Acute glaucoma
Chronic glaucoma
Visual field defects

UKMLA Presentations
Acute change in or loss of vision
Eye pain/discomfort
Gradual change in or loss of vision
Red eye

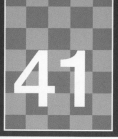
INTRODUCTION

The retina is part of the eye responsible for converting light energy into a nerve impulse (i.e., phototransduction) which is conducted along the optic nerve, chiasm, tracts to the lateral geniculate nucleus and then onwards to the visual cortex in the occipital lobe of the brain.

The retina is a 10-layered structure that essentially follows the rules of all sensory nerve pathways (i.e., three orders). The sensory neuron is the photoreceptor cell (cone and rod cells: nuclei in the outer nuclear layer), the secondary neuron is the bipolar cell (nuclei located in the inner nuclear layer) and the tertiary neuron is the ganglion cell axon – grouped together they make up the optic nerve (see Fig. 41.1).

The retinal vasculature comprises a central retinal artery and vein at the optic disc (see Fig. 41.2).

RETINAL VASCULAR DISEASE

Many conditions that affect the retina primarily affect the retinal vessels, leading to retinal vessel leakage initially (usually due to pericyte loss in diabetes). Eventually the retinal vessels (capillaries) close off, leading to local ischaemia. This results in a rise in vascular endothelial growth factor (VEGF) stimulating abnormal blood vessel growth (neovascularization). Neovascularization can lead to many complications including:

- haemorrhage:
  I. vitreous
  II. preretinal
- tractional detachment
- rhegmatogenous retinal detachment (RRD)

DIABETES

Diabetes is a potentially devastating systemic disease with many organ complications. The onset of ocular complications in diabetic patients is variable and is dependent on systemic control.

Retinal effects of diabetes are divided into maculopathy and retinopathy.

Diabetic maculopathy

These patients may be asymptomatic or present with a gradual (over months) deterioration of vision (Fig. 41.3). Risk factors for diabetic maculopathy are listed in Table 41.1.

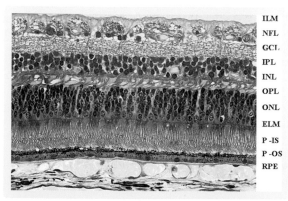

Fig. 41.1 Ten retinal layers: internal limiting membrane (*ILM*); nerve fibre layer (*NFL*); ganglion cell layer (*GCL*); inner plexiform layer (*IPL*); inner nuclear layer (*INL*); outer plexiform layer (*OPL*); outer nuclear layer (*ONL*); external limiting membrane (*ELM*); photoreceptors (inner (*P-IS*) and outer (*P-OS*) segments); and retinal pigment epithelium (*RPE*). (From *Crash Course: Ophthalmology, Dermatology, and ENT*. 3rd ed. Elsevier.)

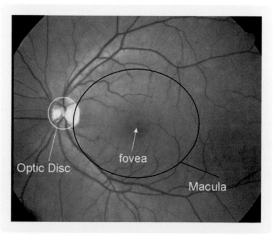

Fig. 41.2 Normal fundus. The fovea is two-disc diameters away from the optic disc (white circle) and also at the centre of the macula area (black circle). (From *Crash Course: Ophthalmology, Dermatology, and ENT*. 3rd ed. Elsevier.)

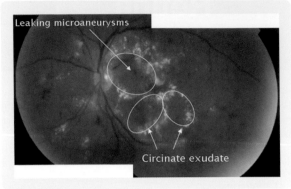

Leaking microaneurysms

Circinate exudate

Fig. 41.3 Diabetic maculopathy, due to leaky blood vessels or microaneurysms in macular region. There is also moderate to severe nonproliferative diabetic retinopathy present. (From *Crash Course: Ophthalmology, Dermatology, and ENT*. 3rd ed. Elsevier.)

Table 41.1 Risk factors for diabetic maculopathy

Risk factors for diabetic maculopathy include:
- Type II > Type I
- Hypertension
- Renal disease
- Hypercholesterolaemia

(From *Crash Course: Ophthalmology, Dermatology, and ENT*. 3rd ed. Elsevier.)

This form is characterized by:

- Microaneurysms.
- Leakage (retinal thickening/oedema, hard exudates) with or without macular ischaemia (seen on fluorescein angiogram).

The prognosis is poor if:

- The leakage is diffuse.
- There is significant ischaemia on fundus fluorescein angiography.
- There is associated cystoid macular oedema.
- There is coexistent renal failure.

Diabetic retinopathy

Diabetic retinopathy patients are usually asymptomatic until very advanced stages (hence the need for a screening programme). With advanced disease (neovascularization), they may present with a sudden painless loss of vision due to haemorrhage. Risk factors for diabetic retinopathy are listed in Table 41.2.

The characteristic changes include:

Nonproliferative diabetic retinopathy (NPDR)

1. Microaneurysms: an indicator of microvascular vessel wall changes/weakness: located deep in the inner nuclear layer.

Table 41.2 Risk factors for diabetic retinopathy

Risk factors for proliferative diabetic retinopathy include:
- Type I > Type II DM
- Poor glucose control
- Ocular surgery (beware postcataract extraction)
- Hypertension
- Renal dysfunction
- Pregnancy
- Anaemia

(From *Crash Course: Ophthalmology, Dermatology, and ENT*. 3rd ed. Elsevior.)

Table 41.3 Nonproliferative diabetic retinopathy classification

- Mild: at least one microaneurysm, and criteria not met for moderate.
- Moderate: intraretinal haemorrhages/microaneurysms, and/or cotton wool spots, venous beading, intraretinal microvascular abnormalities (IRMAs), and criteria not met for severe.
- Severe: at least one of intraretinal haemorrhages in four quadrants, venous beading > in two quadrants, intraretinal microvascular abnormalities >one quadrant and criteria not met for very severe.
- Very severe: at least two of criteria for severe.

(From *Crash Course: Ophthalmology, Dermatology, and ENT*. 3rd ed. Elsevier.)

2. Haemorrhages: flame: in superficial retinal nerve fibre layer; dot and blot: in deeper retinal outer and inner plexiform layers.
3. Thickening/oedema: intraretinal fluid: a sign of leakage.
4. Hard exudates: intraretinal lipoprotein deposits: a sign of leakage. They are sharp, well-demarcated yellow blobs, which are deeper to superficial retinal blood vessels.
5. Cotton wool spots: reflect leakage of axoplasmic fluid: a sign of ischaemia. They are superficial white fluffy retinal blobs and are not usually crossed by retinal blood vessels.
6. Venous beading: a sign of ischaemia. They are sausage-like venules of changing calibre along their length.
7. Intraretinal microvascular abnormalities (IRMA): a sign of intraretinal shunts, another feature of ischaemia.

See Fig. 41.4.

Proliferative diabetic retinopathy (PDR)

All of the above (i.e., NPDR), plus:

1. Neovascularization of the disc (NVD)
2. Neovascularization elsewhere (NVE)
3. Preretinal or vitreous haemorrhage
4. Vitreoretinal traction: adhesion between vitreous and retina leading to retinal elevation.

See Table 41.3 to classify the severity of NPDR.

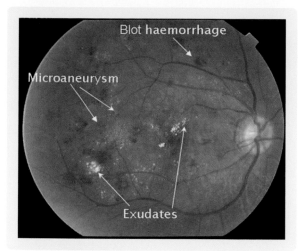

Fig. 41.4 Background diabetic retinopathy or mild nonproliferative diabetic retinopathy. Macular region changes imply the presence of diabetic maculopathy, but it is not clinically significant diabetic macular oedema. (From *Crash Course: Ophthalmology, Dermatology, and ENT*. 3rd ed. Elsevier.)

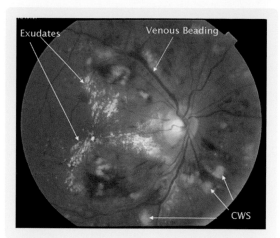

Fig. 41.5 Preproliferative or severe nonproliferative diabetic retinopathy. Signs include cotton wool spots *(CWS)* and venous beading. (From *Crash Course: Ophthalmology, Dermatology, and ENT*. 3rd ed. Elsevier.)

Screening

Prevalence rates of diabetes are now estimated to be between 5% and 10% in Western societies, so there is a need to screen large populations of at-risk individuals in order to detect early changes.

The role of screening is to pick up preclinical (presight threatening) disease and implement appropriate therapy. Patients with suspicious features should be referred to an ophthalmologist for assessment.

Treatment

In all patients, first step in management should be optimizing glycaemic control, blood pressure and hyperlipidaemia.

Maculopathy

If a patient has clinically significant macular oedema (CSMO), then intravitreal anti-VEGF treatment (e.g., bevacizumab or ranibizumab) is found to be most effective in preserving and restoring vision. Macular laser can be performed if patients do not meet the retinal thickness treatment threshold.

Retinopathy

Nonproliferative diabetic retinopathy

NPDR is usually not treated but regular observation is carried out in order to monitor the progression of disease. If severe/

very severe NPDR is present, then pan retinal photocoagulation (PRP) can be considered.

If a patient develops high-risk PDR, then PRP is applied. Some ophthalmologists treat any new vessels, low or high risk. Coexistent maculopathy should be treated first, since PRP itself may exacerbate maculopathy (Fig. 41.5).

Proliferative diabetic retinopathy

PDR is treated with PRP and intravitreal anti-VEGF treatment (e.g., bevacizumab or ranibizumab). The treatment consists of up to 2000 burns during each of three sessions, to minimize cystoid macular oedema. The response to treatment is assessed at 6 to 8 weeks.

The aim of laser in PDR is to ablate and destroy the ischaemic retina, which produces VEGF stimulus to induce neovascularization (Figs 41.6 and 41.7).

Management of other complications

Persistent vitreous haemorrhage, where duration is over 3 months, may require a vitrectomy (removal of vitreous and blood) with internal laser.

A tractional retinal detachment (RD) involving the macula would require a vitrectomy and relieving of traction.

Differential diagnoses

Vascular conditions that may present like diabetic retinopathy include (TIP: Acronym SCORE):

- **S**ickle **c**ell retinopathy: usually SC disease.

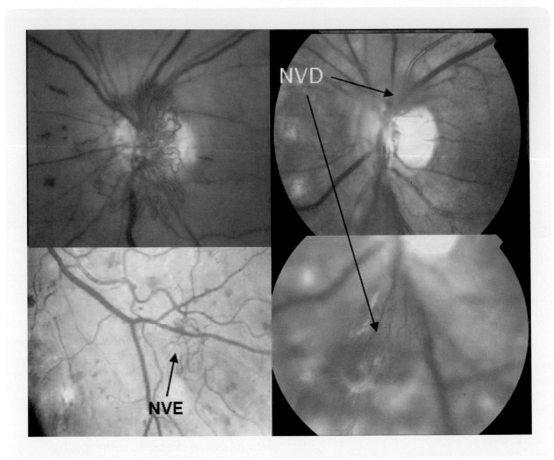

Fig. 41.6 Proliferative diabetic retinopathy (PDR). Signs include new vessels at disc *(NVD)* and elsewhere *(NVE)*. (From *Crash Course: Ophthalmology, Dermatology, and ENT*. 3rd ed. Elsevier.)

- Ocular ischaemic syndrome: reduced carotid blood flow.
- Radiation retinopathy: history of orbital/cranial radiation.
- Eales disease.

RETINAL VEIN OCCLUSION

Retinal vein occlusions can be either central retinal vein occlusion (CRVO) or branch retinal vein occlusion (BRVO). These are relatively common events leading to a painless reduction in vision (mild–severe) (see Fig. 41.8).

Vein occlusions usually occur in the elderly (>55 years) population and can usually be attributed to raised intraocular pressure and/ or arteriosclerosis. However, vascular occlusions may be an indicator of underlying systemic disease such as diabetes,

hypercholesterolaemia or autoimmune disease, thus all patients must be investigated appropriately.

Central retinal vein occlusion

The critical signs of CRVO are diffuse haemorrhages in all four quadrants and dilated tortuous veins. It causes sudden, painless reduction/loss of visual acuity, usually unilateral.

Other signs include:

- Cotton wool spots (a sign of ischaemia)
- Disc swelling
- Macular oedema
- Neovascularization of disc, retina and/or iris – a late feature of ischaemic CRVO
- Severe retinal haemorrhages – 'stormy sunset'

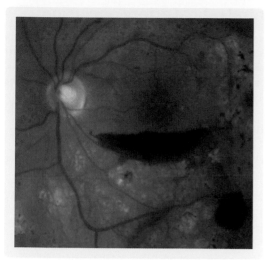

Fig. 41.7 Proliferative diabetic retinopathy. Preretinal haemorrhage secondary to new vessels elsewhere (NVE) inferotemporally. (From *Crash Course: Ophthalmology, Dermatology, and ENT*. 3rd ed. Elsevier.)

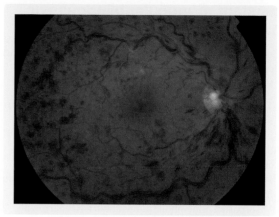

Fig. 41.8 Central retinal vein occlusion (CRVO). Note the four quadrant (flame) haemorrhages and tortuous vessels. Right swollen optic disc and two cotton wool spots (superior to fovea) are visible. (From *Crash Course: Ophthalmology, Dermatology, and ENT*. 3rd ed. Elsevier.)

There are two types of CRVO, ischaemic and non-ischaemic.

Ischaemic

This type characteristically has a greater reduction in vision (6/60) with an afferent pupil defect (RAPD). There is much retinal damage.

On fluorescein angiogram, there are large areas of non-perfusion. Seventy-five percent develop neovascularization if untreated and 50% develop neovascular glaucoma within 3 months. They invariably develop macular oedema.

Follow-up should be frequent (every 2–4 weeks) for the first 6 months.

Treatment: if iris vessels develop (rubreosis) then PRP laser treatment should be applied, and if macular oedema is present then the ophthalmologist would add intravitreal anti-VEGF agents (e.g., ranibizumab and bevacizumab), as part of the management (Fig. 41.9).

Non-ischaemic

These patients have vision better than 6/60 and no relative afferent pupil defect. They usually have milder maculopathy that may resolve spontaneously.

Follow-up is every 4 to 8 weeks for 18 months, since 10% to 15% may convert to ischaemic type.

Treatment: none required unless converts to ischaemic type.

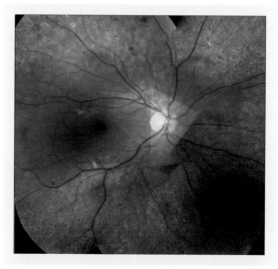

Fig. 41.9 Pan retinal photocoagulation laser scars (mildly pigmented). New vessels at disc have regressed and vitreous haemorrhage has resolved. (From *Crash Course: Ophthalmology, Dermatology, and ENT*. 3rd ed. Elsevier.)

Retinal arterial occlusion

These may be transient (amaurosis fugax) or permanent (central/branch retinal artery occlusion).

Transient monocular blindness or amaurosis fugax

Patients complain of transient (<24 hours) monocular loss of vision.

The causes of transient monocular blindness (TMB) are:

- Thrombotic: cholesterol deposition and atheroma formation within vessel lumen (e.g., carotid artery disease).
- Embolic: platelet, cholesterol, calcific (e.g., carotid artery disease or subacute bacterial endocarditis (SBE) from cardiac valve disease).
- Haematological: sickle cell disease, polycythaemia, anaemia, hyperviscosity states.
- Vasospastic: nonembolic idiopathic arterial narrowing.

Emboli typically cause black loss of vision (i.e., 'negative' visual symptom). Grey, white, patchy (i.e., 'positive' visual symptoms) loss of vision or recovery usually indicates nonembolic loss of vision (e.g., vasospasm).

Signs

There is often no evidence of an embolic event in the retina and the physician relies on the clinical history. Occasionally one can see an embolus (usually at a branching point or arterial bifurcation).

Retinopathy due to poor ocular circulation (e.g., ocular ischaemia) is characterized by multiple mid-peripheral haemorrhages with or without cotton wool spots. Rarely do they develop neovascularization.

Investigation

It is important to assess the presence of treatable carotid artery stenosis (>70%) or cardiac disease.

These patients should be referred for:

- Cardiac workup.
- Carotid Doppler studies.
- ECHO studies.
- Neurological examination (if associated neurological symptoms, e.g., paraesthesia/paresis).
- Bloods: FBC, U&E, lipids, blood glucose, ESR and CRP.
- Autoantibody screen: serum protein electrophoresis (SPEP).

Treatment

Treat the underlying risk factors (e.g., hypertension or diabetes).

Amaurosis fugax may represent a form of a transient ischemic attack (TIA) and so should be treated in similar fashion; give 300 mg of aspirin. Then patients may be required to start clopidogrel if there is a cardiac cause of emboli (e.g., atrial fibrillation). If symptomatic patients have >70% carotid stenosis, then carotid endarterectomy is indicated.

Central retinal artery occlusion

Central retinal artery occlusion (CRAO) is an uncommon but devastating event, usually leading to irreversible blindness in the affected eye. It is usually due to thrombus or embolus. This can only be effectively treated if the patient presents within the first 4 hours of the onset of the visual loss (Fig. 41.10).

Symptoms

- Severe unilateral sudden loss of vision.
- A past history of recurrent transient visual loss may also be present.

There are no systemic symptoms associated with CRAO.

Signs

- Visual acuity is grossly reduced.
- Relative afferent pupil defect (RAPD) is present.
- The classic retinal appearance is of a pale (swollen) retina with a (foveal) cherry red spot.

Occasionally there is central sparing (25%) due to a patent cilioretinal artery. Occasionally it can be bilateral (1%–2%); if so, think of systemic causes such as giant cell arteritis (GCA) or vasculitis.

Investigation

- ESR (urgent to rule out GCA).
- CRP, FBC, U&E.
- Blood pressure.
- Fluorescein angiogram.
- VDRL, SPEP.
- Cardiovascular workup (see above).
- ERG (to determine prognosis).

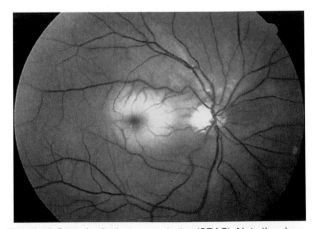

Fig. 41.10 Central retinal artery occlusion (CRAO). Note the cherry red spot in the centre of the macula, with surrounding whitening of the retina. (From Jankovic J et al. *Bradley and Daroff's Neurology in Clinical Practice.* 8th ed., Philadelphia: Elsevier; 2022.)

Treatment

Treatment must be instigated immediately (<4 hours) post CRAO. Ideally, transfer immediately to the eye department. The aim of treatment is to dislodge a presumed embolus (by reducing intraocular pressure).

This is attempted by:

- Ocular massage (exert firm pressure for 10 s, stop for 10 s).
- IV acetazolamide (Diamox) 500 mg stat.
- Anterior chamber paracentesis.
- Rebreathing CO_2 (from a paper bag) – raises carbon dioxide levels in the blood and may help to improve blood flow.
- ESR needs to be checked anyway to exclude giant cell arteritis (particularly over 65 years).

Management is difficult and the prognosis is poor; any underlying conditions should be identified and treated.

These patients, if untreated, are at high risk of subsequent stroke and myocardial infarction.

HYPERTENSIVE RETINOPATHY

This describes a series of classic changes that occur in patients with high blood pressure (a simplified classification is presented in Table 41.4).

They include:

- Haemorrhages.
- Cotton wool spots (CWS).
- AV (arteriovenous) nipping – a specific feature of hypertensive retinopathy (HR) and not DR.
- Copper/silver wiring (a sign of arteriolar sclerosis).
- Macular oedema/exudates (in a circinate/star pattern).
- Disc swelling (indicator of malignant hypertension).
- Arterial macroaneurysms.
- Choroidal ischaemia (sign of severe hypertension) with patchy infarction (due to preeclampsia, DIC or collagen vascular disease).
  See Fig. 41.11 to see features of hypertensive retinopathy.

Table 41.4 Simplified classification of hypertensive retinopathy

Mild HR	Arteriovenous (AV) nipping
Moderate HR	AV nipping and cotton wool spots (CWS)
Severe HR	Disc swelling and other features (e.g., AV nipping and CWS)

(From *Crash Course: Ophthalmology, Dermatology, and ENT.* 3rd ed. 3rd ed. Elsevier.)

Investigations

- Blood pressure.
- Blood glucose.
- Bloods: FBC, U&E.
- Fluorescein angiogram.

Treatment

Treat the blood pressure and observe the retinal changes over a period of weeks. Haemorrhages and cotton wool spots should resolve.

AGE-RELATED MACULAR DEGENERATION

Age-related macular degeneration (ARMD) is the largest single cause of blind registration in the Western world. The disorder is felt to be a combination of inherited and environmental factors. It is a disorder of the retinal pigment epithelium (RPE) with secondary neural retinal degeneration.

Classification

Ten percent of the UK population has ARMD; this is categorized into 'dry' and 'wet' ARMD. 'Dry' ARMD is more common and affects around 90% of patients and 'wet' ARMD affects 10%.

Dry ARMD

The patient present with a gradual painless reduction in vision often over many years (see Figs 41.12 and 41.13).

Characteristically:

- Drusen: yellow round spots in Bruch membrane.
- Pigment clumping.
- Macular atrophy.

Wet ARMD

The patient presents with a sudden loss or distortion of vision which occurs secondary to the formation of a subretinal neovascular membrane (SRNVM, also known as choroidal neovascular membrane – CNVM), haemorrhage or subretinal fluid (SRF) leakage (Fig. 41.14).

Characterized by choroidal neovascularization.

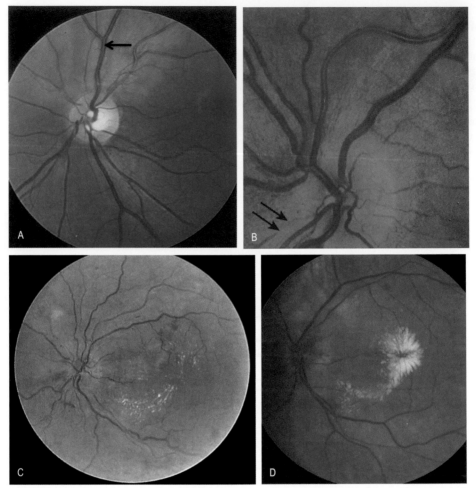

Fig. 41.11 Hypertensive retinopathy. (A) Increased reflectance, giving a silver wiring appearance to the arteriole (arrow). (B) Focal arteriolar narrowing (double arrows) seen in grade 2 disease. (C) Exudates and flame haemorrhages in grade 3 retinopathy. (D) Signs of malignant hypertension in grade 4 disease with a swollen optic disc and macular exudate. (From Dover A, et al.. *Macleod's Clinical Examination.* 15th ed. Elsevier; 2024.)

Investigation

- Full ocular examination. Signs include drusen (small yellowish deposits), pigment clumps, atrophy, haemorrhage, SRF, exudates.
- Amsler grid.
- Fluorescein angiogram (to detect and delineate a neovascular membrane and leakage; hyperfluorescence).
- Ocular coherence tomography (OCT).

Treatment

Treatment for wet ARMD is regular intravitreal anti-VEGF agents (e.g., ranibizumab, bevacizumab, brolucizumab) as numerous trials have shown that the use of anti-VEGF treatments can limit or reverse neovascular membrane growth and preserve vision. This should be initiated within the first two weeks of diagnosis of wet ARMD. Injections are usually administered every four weeks for three months as a loading dose and then adjusted according to response.

Pharmacological treatments aimed at preventing visual loss in patients with dry ARMD include multivitamins and antioxidants (vitamins A, E and zinc), where there is a 40% risk reduction of having severe visual loss. Other agents include dietary components that are macular pigments (lutein and zeaxanthin) which act as antioxidants and are felt to play a role in maintaining retinal health. Patients with extensive drusen's seem to benefit the most from this treatment.

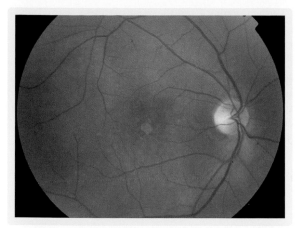

Fig. 41.12 Geographic atrophy or dry age-related macular degeneration. (From *Crash Course: Ophthalmology, Dermatology, and ENT*. 3rd ed. Elsevier.)

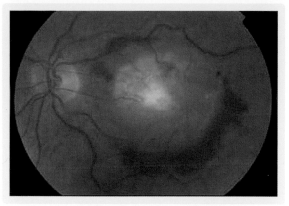

Fig. 41.14 Wet age-related macular degeneration (left eye). Subfoveal choroidal neovascular membrane with circumferential subretinal haemorrhages at the edge of a dome-shaped subretinal fluid collection. (From *Crash Course: Ophthalmology, Dermatology, and ENT*. 3rd ed. Elsevier.)

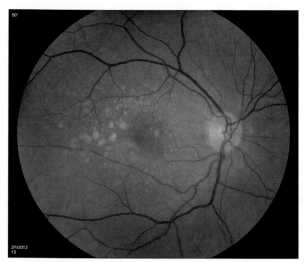

Fig. 41.13 Age-related macular degeneration consists of drusen (round, yellow lesion located at the level of the retinal pigment epithelium). (From Kimmel P, Rosenberg M, et al. *Chronic Renal Disease*. 2nd ed. Academic Press; 2020.)

Floaters: these are black or opaque objects that float across the line of vision and are usually less noticeable with time. Patients can describe them as cobwebs, flies, hairs or nets. They change position with eye movements and are seen most clearly against a white or bright background. Floaters occur because of a change in vitreous gel consistency.

Flashing lights (photopsia): these are lights that flicker in the patient's peripheral field of vision. The cones ('c for central, colour vision') and rods ('peripheral motion or night vision') perform phototransduction (i.e., convert light signals to electrical impulses). Tugging and stretching of the photoreceptor layer by the vitreous causes monocular photopsia due to stimulation of rods and cones. It does not matter if the eye is open or closed.

Important sign to consider on ophthalmoscopy is the presence of Weiss ring – detachment of vitreous membrane around optic nerve to form ring-shaped floater.

Management

Management would be to rule out any retinal tears/detachment by an ophthalmologist; if none, then reassurance to the patient that PVD doesnot cause any permanent loss of vision and no treatment is necessary.

POSTERIOR VITREOUS DETACHMENT

Posterior vitreous detachment (PVD) is the separation of the vitreous membrane from the retina.

Floaters and flashing lights are the two most common symptoms.

RETINAL DETACHMENT

Retinal detachment (RD) occurs when the (top nine layers of the) retina is separated from the 10th retinal layer, the RPE, by SRF. There are three types of RD:

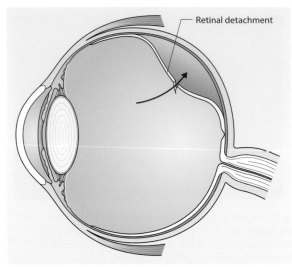

Fig. 41.15 Rhegmatogenous retinal detachment. The *arrow* depicts fluid entering the subretinal space through a retinal tear. (From *Crash Course: Ophthalmology, Dermatology, and ENT*. 3rd ed. Elsevier.)

1. Rhegmatogenous: retinal tear allows liquid from vitreous cavity to form SRF.
2. Exudative: inflammatory and neoplastic lesions (e.g., metastasis, posterior scleritis) lead to serous exudation from leaky blood vessels.
3. Tractional: fibrotic or vascular membranes along the posterior vitreous can contract and pull on the retina. Risk factors include diabetes, CRVO, sickle cell retinopathy and retinopathy of prematurity.

Rhegmatogenous retinal detachment

If the vitreous gel pulls too hard on the retina (in 10%–15% of cases), a tear can develop anteriorly near the firm adhesions of the ora serrata. As fluid from vitreous cavity goes through the retinal tear, the retina (top 9 layers usually) lifts off or detaches from the 10th retinal layer, the RPE.

This SRF leads to rhegmatogenous retinal detachment (RRD).

Symptoms

- Sudden increase in number of floaters and persistent flashing lights (photopsia).

- Curtain coming across the vision of either eye, from any direction; may be black or grey and is persistent.

Around 60% of RRD patients have all TRIAD of symptoms.

A retinal tear commonly occurs in the superotemporal region because gravity causes the superior part of the retina to fall down in the eye and the vitreous gel is anchored firmly more nasally at the optic disc. Therefore, a dark or black curtain or inferonasal field defect can occur which enlarges towards the centre of the field of vision.

Sign

- Visual acuity may be normal or grossly reduced.
- Visual field loss.
- RAPD – if the optic nerve is involved.
- Absent red reflex.

Brown RPE pigment and red blood cells from torn or avulsed blood vessel can be released into vitreous cavity. This very useful and important clinical sign on slit lamp examination is called tobacco dust or Shafer sign.

Macular or foveal vision corresponds to central vision. It is therefore important to note whether the loss of field is small with good central vision (e.g., 6/9 vision) or huge with poor central vision (e.g., CFs vision).

Risk factors

- Diabetes mellitus.
- Age.
- Acute PVD.
- High myopia.
- Trauma.
- Previous complicated/multiple intraocular surgery.

Treatment

Although SRF is present in all three types of RD, the treatment differs:

- Rhegmatogenous: laser, cryotherapy (to seal up or glue down the original tear) with either scleral buckle or vitrectomy.
- Exudative: treat the underlying cause (e.g., metastasis, posterior scleritis).
- Tractional: relieve traction by vitrectomy.

Chapter Summary

- The retinal effects of diabetes can be split into maculopathy and retinopathy; the presentation is usually asymptomatic and often patients present at the late stage of the disease. This signifies the importance of screening populations of high-risk individuals (e.g., diabetic patients) in order to detect early changes to slow the progression of disease and to prevent vision loss.
- In patients with diabetic retinopathy, the first step in management should be optimizing glycaemic control, blood pressure and hyperlipidaemia.
- Nonproliferative diabetic retinopathy usually requires no treatment, but regular monitoring should be carried out to monitor progression of disease.
- Proliferative diabetic retinopathy can be treated with panretinal photocoagulation. Other options could include intravitreal anti-VEGF, particularly if there are other issues such as macular oedema or rubeosis.
- On fundoscopy CRVO = disc swelling, cotton wool spots and retinal haemorrhages ('stormy sunset'), CRAO = pale retina with cherry red spot.
- 'Dry' ARMD is more common and characterized by presence of drusen (yellow round spots in Bruch membrane) and macular atrophy. 'Wet' ARMD is characterized by choroidal neovascular membranes.
- PVD's most common symptoms are flashes and floaters. No specific treatment required, reassurance to patient that symptoms will improve in several months. Ophthalmologist should examine for retinal tears detachment which requires treatment.
- In retinal detachment patient will often describe 'black curtain' falling down.

UKMLA Conditions
Central retinal arterial occlusion
Diabetic eye disease
Macular degeneration
Retinal detachment
Visual field defects

UKMLA Presentations
Acute change in or loss of vision
Flashes and floaters in visual fields
Gradual change in or loss of vision
Loss of red reflex

Medical ophthalmology and uveitis

CONNECTIVE TISSUE DISEASES

Rheumatoid arthritis

Rheumatoid arthritis (RA) is a chronic systemic inflammatory condition characterized by a persistent, peripheral, symmetrical polyarthritis. It is a common disease affecting females more than males (F>M).

General, neuromuscular and ocular features are shown in Table 42.1.

Systemic lupus erythematosus

Systemic lupus erythematosus (SLE) is a multisystem autoimmune condition characterized by autoantibodies to double-stranded DNA (dsDNA). Antigen–antibody complex deposition may result in the kidneys being affected. Females are affected more than males (F>M).

General, renal, ocular and retinopathy features of SLE are shown in Table 42.2.

Table 42.1 General, neuromuscular, and ocular features of rheumatoid arthritis (TIP: ACRONYMS: RUN, VAN, LAP, MAN.SPEK.)

General features	Neuromuscular		Ocular
Vascular: (RUN) • Raynaud phenomenon • Ulceration of skin • Nailfolds splinter haemorrhages	Lung nodules and fibrosis	Proximal myopathy	Scleritis (MCQ: not iritis)
Arthritis: predominately peripheral and symmetrical	Amyloidosis of kidneys	Atlantoaxial subluxation (cervical vertebra level 1 and 2) may result in spinal cord compression	Peripheral corneal thinning may perforate if very severe
Nodules: tendons, internal organs and pressure points (TIP)	Pericarditis	Sensory neuropathy	Episcleritis
Keratoconjunctivitis sicca – 'dry eyes', also associated with Sjogren syndrome			

(From *Crash Course: Ophthalmology, Dermatology, and ENT*. 3rd ed. Elsevier.)

Table 42.2 General, renal, ocular and retinopathy features of systemic lupus erythematosus (TIP: ACRONYMS: BRAN, Renal PRHO, PEN.SPEK.)

General features		Kidneys	Ocular features	Retinopathy
Facial butterfly rash	Pericarditis	Proteinuria	Scleritis	'Primary' retinal vasculitis (with cotton wool spots – disc oedema and haemorrhages)
Raynaud phenomenon	Lungs: pleurisy, effusions and fibrosis	Chronic renal failure	Peripheral corneal thinning	
Polyarthralgia symmetrical	Peripheral	Hypertension	Eyelid erythema	
and migratory	Neuropathy			
Nailfold infarcts	Psychosis	Nephritic syndrome	Keratoconjunctivitis	'Secondary' to hypertension
		(i.e., oedema)	Sicca	

(From *Crash Course: Ophthalmology, Dermatology, and ENT*. 3rd ed. Elsevier.)

Scleroderma

Chronic disease dominated by cutaneous manifestations. Females are affected more than males (F>M). SCL70, anti-centromere antibody blood tests. It can be part of CREST syndrome.

General, CREST syndrome and ocular features are shown in Table 42.3.

Polymyositis and dermatomyositis

Insidious, symmetrical, proximal muscle weakness results from muscle inflammation. This is a rare condition more common in females than males (F>M). Blood tests: CK, ANA, smooth muscle and Jo1 autoantibodies.

General and ocular features are listed in Table 42.4.

VASCULITIDES

Giant cell arteritis

Giant cell arteritis (GCA) or temporal arteritis is an arteritis affecting any extracranial medium and large muscular arteries. GCA is an ophthalmic emergency as permanent vision loss is a feared complication of GCA. Patients are usually more than 50 years old.

Symptoms

The main symptoms that should raise suspicious of GCA include:

- Headache

Table 42.3 General, CREST syndrome and ocular features of scleroderma (TIP: ACRONYM: MI. renal PRHo. CREST. SPEK, LER.)

General features	CREST syndrome	Ocular features
Microstoma – 'purse string mouth'	Calcinosis	Tight skin over eyelids causing punctal ectropion
Nailfold infarcts	Raynaud phenomenon	Keratoconjunctivitis sicca
Lungs: fibrosis	Oesophageal and small intestine fibrosis, causing dysphagia and malabsorption	Lagophthalmos
Heart: myocarditis and pericarditis	Sclerodactyly	Epiphora
Kidneys: renal failure and hypertension	Telangiectasia	Retinopathy usually caused by renal hypertension

(From *Crash Course: Ophthalmology, Dermatology, and ENT*. 3rd ed. Elsevier.)

Table 42.4 General and ocular features of polymyositis and dermatomyositis (TIP: ACRONYM: CREST.FANISH.ROPED. N.B. Scleroderma CREST syndrome is different.)

General features		Ocular features
Cardiomyopathy		
Raynaud phenomena	Lung fibrosis	Retinopathy with cotton wool spots
Oesophageal dysphagia and dysphonia from laryngeal and pharyngeal muscle involvement	Arthralgia	Periorbital oedema
(Shoulder and hip) muscular girdle weakness	Nailfold infarcts	Purple eyelids – or a heliotrope rash
Telangiectasia	Skin: purple (heliotrope) rash (in 25% patients)	Diplopia – resulting from ocular myopathy

(From *Crash Course: Ophthalmology, Dermatology, and ENT*. 3rd ed. Elsevier.)

- Jaw claudication.
- Tender, palpable temporal artery.
- Systemic symptoms: lethargy, depression, anorexia and night sweats.

Main ocular complication is anterior ischemic optic neuropathy, which arises from the occlusion of the posterior ciliary artery, leading to ischemia of the optic nerve head (Fig. 42.1).

Investigations

- ESR is elevated (CRP may also be elevated).
- Fundoscopy: swollen pale disc and blurred margins.
- Temporal artery biopsy is usually performed within 1 week to confirm diagnosis.

Histology shows:

- Artery wall thickened by inflammatory cells (histiocytes, lymphocytes, and giant cells, fibrinoid necrosis); skip lesions.
- Discontinuous internal elastic lamina (IEL) can be detected not just within 1 week, but as long as 28 days later.

Treatment

If GCA is suspected in a patient, you should administer treatment prior to sending the patient for a temporal biopsy.

- High-dose prednisolone should be used if there is no visual loss.
- Evolving visual loss: IV methylprednisolone should be administered.

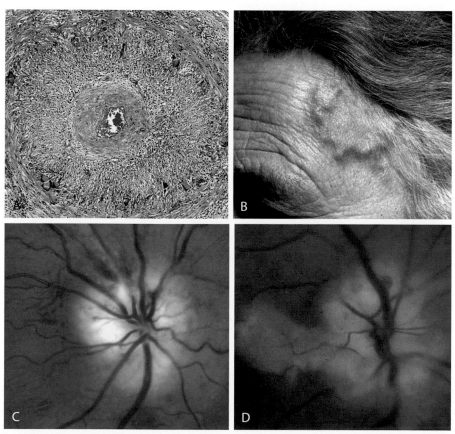

Fig. 42.1 Giant cell arteritis. (A) Histology shows transmural granulomatous inflammation, disruption of the internal elastic lamina, proliferation of the intima and gross narrowing of the lumen. (B) The superficial temporal artery is pulseless, nodular and thickened. (C) Ischemic optic neuropathy. (D) Ischemic optic neuropathy and cilioretinal artery occlusion. (From Kanski JJ, Bowling B. *Clinical Ophthalmology: a Systematic Approach*. 7th ed. Philadelphia: Saunders; 2010.)

UVEITIS

Uveitis is a term used to describe inflammation of the uveal tract. The uveal tract is comprised of the iris, ciliary body and choroid. Uveitis may occur in isolation, secondary to another intraocular problem or as part of systemic disease (Fig. 42.2). The systemic causes of uvetits and treatment is outlined in Table 42.6.

Classification of uveitis

Uveitis may be classified in a number of different ways.
See Table 42.5.

HINTS AND TIPS

There are three types of uveitis: anterior, intermediate or posterior. It is therefore important to dilate the pupil, view the retina and check whether cells are present in the vitreous cavity and to ascertain if the posterior segment is involved.

Anterior uveitis

This refers to iritis or iridocyclitis and is the most common form. The majority of patients only ever have one episode with no recurrences. The cause is usually idiopathic but has an association with HLA-B27 (Fig. 42.3).

Patients typically complain of an acutely painful, red eye with photophobia, because the iris is moving in a sticky environment.

Other symptoms may include:

- blurred vision
- ciliary flush
- impaired visual acuity

The signs of uveitis are listed below:

- Cells/flare in the anterior chamber
- Hypopyon
- Keratic precipitates (KP) fine or 'mutton fat', i.e., granulomas
- High/low or normal IOP
- Posterior synechiae (PS)
- Peripheral anterior synechiae (PAS)
- Iris bombé
- Angle closure glaucoma
- Cataract

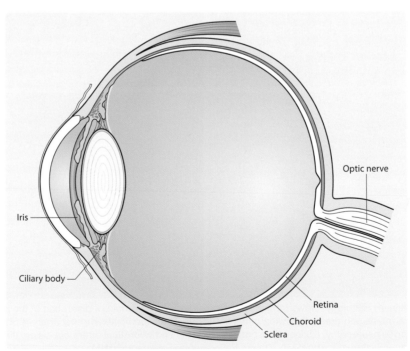

Fig. 42.2 Anatomy of the uveal tract: iris, ciliary body and choroid. (From *Crash Course: Ophthalmology, Dermatology, and ENT*. 3rd ed. Elsevier.)

Investigation

Do not forget a dilated fundus examination to exclude any posterior segment involvement. Granulomatous, recurrent or bilateral uveitis episodes warrant referral to ophthalmologists and further investigations.

> **HINTS AND TIPS**
>
> When all parts of the uveal tract are inflamed, it is referred to as panuveitis and may be an indicator of underlying systemic disease.

Treatment

- Cycloplegia (pain relief and to prevent posterior synaechiae), e.g., cyclopentolate or atropine.
- Antiinflammatory drops (steroids).
- Control any rise in IOP (avoid prostaglandin analogues).
- Add systemic/local steroid if indicated (see text).
- Treat any underlying cause, e.g., sarcoidosis.

Table 42.5 Classification of uveitis

Anatomy
- Anterior
- Intermediate
- Posterior
- Panuveitis

Duration
- Acute
- Chronic

Age of onset
- Infantile
- Juvenile
- Adult

Granulomas
- Granulomatous
- Nongranulomatous

(From *Crash Course: Ophthalmology, Dermatology, and ENT.* 3rd ed. Elsevier.)

Specific causes of anterior uveitis

HLA-B27 +ve

Patients with this particular haplotype are more susceptible to iritis. There is no specific treatment other than for the iritis. They should be investigated for ankylosing spondylitis.

Below is a list of HLA-B27 +ve conditions:

- ankylosing spondylitis
- reactive arthritis
- psoriatic arthritis

Autoimmune conditions

- Juvenile idiopathic arthritis-associated uveitis
- Inflammatory bowel disease – which includes Crohn disease and ulcerative colitis
- Behçet disease
- Sarcoidosis
- Systemic lupus erythematous

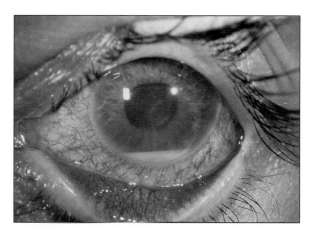

Fig. 42.3 HLA-B27–related acute anterior uveitis. This severe case of anterior uveitis demonstrates fibrin clot formation and hypopyon in the anterior chamber. (From Yanoff M, Duker J. *Ophthalmology.* 6th ed. Elsevier; 2023.)

Table 42.6 Identification of systemic cause of uveitis and treatment modification

Systemic cause of uveitis	Modification of therapy
Sarcoidosis	Respiratory physician referral and systemic steroids +/– disease modifying agent may be added later
Ankylosing spondylitis	Rheumatology physician referral and may require systemic nonsteroidal antiinflammatory drug
Reiter syndrome	Treat the urethritis, e.g., with doxycycline Rheumatology physician referral for arthritis
Juvenile idiopathic arthritis (JIA)	Rheumatology referral and systemic steroids +/– disease modifying agent may be added later

(From *Crash Course: Ophthalmology, Dermatology, and ENT.* 3rd ed. Elsevier.)

Infectious causes of uveitis

Tuberculosis

Tuberculosis is a granulomatous disease and about 2% to 5% of patients have ocular uveitic manifestations, including:

- mutton fat keratic precipitates
- panuveitis
- choroidal granulomas
- multifocal choroiditis
- retinal ischaemia/neovascularization
- optic disc oedema

One should always test for TB – Mantoux test. Treatment is with (ACRONYM: RIPE):

- **R**ifampicin
- **I**soniazid
- **P**yrazinamide
- **E**thambutol

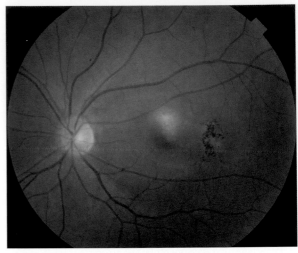

Fig. 42.4 Necrotizing retinochoroiditis satellite to old hyperpigmented scars in ocular toxoplasmosis. (From Sadda SR, et al. *Ryan's Retina*. 7th ed. Elsevier; 2023.)

Syphilis

The eye can be involved in syphilis (secondary and tertiary disease).

Secondary syphilis can lead to:

- Iridocyclitis (granulomatous (gumma)/nongranulomatous).
- Cornea (interstitial keratitis).
- Chorioretinitis:
    1. Multifocal or diffuse.
    2. Massive pigmentary change.
    3. Neuroretinitis (disc and macular oedema, cotton wool spots and haemorrhages).

Syphilis can be diagnosed with an FTA-Abs test. Treatment is with penicillin or doxycycline.

Toxoplasmosis

Toxoplasmosis is a parasitic infection that can infect the eye in utero (congenital) and postnatally. Congenital toxoplasmosis can affect the eye (e.g., choroid and then retina) and the rest of the embryo (e.g., brain and chest). Infected children may be normal or have multiple birth defects depending on the age of inoculation.

Adult toxoplasmosis may be primary (rare) or a reactivation of an old locus of infection.

Primary toxoplasmosis is usually acquired from the ingestion of undercooked/raw meat. These patients have an ill-defined pale chorioretinitis with a mild-to-moderate amount of vitreous activity (Fig. 42.4).

Secondary/reactivated toxoplasmosis has a classic appearance of a pigmented scar with adjacent white fluffy infiltrate.

There is often an intense vitritis making the view of the retina difficult. Vision may be reduced from cystoid macular oedema, direct or indirect foveal involvement (e.g., branch retinal artery or vein occlusion).

Patients are treated if they have:

- Lesions within the macula (particularly between disc and fovea).
- Lesions adjacent to the disc.
- Lesions overlying a major vessel (risk of vein occlusion).

Treatment

Treatment is with one of two regimens:

1. Pyrimethamine, sulphadiazine, folinic acid and oral steroid.
2. Clindamycin and oral steroid.

Herpes zoster

Herpes zoster can affect any part of the eye. It is a DNA virus that lies dormant on the ganglia of sensory nerves (e.g., trigeminal ganglion in herpes zoster ophthalmicus (HZO) or the dorsal root ganglion in shingles).

HZO classically presents with a tingling sensation over the scalp and forehead of affected patients. The rash subsequently develops, not crossing the mid-line. Direct ocular involvement may follow any time after the appearance of the rash. There is increased likelihood of intraocular involvement if there are vesicles on the tip of the nose (Hutchinson's sign) or lid margin.

The diagnosis tends to be made clinically, though antibodies may be tested.

The consequence of a herpes zoster infection to the eye are shown in Table 42.7.

Treatment

If patients have posterior segment disease or an orbital apex syndrome, systemic antiviral treatment should be commenced immediately, as there is a risk of developing encephalitis. IV aciclovir 800 mg for five days can be given.

Cytomegalovirus

Cytomegalovirus (CMV) is a ubiquitous virus that is usually nonpathogenic. However, in immunocompromised individuals (e.g., AIDS or posttransplant), CMV retinitis may occur.

This is seen clinically as a progressive retinitis (see Fig. 42.5) with cotton wool spots and haemorrhages. Retinal thinning and secondary rhegmatogenous retinal detachment may develop (Fig. 42.5).

The diagnosis is made clinically or with vitreous biopsy and PCR.

Treatment is with systemic and intraocular antiviral agents (e.g., ganciclovir, foscarnet, cidofovir). If retinal detachments develop, they usually require silicone oil insertion.

HIV

HIV infection may affect the eye directly, or secondary opportunistic infections may cause problems.

See Tables 42.8 and 42.9 for some HIV-related eye signs and a list of opportunistic diseases affecting the retina in HIV patients.

Endophthalmitis

This term describes inflammation of one or more coats of the eye with contiguous cavity inflammation. It is usually reserved for infections of the eye and can be classified according to cause, onset or causative organism. Acute causes are usually caused by a *Staphylococcus* infection (e.g., *Staphylococcus epidermidis* or *Staphylococcus aureus*) (Fig. 42.6).

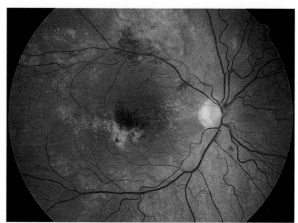

Fig. 42.5 Cytomegalovirus (CMV) retinitis with haemorrhagic areas is seen superior to the fovea and a denser area just below the fovea. Borders are opaque and associated with variable amounts of haemorrhage. (From Sadda SR, et al. *Ryan's Retina*. 7th ed. Elsevier; 2023.)

Table 42.7 Consequences of herpes zoster infection to the eye

Region of the eye affected	Features
Lids	Rash Ptosis (isolated or part of a cranial nerve III nerve palsy or Horner syndrome)
Extraocular muscle	Motor nerve palsy, single or multiple
Conjunctiva	Follicular conjunctivitis
Scleritis	Necrotizing scleritis Sclerokeratitis
Cornea	Epitheliopathy with reduced sensation (small erosions) Stromal disease including interstitial keratitis. Endotheliitis
Iris	Iritis Ischaemia (iris sector atrophy)
Lens	Cataract formation
Vitreous	Vitritis
Retina	Retinitis Central/branch vein occlusion Retinal detachment
Optic nerve	Optic neuritis Ischaemic optic neuropathy

Endophthalmitis may occur following:

- Intraocular surgery (risk is about 0.1%–0.2%).
- Penetrating trauma (up to 10% risk of endophthalmitis).
- Draining glaucoma bleb (increased risk in mitomycin C blebs).
- Endogenous (very rare, occurs in septic patients).

Patients presenting soon after surgery or following trauma with very painful red eyes should be referred urgently. If they develop a hypopyon, they should be managed as an endophthalmitis. The prognosis is often poor for these patients, especially if there is any delay in diagnosis.

Investigation and management of endophthalmitis

- Appropriate history and ocular examination performed (check for hypopyon).
- Patients should be prepared for aqueous and vitreous tap and intravitreal antibiotic injection.
- Vitreous tap performed with local anaesthesia (topical and subtenon injection). 0.1 mL of aqueous and 0.1 mL of vitreous aspirated.
- Intravitreal vancomycin (1 mg/0.1 mL) with either ceftazidime (2 mg/0.1 mL) or amikacin (0.4 mg/0.1 mL). If fungal infection suspected intravitreal amphotericin (10 μg) is also given.
- Topical and oral ciprofloxacin (good intraocular penetration) commenced.

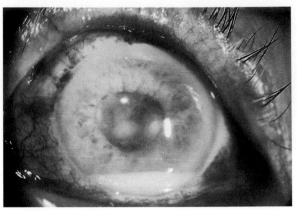

Fig. 42.6 Hypopyon in patient with postoperative endophthalmitis. (From Garg S, Koch D. *Steinert's Cataract Surgery*, 4th ed. Elsevier; 2023.)

HINTS AND TIPS

Any postoperative acute red eye (e.g., cataract surgery in past 2 weeks) with increasing pain and/or decreased vision is suggestive of infection and should be referred immediately for ophthalmic review. Always check the vision to have an early point of reference.

Table 42.8 A small selection of HIV-related eye signs

Part of eye	Some HIV-related eye signs
Conjunctiva	Conjunctivitis Kaposi sarcoma (may be hidden in fornix)
Retina	Mild retinitis with occasional haemorrhages and/or cotton wool spots

(From *Crash Course: Ophthalmology, Dermatology, and ENT*. 3rd ed. Elsevier.)

Table 42.9 Opportunistic diseases affecting the retina in HIV patients

Part of eye	Opportunistic diseases
Retina	Cytomegalovirus
	Herpes zoster/simplex
	Toxoplasmosis
	Syphilis

(From *Crash Course: Ophthalmology, Dermatology, and ENT*. 3rd ed. Elsevier.)

● Chapter Summary

- Giant cell arteritis is an ophthalmic emergency as permanent vision loss is a feared complication. If GCA is suspected in a patient, you should give high-dose steroids as treatment prior to confirmation of diagnosis.
- The uveal tract consists of the iris, ciliary body and choroid. Anterior uveitis refers to inflammation of the iris and is the most common subtype. The cause is usually idiopathic but can be associated with HLA B27.
- Anterior uveitis presents with an acutely painful red eye with photophobia. Treatment includes cycloplegics (e.g., atropine) and steroids eye drops.
- Infective causes of uveitis include tuberculosis, syphilis, toxoplasmosis, herpes zoster virus and cytomegalovirus.
- Patients presenting with acute painful red eye following intraocular surgery should raise suspicion on endophthalmitis and should be referred urgently to an ophthalmologist.

UKMLA Conditions
Iritis
Uveitis

UKMLA Presentations
Acute change in or loss of vision
Diplopia
Eye pain/discomfort
Ptosis
Red eye

Neuro-ophthalmology

INTRODUCTION

Neuro-ophthalmology describes the interaction between the eye and the rest of the nervous system. Broadly, the eyes can be directly affected in neurological disease or act as an indicator of central nervous system problems such as tumours or vascular events such as stroke.

ANATOMY

Neuro-ophthalmic diagnosis relies on a good knowledge of anatomy. This relates in particular to the optic nerve pathway, pathways governing eye movement and control of the pupil. See Fig. 43.1 and Table 43.1 for the visual pathway and the characteristic field defects produced.

Optic nerve

The optic nerve is made up of approximately 1.5 million ganglion cell axons (first-order neurons). The nerve courses posteriorly and medially through the orbit to enter the anterior cranial fossa through the optic canal and then onwards to the optic chiasm. Fibres derived from the nasal retina decussate at the chiasm while temporal fibres remain ipsilateral. The chiasm lies above the pituitary gland and is thus the portion of the pathway affected by pituitary tumours.

Optic tract

Fibres run from the optic chiasm to the lateral geniculate body to synapse with the second-order neurons, which then form the optic radiations. A group of fibres (about 10%) leave the tract to synapse directly in the pretectal nucleus (part of the autonomic system) which drives pupillary responses via the third cranial nerve.

Optic radiations

Following synapse in the lateral geniculate body, the nerve fibres fan out and run through the parietal and temporal lobe. These fibres then recongregate within the occipital lobe cortex.

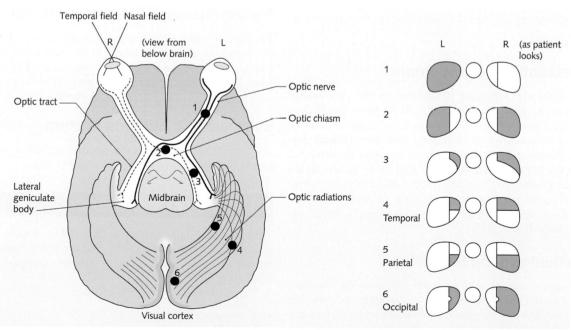

Fig. 43.1 Lesions of different parts of the visual pathway produce characteristic field defects. (From *Crash Course: Neurology*. 4th ed. Elsevier; 2016.)

Table 43.1 Visual field defects according to location of lesion along visual pathway

Location of lesion	Type of field defect
Optic nerve	Complete monocular
Optic chiasm	Bitemporal hemianopia
Optic tract	Homonymous hemianopia
Optic radiations (temporal lobe)	Homonymous superior quadrantanopia ('pie in the sky')
Occipital lobe (visual cortex)	Homonymous hemianopia
Occipital cortex macular sparing	Homonymous hemianopia with macula sparing

(From *Crash Course: Ophthalmology, Dermatology, and ENT*. 3rd ed. Elsevier.)

HINTS AND TIPS

The patient's right visual field projects to the left occipital cortex and vice versa. Try not to get confused between the examiners and the patient's perspective of left or right.

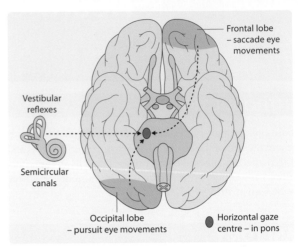

Fig. 43.2 The horizontal gaze centre, which lies in the pons, coordinates signals originating from the vestibular system, frontal and occipital lobes. (From *Crash Course: Ophthalmology, Dermatology, and ENT*. 3rd ed. Elsevier.)

EYE MOVEMENTS

Eye movements are controlled by various intraocuular muscles (see Fig. 43.3).

Horizontal eye movement

Horizontal eye movement is mediated via the para-median pontine reticular formation (PPRF) in the pons. This nucleus lies in the pons adjacent to the sixth nerve nucleus. The PPRF also coordinates signals originating from the vestibular system, frontal and occipital lobes. Communicating fibres run from the PPRF to the contralateral third nerve nucleus via the medial longitudinal fasciculus (MLF). Effectively the contralateral medial rectus activity is driven at the same time as the ipsilateral lateral rectus; thus, we have 'comitant', i.e., linked, eye movement (Fig. 43.2).

Vertical eye movement

Vertical eye movement is mediated higher up the brainstem in the rostral interstitial (ri) MLF in the upper midbrain. The communication is via posterior commissure fibres which run behind the aqueduct of Sylvius. These fibres extend to both third nerve nuclei and drive vertical gaze.

AUTONOMIC CONTROL OF THE PUPIL

The pupil size is controlled by the autonomic nervous system (there is both parasympathetic and sympathetic innervation).

Parasympathetic nervous system

The parasympathetic fibres originate in the Edinger–Westphal (EW) nucleus which sits adjacent to the third nerve nucleus. Fibres (10%) from the optic tract synapse in the EW nucleus. Fibres from the EW nucleus run with the third nerve and innervate the ciliary muscle and constrictor pupillae.

Sympathetic nervous system

The sympathetic fibres innervate the dilator pupillae, Müller's muscle (in lid), lacrimal glands and orbital vessels.

PUPILLARY DISORDERS

The pupil reacts (gets smaller) to light and convergent stimulus. Light induces pupillary constriction through the light reflex mediated through the optic nerve (afferent) and parasympathetic fibres (efferent).

The accommodation reflex is a triad of:

- convergence
- lens thickening
- miosis

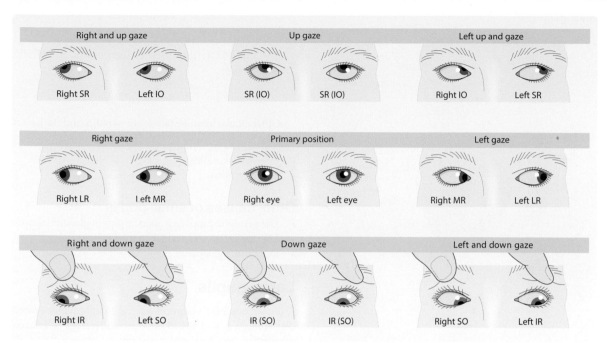

Fig. 43.3 Muscles responsible for eye movements. The primary position refers to the position of the eyes when looking straight ahead. IO, *Inferior oblique;* IR, *Inferior rectus;* LR, *Lateral rectus;* MR, *Medial rectus;* SO, *Superior oblique;* SR, *Superior rectus.* (From Yogarajah M. *Crash Course: Neurology.* 4th ed. Elsevier; 2016.)

The accommodation reflex is mediated through the parasympathetic system; however, the centre mediating the response is poorly defined, thus some conditions affecting the parasympathetic fibres between the pretectal nucleus and EW nucleus lead to 'light-near dissociation', i.e., they can still accommodate but cannot react to light. This is classically seen with Argyll Robertson pupils in syphilis and Parinaud (dorsal midbrain) syndrome (Fig. 43.4).

Specific conditions affecting the pupil

Before considering a pathological cause of anisocoria, it must be remembered that up to 10% of the population have physiological anisocoria (pupil difference >2 mm that is constant in light or dark conditions).

Relative afferent pupillary defect

A lesion of the visual pathway anterior to the lateral geniculate body may result in an afferent pupillary defect. If a light is shone into the normal eye, the direct and consensual responses are normal; if a light is shone into the affected eye, pupil constriction is slow and may be incomplete.

If the light is swung from one eye to the other (3–4 s on each eye), both pupils will constrict appropriately during illumination of the normal eye but both will then dilate as the light shines into the abnormal visual pathway; this results from impairment of the afferent arc of the light reflex on the abnormal side.

The most common cause of a relative afferent pupillary defect (RAPD) is optic neuritis.

Small pupils

Horner syndrome

This is characterized by the classic clinical triad of PAM (ptosis, anhidrosis, miosis) (see Fig. 43.5), or for multiple choice questions try PACME(H):

- **P**tosis (slight due to paralysis of Müller muscle).
- **A**nhidrosis (ipsilateral decreased sweating in post-ganglionic lesion).
- **C**iliospinal reflex (lost; a rarely known vestigial reflex).
- **M**iosis.
- **E**nophthalmos (apparent; not true if lid elevated by 1 mm).
- **H**eterochromia (in congenital cases).

> **HINTS AND TIPS**
>
> Painful (i.e., headache) Horner syndrome is an emergency and the patient should be referred for investigation of a carotid artery dissection.

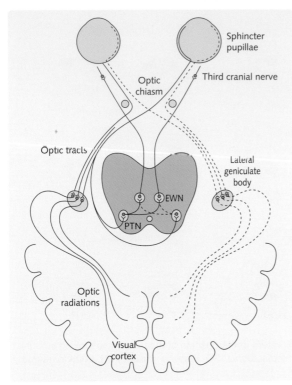

Fig. 43.4 Schematic of light reflex and visual field pathway. Pretectal area *(PTN)* and Edinger–Westphal nucleus *(EWN)* are both at the level of the midbrain. (From *Crash Course: Ophthalmology, Dermatology, and ENT.* 3rd ed. Elsevier.)

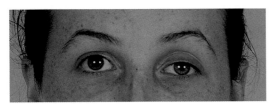

Fig. 43.5 Left-sided Horner syndrome with ptosis (drooped eyelid) and miosis (constricted pupil). In addition, Horner syndrome can lead to different eye colours (heterochromia). (Courtesy of Shriners Hospital for Children, Philadelphia.)

Argyll Robertson pupil

This is a small, irregular pupil that reacts poorly to light. The near reflex is intact.

Argyll Robertson pupil (ARP) is usually seen in neurosyphilis and can occur in diabetes mellitus.

Other ocular manifestations of syphilis should be sought, such as:

- interstitial keratitis
- chorioretinitis

Other causes of small pupils
- Use of miotic drops (e.g., pilocarpine in glaucoma patients).
- Due to posterior synechiae in iritis patients.
- Drug use, e.g., opiates.

Large pupils

A dilated pupil is a common referral to ophthalmic emergency departments and is usually due to inadvertent pharmacological dilation which should be sought on history. It can also be a marker for serious conditions such as an intracerebral aneurysm or haemorrhage causing a third nerve palsy.

Holmes–Adie pupil

Patients present with a dilated pupil and often blurred vision. This may come on after a viral illness which affects the ciliary ganglion. There is a very slow reaction to light and slow reaction to accommodation.

If there is associated loss of deep tendon reflexes it is referred to as Holmes–Adie syndrome.

Trauma

Following globe trauma, the iris sphincter may be damaged leading to a large pupil that reacts poorly. Clinically there may be iris transillumination defects seen and angle recession on gonioscopy. These patients are at risk of developing glaucoma.

MOTILITY DISORDERS

Motility disorders refer to any disorder of eye movement. This includes extraocular muscles (isolated nerve palsies, multiple nerve palsies or myogenic causes), brainstem lesions, central brain lesions and nystagmus.

Third cranial nerve palsy

The third cranial nerve innervates the superior, inferior and medial recti, inferior oblique and levator palpebrae superioris (LPS), which opens the eyelid. The parasympathetic third nerve, from the EW nucleus, supplies the pupil and ciliary body. See Table 43.2 for summary of third cranial nerve lesions.

Clinical appearance

The key discerning feature in assessing patients with third nerve palsy is the presence or absence of pupil involvement (dilated).

Should the pupil be involved there is a greater likelihood of a compressive lesion (such as an aneurysm of the posterior communicating artery) and a CT scan or MRI angiogram should be attained immediately.

In third nerve palsy without pupil involvement the incidence of a compressive lesion is far less and the usual cause is microvascular disease in patients over 50 years old.

The affected eye is exotropic, intorted and hypotropic (i.e., 'down and out'), due to unopposed action of the fourth and sixth cranial nerves. There may be:

- Ptosis (a droopy lid)
- Diplopia (horizontal and vertical) due to limited ocular movements
- Abnormal head posture (chin elevation and face turn in direction of palsy)
- Dilated pupil

There may or may not be all of these features, depending on the extent of palsy (i.e., complete or incomplete palsy).

Causes of a third nerve palsy

Aetiology

Pupil-involving: compression from posterior communicating artery aneurysm, intracranial tumours, closed head trauma.

Pupil-sparing: microvascular (ischaemia from diabetes and hypertension), giant cell arteritis, multiple sclerosis and cavernous sinus disease.

Differential diagnosis of third nerve palsy

- Myasthenia gravis (classically a fluctuating diplopia, fatiguability).
- Orbital inflammatory lesions (e.g., orbital lymphoma, orbital myositis, thyroid eye disease).
- Chronic progressive external ophthalmoplegia.
- Midbrain disease (abnormal ocular motility, e.g., with an internuclear ophthalmoplegia that looks like a medial rectus weakness).

Table 43.2 Third (oculomotor) cranial nerve lesions

3rd nerve and nucleus lesions give rise to
- Diplopia in all directions of gaze
- Lateral and downward deviation of the eye
- Ptosis (partial or full)
- A dilated pupil unresponsive to light and accommodation
- (There is often only partial involvement, and therefore the clinical signs may not include all of the features indicated above: e.g. partial ptosis, pupil-sparing, not all muscles supplied by the 3rd nerve affected)

Causes

3rd nerve lesions
- ICA/PcomA/Basilar/PCA/SCA aneurysm
- Cavernous sinus thrombosis
- Lesions of the superior orbital fissure (malignant infiltration)
- Microvascular - diabetes or vasculitis

Midbrain lesions affecting the 3rd nucleus
- Infarction
- Demyelination
- Glioma
- Metastasis

In midbrain lesions, also look for:
- A contralateral hemiplegia
- Ipsilateral limb ataxia
- Coarse rubral tremor (involvement of cerebellar and red nuclear fibres)

Patient looking forwards

Patient looking in the direction of the arrow

ICA, internal carotid artery; PcomA, posterior communicating artery; PCA, posterior cerebral artery; SCA, superior cerebellar artery

(From *Crash Course: Neurology.* 4th ed. Elsevier; 2016.)

Fourth cranial nerve palsy

Fourth nerve palsy affects the superior oblique muscle (SOM) leading to its paresis. The SOM is responsible for intorsion, abduction and downgaze. SOM is the major intorter, i.e., rotational movement around the z-axis such that the superior globe rotates medially and the inferior globe rotates laterally. The superior rectus has a limited intorting role. See Table 43.2 for summary of fourth cranial nerve lesion.

Causes

The nerve is fine with a long intracranial course and is thus susceptible to damage from head trauma. Other causes of palsy are:

- Congenital. Patients may be asymptomatic for years. They typically have large vertical fusional amplitudes, tested with a synoptophore, unlike traumatic fourth nerve palsies.
- Vascular (diabetes, hypertension).
- Demyelination.
- Tumour (intracranial).
- Giant cell arteritis.
- Aneurysm.

Clinical features

The features/signs of a fourth nerve palsy can be quite subtle and unless specifically tested for may not be detected.

- Diplopia (on depression, mainly vertical and torsional).
- Abnormal head posture (head tilt and face turn to unaffected eye and chin depression).
- Diagnosis is made with a head tilt test (tilting the head to the ipsilateral side induces an upward movement of the globe. This is due to unopposed superior rectus action: the other intorter of the eye).

Sixth cranial nerve palsy

This is probably the most commonly recognized nerve palsy and can be quite dramatic for the patient and their family. The sixth nerve innervates the lateral rectus muscle responsible for abduction of the eye. See Table 43.4 for summary of sixth cranial nerve lesion.

Causes

Causes of sixth nerve palsies depend on site of the lesion and are largely the same as those causing third and fourth nerve palsy. The sixth nerve is particularly vulnerable to damage caused by raised intracranial pressure (ICP) and is therefore often described as a 'false localizing sign' because it provides no information as to the site of the lesion.

Clinical features

Sixth nerve palsies are often quite apparent with an obvious ipsilateral convergent squint due to unopposed medial rectus action. This esotropia deviation is worse on distance fixation. Horizontal diplopia and abnormal head posture (face turn towards affected eye) may also be present.

Table 43.3 Fourth (trochlear) cranial nerve lesions

4th nerve and nucleus lesions give rise to paralysis of the superior oblique muscle:
- Vertical and oblique diplopia on looking down and inwards
- The eye sits rotated slightly outwards and upwards (extorsion)
- The patient tries to compensate by tilting the head away from the affected eye

Causes

4th nerve lesions
- Isolated 4th nerve lesions are rare and usually due to diabetes (ischaemic infarction of the nerve) or trauma
- Lesions of the cavernous sinus and superior orbital fissure will involve the 3rd and 6th nerves, and branches of the 5th nerve

Midbrain lesions affecting the 4th nucleus
- Infarction
- Demyelination
- Glioma
- Metastasis

Patient looking forwards

Patient looking in the direction of the arrow
- The right eye fails to depress and adduct.

Note: The weakness of the superior oblique muscle is contralateral to the side of a lesion at nuclear level. Many patients show a head tilt to the side opposite to that of the defective eye

(From *Crash Course: Neurology.* 4th ed. Elsevier; 2016.)

Nystagmus

Nystagmus is repetitive involuntary to and fro oscillation of the eyes. An ophthalmological referral should be made. It may be horizontal, vertical or torsional.

The most common type seen is horizontal nystagmus. Note the description of the direction of the nystagmus is based on the fast phase (jerk) component (e.g., downbeat nystagmus has a slow upward drift with a rapid downward movement). Occasionally there is no fast and slow phase, but phases of equal speed; this is pendular nystagmus.

Table 43.4 Sixth (abducens) cranial nerve lesions

6th nerve and nucleus lesions give rise to paralysis of the lateral rectus muscle:
- Horizontal diplopia maximal on lateral gaze to the side of the lesion. A convergent strabismus may be evident in the primary position, but becomes more apparent on abduction of the affected eye

Causes

6th nerve lesions
- Microvascular - diabetes or vasculitis
- Trauma
- Vertebral or basilar aneurysm
- Gradenigo's syndrome - due to infection of the petrous temporal bone
- Cavernous sinus thrombosis
- Fracture or malignant infiltration (nasopharyngeal carcinoma) of the skull base
- Lesions of the superior orbital fissure

Pontine lesions affecting the 6th nucleus
- Infarction
- Demyelination
- Glioma
- Metastasis

In pontine lesions, also look for:
- A contralateral hemiplegia
- Ipsilateral weakness of the upper and lower face (7th nerve fibres hooking around the 6th nucleus)

Patient looking forwards

Patient looking in the direction of the arrow

(From Crash Course: Neurology. 4th ed. Elsevier; 2016)

Types

Nystagmus can be physiological (i.e., may be induced in normal individuals) or pathological (i.e., exist as a specific entity or part of an associated condition).

Physiological nystagmus

In certain situations or conditions, it is normal to have mild nystagmus.

- Caloric testing refers to the instillation of warm and/or cold water into the ear of patients to induce a nystagmus.
- Gaze-evoked nystagmus. It is normal to have a mild nystagmus on extreme left or right gaze. When testing eye movements with nystagmus, just move the eye about 30 degrees from the midline.

Acquired nystagmus

Unlike congenital nystagmus patients, those with recent onset nystagmus may complain of oscillopsia, i.e., 'everything moves around'. This may be seen with:

- Recent visual loss (e.g., trauma).
- Toxicity (e.g., alcohol, phenothiazines or Wernicke encephalopathy).
- Cerebral disease (stroke, MS or tumour).

Management: patients presenting with recent onset nystagmus need to have full history, full physical examination (especially neurological system), toxicity screen if history is indicative and neurological imaging.

Once identified, the cause should be treated, as appropriate.

OPTIC NERVE DISEASE

A number of clinical features should be sought if optic nerve dysfunction is suspected. See Table 43.5 for various causes of optic neuropathy. They include:

- Reduced visual acuity.
- Abnormal visual field (constricted in glaucoma, caecocentral (scotoma between central fixation and the blind spot) field loss).
- Reduced pupillary response (afferent pupil defect).
- Poor colour vision (tested with Ishihara plates or red desaturation test).

Clinical features

When examining an optic nerve, the following features of the disc should be observed and commented on:

- Neuroretinal rim.
- Swelling (may just be apparent as a hyperaemic disc initially).
- Haemorrhages.
- Atrophy.
- Notches.
- Cup/disc ratio (CDR).
- Glaucoma.
- Disc vessels.
- Retinal vessels.

Table 43.5 Causes of optic neuropathy

Mechanism	Examples
Inflammatory (optic neuritis)	Demyelination associated with multiple sclerosis - most common but others include: • acute disseminated encephalomyelitis (ADEM) • sarcoidosis • systemic autoimmune disease (e.g., SLE, Wegener's granulomatosis) • infection (e.g., toxoplasmosis, cat scratch fever, syphilis, Lyme disease)
Vascular	Ischaemic optic neuropathy - can be associated with vasculitis (e.g. giant cell arteritis) or associated with small vessel disease due to age, hypertension or diabetes
Space-occupying lesions	Compressive optic neuropathy due to optic nerve or orbital neoplasm (e.g., meningioma or glioma)
Toxins/drugs	Alcohol overuse, methanol, tobacco, amiodarone, ethambutol, post-radiotherapy
Nutritional deficiencies	Vitamins B_{12} and B_1, folate
Genetic	Leber's hereditary optic neuropathy- presents with subacute painless, sequential optic neuropathy over weeks to months
Raised intracranial pressure	Long-standing papilloedema can cause optic neuropathy
Trauma	

(From *Crash Course: Neurology*. 4th ed. Elsevier; 2016.)

- Peripapillary (area adjacent to the disc) zones.

Examples of different types of optic neuropathy include:

Management

If an optic neuropathy is suspected the following investigations should be performed:

- ESR (especially in a patient >50 years old with ION to exclude GCA).
- FBC.
- Visual field test (identify caecocentral field loss or associated bitemporal loss seen with pituitary tumours).

- Vitamin B_{12} and folate levels.
- Autoantibody screen.
- Orbital and brain imaging if a compressive optic neuropathy is suspected.
- Temporal artery biopsy is performed in cases of suspected GCA.

Once an underlying diagnosis is made, appropriate treatment can be implemented.

OPTIC DISC SWELLING

Optic disc swelling is a common referral to ophthalmologists and there are many causes. They can be broadly divided into:

- intracranial (papilloedema)
- ocular
- systemic

Papilloedema

Papilloedema is bilateral disc swelling due to raised ICP.

Symptoms

These patients may be asymptomatic or present with one or more of the following:

- Visual obscurations (transient loss of vision on standing up).
- Headache, nausea, vomiting or double vision (sixth nerve palsy).
- Reduced visual acuity.
- Reduced colour vision.

Signs

The signs of papilloedema are:

- Bilateral swollen hyperaemic discs.
- Disc haemorrhages.
- Visual field defect (specific if lesion affects optic pathway, enlarged blind spot initially or constricted field if papilloedema is longstanding).
- Absent spontaneous venous pulsations at the disc.
- 'Champagne cork' appearance in chronic papilloedema.
- Optic atrophy.

Causes

The common causes are:

- Idiopathic intracranial hypertension (IIH), an idiopathic condition affecting young overweight females, classically). They usually have a normal CT scan (+/− dilated ventricles).
- An intracranial tumour.

- Meningitis (patients have a fever +/− neck stiffness).
- Brain abscess (patients are moribund with a high fever).
- Sagittal sinus thrombosis.

The differential diagnosis for papilloedema is lengthy and is covered in the following sections on ocular and systemic causes of optic disc swelling.

Investigation

The investigations required are:

- Urgent CT scan to assess presence of a mass lesion.
- MRI scan may also be indicated to aid specific diagnosis.
- Lumbar punctures (high opening pressures in the presence of a normal CT scan may indicate IIH).

The management of papilloedema is directed towards the underlying cause and its treatment.

HINTS AND TIPS

Optic disc swelling is not the same as papilloedema. Papilloedema is bilateral swollen discs due to raised intracranial pressure (ICP).

Ocular causes

Many intrinsic ocular conditions may lead to disc swelling and are covered in more detail in other parts of the book. They include:

- Central retinal vein occlusion (retinal haemorrhages are also present in all four retinal fundus quadrants).
- Uveitis (particularly with posterior uveitis or scleritis; there may be contiguous optic nerve inflammation and swelling).
- Anterior ischaemic optic neuropathy (AION).
- Optic disc infiltration (can be granulomatous as in sarcoidosis or malignant as with leukaemia or metastases).
- Optic nerve tumours (e.g., glioma or meningioma; disc is swollen if there is rapid growth).
- Orbital thyroid disease (due to acute inflammation and swelling of the orbit).

Systemic causes

The most common and serious systemic condition associated with disc swelling is hypertension. Disc swelling indicates grade IV (or severe) hypertensive retinopathy and urgent treatment is required.

Thus, investigation of disc swelling should include blood pressure measurement and a full blood count.

CHIASMAL DISEASE

Symptoms

Disorders near the chiasm can affect the visual system, with patients complaining of:

- Blurred vision.
- Constricted field (bitemporal hemianopia – 'I bump into things doctor').
- Headache.

Ocular signs of chiasmal disease

- Bitemporal hemianopia.
- See-saw nystagmus.

Causes

- Pituitary tumour (compresses from below, thus supero-temporal field affected first).
- Meningioma.
- Craniopharyngioma (compresses from above, thus infero-temporal field affected first). Usually seen in younger patients.

Types of pituitary tumour

Adenomas

A detailed description of pituitary adenomas can be found in the Crash Course book on Medicine.

Pituitary apoplexy

This is a rare and potentially life-threatening condition. It is due to haemorrhage into a pituitary adenoma, often occurring in pregnancy. Patients present with severe headache +/− multiple motor nerve palsies.

Investigation of pituitary tumours

Imaging
- CT scan.
- MRI scan (better at detailing the relationship of the enlarged gland to the surrounding structure).

Endocrine tests
- Serum prolactin.
- FSH.
- TSH.
- Growth hormone.

These tests help identify the cell type in the tumour, explain systemic effects of the tumour (e.g., acromegaly) and monitor response to treatment.

Treatment

Pharmacological
Bromocriptine is used to treat prolactinomas.

Surgery
Patients may have their tumours removed by a transsphenoidal approach.

Radiotherapy
Meningiomas are slowly growing, histologically benign tumours which may affect any part of the meninges.

These lesions are treated by resection when accessible, with or without radiotherapy.

Chapter Summary

- The accommodation reflex is a triad of convergence, lens thickening and pupil constriction (miosis).
- Small pupils can be caused by: Horner syndrome is characterized by a clinical triad consisting of ptosis, anhidrosis, and miosis. Or Argyll Robertson pupil (ARP), which is usually seen in tertiary syphilis – remember acronym ARP: Accommodation Reflex is Preserved.
- Third cranial nerve palsy causes the affected eye to be 'down and out'.
- Fourth cranial nerve supplies the superior oblique extra ocular muscle, and clinical features of cranial nerve palsy are subtle – causes diplopia (on depression, mainly vertical and torsional) and abnormal head posture.
- Sixth cranial nerve supplies the lateral rectus extra ocular muscle – sixth cranial nerve palsy causes an obvious ipsilateral convergent squint.
- Optic disc swelling is not the same as papilloedema. Papilloedema is bilateral swollen discs due to raised intracranial pressure (ICP). Optic disc swelling is most commonly caused by hypertension.
- If bitemporal hemianopia present, think pituitary tumour; most common pituitary tumour is a pituitary adenoma.

UKMLA Conditions
Optic neuritis
Squint
Visual field defects

UKMLA Presentations
Diplopia
Ptosis

Self-Assessment

UKMLA High Yield Association Table

Key findings	Diagnoses
Three-per-second spike and wave discharge on electroencephalogram	Absence seizures
'Fencing posture' during a seizure	Frontal lobe seizure
Lip-smacking and chewing automatisms	Temporal lobe seizure
Severe headaches with orbital, retro-orbital pain, autonomic symptoms and restlessness	Cluster headache
Headaches with tenderness on combing hair and tender temple	Giant cell arteritis
Headache with swollen optic discs and reduced retinal vein pulsations	Raised intracranial pressure
Stabbing paroxysmal pain in face triggered by touching face and mouth	Trigeminal neuralgia
Sudden onset vertigo lasting seconds upon turning in bed	Benign paroxysmal positional vertigo
Tremor worse on performing a task and holding arms outstretched, improving with alcohol	Essential tremor
Fluctuating memory loss with prominent visual hallucinations	Lewy body dementia
Pregnant and requiring treatment for epilepsy	Lamotrigine
Episodes of relapsing-remitting neurological symptoms and episode of optic neuritis	Multiple sclerosis
Ascending progressive weakness and sensory loss in limbs after an infective illness	Guillain–Barré syndrome
Progressive weakness since childhood with pes cavus, symmetrical sensory loss to the knees and symmetrical wasting in the distal legs	Charcot–Marie–Tooth disease
Weakness in a patient with small cell lung cancer	Lambert–Eaton syndrome
Confusion, falls, nystagmus, ophthalmoplegia	Wernicke encephalopathy
Vomiting blood after a head injury	Cushing ulcer
Amyloid plaques and neurofibrillary tangles on neuropathology	Alzheimer's disease
Memory loss, falls and incontinence	Normal pressure hydrocephalus
Stepwise deterioration of cognitive function	Vascular dementia
Memory loss, disInhibition, behaviour change, apathy	Frontotemporal dementia
Crescent-shaped bleed on CT	Subdural haemorrhage
Loss of facial movements, with sensation intact	Bell palsy
Fatigue with repetitive movements	Myasthenia gravis
Sudden severe headache, known polycystic kidney disease	Subarachnoid haemorrhage
Head trauma, lucid interval, then drowsy, biconvex bleed on CT	Extradural haematoma
Tinnitus and deafness	Ménière's disease
Facial weakness and vesicles in ear	Ramsay Hunt syndrome
Motor loss in one limb with sensory loss to pain and temperature in the other leg	Brown–Séquard syndrome
Loss of pain and temperature sensation with intact proprioception and vibration	Syringomyelia
Reduced adduction of affected eye, and abduction nystagmus of contralateral eye	Internuclear ophthalmoplegia

Continued

Key findings	Diagnoses
Weakness of shoulder abduction and external rotation	Suprascapular nerve lesion
Weakness of thumb adduction (Froment sign)	Ulnar nerve lesion
Most common benign CNS tumour in adults	Meningioma
Weather, exercise, fever and hot showers leading to worsening symptoms in multiple sclerosis	Uhthoff phenomenon
Sensation of shooting electrical pain elicited by neck flexion that radiates down the body	Lhermitte sign
Rapidly progressive dementia with myoclonus	Creutzfeldt–Jakob disease (CJD)
Rapidly progressive demyelinating disease caused by reactivation of a latent JC virus infection in immunosuppressed individuals	Progressive multifocal leucoencephalopathy (PML)
Movement disorder with reduced caeruloplasmin and increased urine copper excretion	Wilson disease
Overweight young woman with headaches, visual loss and papilloedema	Idiopathic intracranial hypertension
Mild pain/painless red-eye with mobile vessels and blanching after the application of phenylephrine drops	Episcleritis
Acute onset painful red eye with blurred vision, photophobia and small, fixed irregular pupil	Anterior uveitis
Acute onset severely painful red eye with decreased visual acuity, halos, semidilated pupils and hazy cornea	Acute angle-closure glaucoma
Sudden painless loss of vision with a 'cherry-red' spot on a pale retina, and relative afferent pupillary defect	Central retinal artery occlusion
Sudden painless loss of vision with severe retinal haemorrhages on fundoscopy – 'stormy sunset' appearance	Central retinal vein occlusion
Sudden onset of flashes and floaters	Posterior vitreous detachment
Sudden change in vision with a 'curtain/veil' originating from the peripheral vision and progressing to central vision	Retinal detachment
Painless, transient monocular loss of vision with a description of a 'black curtain' coming down	Amaurosis fugax
Sudden onset unilateral swelling of the eye, with reduced colour vision/visual acuity, proptosis and severe pain on eye movement	Orbital cellulitis
Dendritic ulcer on fluorescein eye stain	Herpes simplex keratitis
Painful blistering rash on trigeminal nerve dermatome distribution + tip of the nose	Hutchinson sign
Painful red eye with swelling post cataract/ocular surgery	Endophthalmitis
Progressive change in vision with decreased visual acuity and central field loss/distortion	Age-related macular degeneration
Progressive change in vision with decreased visual acuity and peripheral field loss	Primary open-angle glaucoma
Patient with multiple sclerosis with unilateral acute vision changes with painful eye movements	Optic neuritis
Visual field defect presenting with bitemporal hemianopia	Pituitary tumour
Miosis, ptosis, enophthalmos, +/– anhidrosis	Horner syndrome
Eye deviation 'down and out'	Cranial nerve III palsy
Defective downward gaze and vertical diplopia	Cranial nerve IV palsy
Defective abduction of the eye and horizontal diplopia	Cranial nerve VI palsy

UKMLA Single Best Answer (SBA) questions

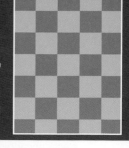

Chapter 2 The examination

1. Which of the following statements are true?
   A Hypotonia, hyporeflexia and plantar extension are signs of a lower motor neuron lesion.
   B Trauma, tumour and stroke are all potential causes of lower motor neuron lesions.
   C Cogwheel tremor is always present with Parkinson's disease.
   D Abnormal eye movements can be expected with motor neuron disease.
   E A feature of Parkinson's disease is not habituating to a glabellar tap.

Chapter 3 Further investigations

1. Fibrillation potentials in electromyography are due to activity of:
   A Individual muscle fibres.
   B At least five muscle fibres.
   C Individual motor units.
   D At least five motor units.
   E Neuromuscular junction.

2. Anti-Jo antibodies are positive in:
   A Systemic lupus erythematosus (SLE).
   B Sjogren syndrome.
   C Myasthenia gravis.
   D Guillain–Barré syndrome.
   E Polymyositis.

3. The best imaging modality for spinal cord pathology is:
   A X-ray of the spine.
   B CT of the spine.
   C CT myelography.
   D MRI of the spine.
   E Spinal arteriography.

4. The cerebrospinal fluid (CSF) glucose is usually 60%–80% that of the plasma glucose. A low CSF glucose may be seen in:
   A Alzheimer's disease.
   B Ischaemic stroke.
   C Multiple sclerosis.
   D Guillain–Barré syndrome.
   E Tuberculous meningitis.

Chapter 5 Disturbances of consciousness

1. On assessment of conscious state a patient opens his eyes to voice, speaks inappropriate words and flexes his elbow when supraorbital pressure is applied. His Glasgow Coma Scale score (GCS) is:
   A 7
   B 8
   C 9
   D 10
   E 11

2. Which of these is NOT routinely tested in confirming brainstem death?
   A Oculocephalic response
   B Corneal response.
   C Cardiological reflex to adrenaline.
   D Respiratory reflex to hypercapnia.
   E Gag reflex.

3. An 85-year-old man presents following a stroke with decreased consciousness and an apneustic breathing pattern. Where is the likely location of the stroke?
   A Midbrain.
   B Pons.
   C Left cerebral hemisphere.
   D Cerebellum.
   E Basal ganglia.

4. A 16-year-old girl is brought to the A&E department after losing consciousness for minutes. She was accompanied by her father who witnessed the event. The following clinical feature may help differentiate between a seizure and a syncopal attack:
   A The patient was lying in bed at the onset.
   B There were brief jerks of the limbs.
   C The tongue was bitten.
   D There was urinary incontinence.
   E There was prolonged malaise after the attack.

5. A primary school teacher noticed that one of his 9-year-old pupils had become less attentive in class and mentioned this to the child's mother, who had also noticed this and had witnessed her daughter have brief blank spells lasting a few seconds up to three times a

day. Absence seizures (formerly known as petit mal) are associated with:

A   Learning difficulty.

B   Prolonged postictal confusion.

C   Distinctive 3-per-second spike and wave discharge on electroencephalogram (EEG).

D   Posttraumatic epilepsy.

E   Structural brain lesion on MRI.

6. A 21-year-old woman was brought to A&E by ambulance after she had a generalized convulsion. Her mother accompanied her and also reported that her daughter often had blank spells and had developed unexplained bouts of fear and anxiety from time to time associated with *déjà vu*. Temporal lobe epilepsy is associated with:

A   Repetitive conjugate eye movements.

B   Lip-smacking and chewing automatisms.

C   Jerking of the upper limbs.

D   Adopting a 'fencing posture' at the start of an episode.

E   Seeing flashes or balls of light.

7. A 27-year-old woman was brought to the A&E department by ambulance after she collapsed to the floor and lost consciousness. The event had been witnessed by a friend who told the ambulance driver that just before collapsing she suddenly developed a severe headache with neck pain. In a subarachnoid haemorrhage:

A   A lumbar puncture (LP) is contraindicated because of the risk of coning.

B   Severe hypertension should be treated immediately with antihypertensive agents.

C   A berry aneurysm is more often found in the posterior rather anterior circulation.

D   CT of the head detects 50% of haemorrhages.

E   There is a 20% chance of rebleed within the first 2 weeks.

8. A 13-year-old girl is noticed by her teacher to be not concentrating on her work. The teacher describes episodes where she stares into space for approximately a minute and rapidly returns to normal. The girl is otherwise very well and has a normal neurological examination. She had one febrile convulsion as a child. What is the most likely diagnosis?

A   Narcolepsy

B   Hypoglycaemia

C   Absence seizure

D   Postural hypotension

E   Subarachnoid haemorrhage

9. An 18-year-old man complains of episodes where he suddenly collapses and both upper limbs start to shake. He feels slightly distant while the shaking occurs but

remembers people around him being concerned. The attacks last between 30 s and 5 minutes and have occurred up to 10 times in a day. When the shaking stops, he complains of feeling slightly tired but can resume his activities. He is due to sit his A-levels in 4 months. There is a family history of epilepsy in his younger sister after she had meningitis as a baby. What is the most likely diagnosis?

A   Vasovagal syncope

B   Cardiogenic syncope

C   Focal onset impaired awareness seizure

D   Tonic–clonic seizure

E   Nonepileptic seizure

10. A 24-year-old woman presents with episodes of loss of consciousness for a few minutes and one of the recent attacks was followed by some mild stiffening in all her limbs and urinary incontinence. The episodes tend to happen at the end of the day when she is standing on the train coming home. She is aware that she feels slightly nauseated before the attacks and feels as if a curtain is coming over her vision before she loses consciousness. Normally, she recovers fully in a few minutes after being given a seat by another passenger. What is the most likely diagnosis?

A   Vasovagal syncope

B   Cardiogenic syncope

C   Focal onset impaired awareness seizure

D   Tonic–clonic seizure

E   Nonepileptic seizure

11. A 25-year-old woman has lapses of consciousness that occur anytime of the day. There are no associated movements or incontinence. She has also found that she has been feeling extremely tired throughout the day, despite having a good night's sleep. The attacks last from seconds to minutes and she does not get any warning they are going to occur. She also describes vivid 'dream-like' images on going to sleep and feels she cannot move her body on waking up for several minutes. What is the most likely diagnosis?

A   Tonic–clonic seizure

B   Nonepileptic seizure

C   Narcolepsy

D   Hypoglycaemia

E   Absence seizure

12. A 35-year-old man complains of episodes of confusion. His wife tells you that he will suddenly 'go blank and stare into space' for several minutes. He often wanders around the room and picks up and puts down objects repeatedly. His wife tells you he does not respond appropriately to her

concerns during the attack and he often feels extremely tired once they have finished. He sometimes gets a 'strange, horrible taste' in his mouth prior to the attacks. What is the most likely diagnosis?

A Vasovagal syncope
B Cardiogenic syncope
C Focal onset impaired awareness seizure
D Tonic–clonic seizure
E Nonepileptic seizure

Chapter 6 Disorders of higher cerebral function

1. Following a stroke, a right-handed patient has difficulties with speech. He can understand questions being asked but is nonfluent in his answers. Where is the lesion?
A Left frontal lobe
B Right frontal lobe
C Left temporal lobe
D Right temporal lobe
E Left parietal lobe

2. Following a stroke, a right-handed patient has visual inattention. Which area of the brain is responsible for visuospatial ability?
A Left temporal lobe
B Right temporal lobe
C Left parietal lobe
D Right parietal lobe
E Left occipital lobe

3. Which arteries supply the majority of the occipital lobes?
A Anterior cerebral arteries.
B Ophthalmic arteries.
C Middle cerebral arteries.
D Posterior cerebral arteries.
E Posterior communicating arteries.

4. A 60-year-old man lives in a nursing home since suffering a severe subarachnoid haemorrhage 5 years ago. Recently, his carers have noticed that his walking is becoming much slower and he is becoming slightly confused and forgetful. They have also noticed that, despite regular toileting, he has urinary incontinence. On examination, he has old left-sided pyramidal signs, but coordination in his right side and sensory examination are normal. When he tries to stand up, he slips backwards into his chair. His mini-mental test score is 21 out of 30, whereas 2 years ago it was noted to be 28. He informs you that he is simply unaware of needing to pass urine. What is the most likely diagnosis?
A Alzheimer's disease
B Frontotemporal dementia
C Normal pressure hydrocephalus

D Acute confusional state
E Nonconvulsive status epilepticus

5. A woman aged 20 years dropped out of university recently because of a depressive illness. She has noticed that in retrospect she has also had strange sensations in her arms and legs over the past 2 months. In spite of treatment for her depression, her parents have noticed that she is becoming forgetful, disorientated and clumsy. What is the most likely diagnosis?
A Multiinfarct dementia
B Subcortical ischaemic leucoencephalopathy
C New variant Creutzfeldt–Jakob disease (CJD)
D Vitamin B_{12} deficiency
E Pseudodementia

6. A 75-year-old patient with hypertension had a minor stroke 1 year ago, from which he made a good recovery although he was left with mild weakness on the left side and mild confusion. Since then, he has had two further acute episodes of slurred speech and then dysphasia, which have partially resolved but have left him functionally disabled. He is now very forgetful and shuffles when he walks. His wife suggests to you in confidence that he is 'not the man I used to know'. On examination, he has a pseudobulbar palsy, brisk but symmetrical reflexes and extensor plantar responses with mild left-sided pyramidal weakness. What is the most likely diagnosis?
A Multiinfarct dementia
B Subcortical ischaemic leucoencephalopathy
C New variant Creutzfeldt–Jakob disease (CJD)
D Vitamin B_{12} deficiency
E Pseudodementia

7. A 70-year-old woman comes to the clinic with her daughter. The patient admits to having problems with her memory, which is frustrating for her, but she is mostly unaware of her difficulties. Her daughter then suggests that actually her mother has been becoming increasingly muddled and forgetful. Two weeks previously, her mother was found wandering lost in her local shops. Two months before that the patient decided to stop attending her social meetings because she found it difficult to keep up with the conversation. She had also forgotten recent family events. Neurological examination was normal apart from a mini-mental test score of 22 out of 30. What is the most likely diagnosis?
A Alzheimer's disease
B Frontotemporal dementia
C Normal pressure hydrocephalus
D Acute confusional state
E Nonconvulsive status epilepticus

8. An 82-year-old man presents to clinic with a 5-month history of 'apathy, loss of interest and forgetfulness'. He has withdrawn from all his social engagements following the death of his wife 6 months previously. He recently had a small house fire because he left a chip pan on, but he was able to call the fire brigade. He has lost a significant amount of weight recently because he claims he is never hungry. He is often seen wandering around his local shops alone but his daughter claims his cupboards are empty and his house is in a bad condition. Neurological examination is normal and his mini-mental test score is 28 out of 30, but he was very slow in giving his answers. What is the most likely diagnosis?
   A Multiinfarct dementia
   B Subcortical ischaemic leucoencephalopathy
   C New variant Creutzfeldt–Jakob disease (CJD)
   D Vitamin B$_{12}$ deficiency
   E Pseudodementia

Chapter 7 Headache

1. A 33-year-old man presents with repeated headaches centred around his right eye, causing it to tear and look red. The headache usually lasts 15 minutes and he has to pace around the room due to the pain. What is the most likely headache diagnosis?
   A Giant cell arteritis (GCA)
   B Tension headache
   C Migraine
   D Glaucoma
   E Cluster headache

2. A 60-year-old patient reports a new onset headache for the last week that has made him feel drained. He finds combing his hair to be painful and on examination he has a tender right temple. What is the most likely headache diagnosis?
   A Giant cell arteritis
   B Tension headache
   C Migraine
   D Glaucoma
   E Cluster headache

3. The aura in a typical migraine should not last longer than:
   A 1 minute
   B 10 minutes
   C 30 minutes
   D 60 minutes
   E 12 hours

4. Which of these is NOT a red flag for new onset headaches?
   A Worse when lying down

   B Ptosis
   C Papilloedema
   D Neck stiffness
   E Age older than 50 years

5. A 54-year-old man presents to the A&E department complaining of a headache, which is prominent on waking in the morning and wakes him from sleep at night. He reports that he has not had headache before and feels unwell. Fundoscopy shows swollen optic discs bilaterally with loss of retinal venous pulsation. The visual examination is likely to demonstrate the following:
   A A loss of colour vision
   B An enlarged blind spot
   C A central scotoma
   D A small pupil
   E A relative afferent pupillary defect

6. A 56-year-old woman is reviewed by her GP as she has expressed concerns about her headaches. She has had headaches for at least 20 years but her sister had recently been diagnosed with a brain tumour and was undergoing cranial radiotherapy under the local oncologists. Her mother died of status epilepticus that was thought to be due to a brain tumour. The headache of raised intracranial pressure is typically associated with:
   A Worsening with coughing, sneezing or bending over
   B Fortification spectra
   C Stabbing or shooting pains
   D Being better on waking first thing in the morning and worse on standing
   E Photophobia and phonophobia

7. A 39-year-old man complains of a throbbing unilateral about once a month and a headache after eating chocolate or drinking red wine. His mother and sister are known to have classical migraine. A diagnosis of migraine headache is also supported by:
   A Continuous daily headache
   B Episodes of loss of consciousness
   C Improved by standing
   D Associated nausea, vertigo and photophobia
   E Tight, band-like pain around the whole of the head

8. A fit and well 30-year-old man presents with a sudden onset severe headache, confusion, photophobia and neck stiffness. What is the most likely diagnosis?
   A Cervical spondylitis
   B Giant cell arteritis
   C Meningitis
   D Migraine
   E Subarachnoid haemorrhage

9. A 45-year-old woman presents with recurrent headaches for the last year. She has no focal neurological deficit or associated symptoms and the headaches have not been worsening. What is the most likely diagnosis?
   A Chronic sinusitis
   B Giant cell arteritis
   C Malignancy
   D Migraine
   E Tension headache

10. An 18-year-old student who has just started university presents with a worsening headache and marked photophobia. What is the most likely diagnosis?
    A Cervical spondylitis
    B Ménière's disease
    C Meningitis
    D Subarachnoid haemorrhage
    E Subdural haematoma

11. A 22-year-old man presents to the A&E department with a severe headache that started 12 hours earlier and is increasingly severe. He has vomited twice. On examination, he is confused, photophobic and has a stiff neck. Kernig sign is positive, but the rest of the neurological examination is normal. His lumbar puncture shows an opening pressure of 23 cm H_2O, 160 polymorphs, 10 red cells, protein of 1.2 g/L and cerebrospinal fluid (CSF) glucose of 2 mmol/L (serum 5.4 mmol/L). What is the most likely diagnosis?
    A Bacterial meningitis
    B Tuberculous meningitis
    C Viral meningitis
    D Low-pressure headache
    E Raised intracranial pressure headache

12. A 68-year-old smoker presents to clinic with a 3-week history of a progressive headache, which is increasing in severity. It is worse in the morning and after his afternoon nap. Over the past few days, he has been feeling increasingly nauseated and his right hand is becoming slow and clumsy. His wife feels that he is 'not himself' and that 'he cannot get his words out'. On examination, he has pyramidal weakness in the right arm and an expressive dysphasia. His optic disc margins are slightly indistinct. What is the most likely diagnosis?
    A Bacterial meningitis
    B Tuberculous meningitis
    C Viral meningitis
    D Low-pressure headache
    E Raised intracranial pressure headache

13. A 24-year-old woman has recently started the contraceptive pill and has noticed that three or four times per month she gets a numbness in her face, which resolves in 20 minutes and is followed by numbness in her arm, which also resolves in 20 minutes. She then develops a bilateral retro-orbital and throbbing headache that makes her feel sick, although she does not usually vomit. She has to return home from work and rest in her bedroom with her curtains drawn, but she usually feels better the next day. Her mother says that she had a few similar attacks in her teens but never as severe as her daughter's. What is the most likely diagnosis?
    A Tension-type headache
    B Migraine with aura
    C Migraine without aura
    D Stroke
    E Subarachnoid haemorrhage

14. A 40-year-old man comes to A&E with a 3-hour history of severe headache, which is now improving slightly. He normally gets headaches when he is stressed, but he has never had anything as bad as this headache. On examination, he has slight neck stiffness, a right-sided ptosis, double vision on looking to the left and up as well as a slightly bigger pupil on the right compared with the left, but he is otherwise well now. His head CT is normal and his lumbar puncture shows an opening pressure of 25 cm H_2O, with 500 red cells and 3 lymphocytes. The protein is 0.8 g/L and the glucose is normal. He is kept in for observation overnight and during the night he alerts the nurses because his severe headache has returned. He subsequently becomes drowsy and has a tonic–clonic seizure. What is the most likely diagnosis?
    A Tension-type headache
    B Migraine with aura
    C Migraine without aura
    D Stroke
    E Subarachnoid haemorrhage

15. A 72-year-old man with diabetes presents to A&E with a 12-hour history of dull right-sided headache associated with acute onset of left-sided weakness. On examination, he is moderately drowsy but has a Glasgow Coma Scale score of 15. He also has left hemiparesis and left homonymous hemianopia. His headache seems to be dull and nagging, but he has no neck stiffness or photophobia. He is apyrexial, with a temperature of 37.0°C. His wife tells you that 2 weeks ago the left side of his body went numb but it went away within a few hours. What is the most likely diagnosis?
    A Tension-type headache
    B Migraine with aura
    C Migraine without aura
    D Stroke
    E Subarachnoid haemorrhage

Chapter 9 Facial sensory loss and weakness

1. A 32-year-old man presents to A&E with facial pain triggered by touching his face and mouth and because of this has been unable to shave or eat properly for 4 days. The casualty officer identifies a normal neurological examination. Trigeminal neuralgia:
   A Is associated with ipsilateral facial weakness.
   B Is usually bilateral.
   C Is a severe, stabbing, paroxysmal pain.
   D Is usually familial.
   E Is associated treated with steroids.

Chapter 10 Deafness, tinnitus, dizziness and vertigo

1. What frequency is the tuning fork used in Rinne test?
   A 100 Hz
   B 200 Hz
   C 256 Hz
   D 512 Hz
   E 600 Hz

2. A patient reports getting sudden onset vertigo lasting seconds when turning over in bed. What is the most likely diagnosis?
   A Vestibular neuritis
   B Benign paroxysmal positional vertigo (BPPV)
   C Acoustic neuroma
   D Glue ear
   E Ménière's disease

3. Which of these conditions does NOT typically affect the cochlear nerve?
   A Acoustic neuroma
   B Sarcoidosis
   C Meningitis
   D Arteriovenous malformation
   E Multiple sclerosis

4. A 35-year-old man had been diagnosed with a vestibular schwannoma (previously referred to as an acoustic neuroma) by a neurologist after he went to his GP complaining of a pressure in his ear and poor balance. MRI of the brain with gadolinium contrast identified an enhancing lesion of the 8th cranial nerve on the right. The clinical features of a lesion of the right cerebellopontine angle (CPA) may include:
   A Conductive deafness on the right side
   B Right-sided cerebellar features
   C Right-sided weakness of the lower face
   D A pseudobulbar dysarthria
   E Vertigo as a prominent early symptom

Chapter 11 Dysarthria, dysphonia and dysphagia

1. Dysphasia may result from a lesion of:
   A The cerebellum
   B Broca area
   C The hypoglossal nerve
   D The basal ganglia
   E The accessory nerve

2. The following may give rise to a pseudobulbar palsy:
   A Poliomyelitis
   B Motor neuron disease
   C Huntington's disease
   D Occlusion of the anterior cerebral artery
   E Myasthenia gravis

Chapter 13 Movement disorders

1. A 50-year-old patient presents with a 5-year history of tremor that is worse when performing a task such as holding a cup or using cutlery. The symptoms improve after he has some alcohol. There is no tremor at rest. What is the most likely diagnosis?
   A Parkinson's disease
   B Essential tremor
   C Alcohol excess
   D Rubral tremor
   E Psychogenic tremor

2. A 21-year-old pianist noticed a fine tremor in both hands that was a little more prominent while playing. His GP informed him that it was a physiological tremor that is:
   A Treated with sodium valproate.
   B Improved by medication containing L-DOPA.
   C Usually treated by deep brain stimulation.
   D Improved by β-blockers.
   E Treated with neuroleptics.

3. A 30-year-old woman presents to clinic with difficulty drinking a cup of tea because of a tremor. It is absent at rest but she also notices it as she is writing. She has noticed that it rarely affects her when she goes out at the weekend for a few drinks. On examination, she has a postural tremor of the upper limbs. What is the most likely diagnosis?
   A Idiopathic Parkinson's disease
   B Multisystem atrophy
   C Huntington's disease
   D Wilson disease
   E Benign essential tremor

4. A 21-year-old man presents with a 1-year history of slurring of his speech and difficulty swallowing. More

recently, he has noticed that his legs and arms can go into spasms and have become tremulous. What is the most likely diagnosis?

A Idiopathic Parkinson's disease
B Multisystem atrophy
C Huntington's disease
D Wilson disease
E Benign essential tremor

5. A patient with Parkinson's disease has been managed successfully by his GP for the past 6 years, but recently he has been experiencing writhing movements of his tongue, face, neck, trunk and limbs that is worst 2 hours after he takes his dose of levodopa but resolves by the time the medication wears off. It is now difficult for him to do anything during these episodes. What is the most likely diagnosis?

A Spasmodic torticollis
B Physiological tremor
C Levodopa-induced dyskinesias
D Hemiballismus
E Pseudoathetosis

6. A 70-year-old woman with hypertension has a sudden onset of wild flailing movements of her right arm and leg. She is otherwise well. What is the most likely diagnosis?

A Spasmodic torticollis
B Physiological tremor
C Levodopa-induced dyskinesias
D Hemiballismus
E Pseudoathetosis

7. A 42-year-old man, who has recently lost contact with his family because of 'differences', has noticed that he has become very fidgety. He functionally copes with constant fidgety movements but finds it frustrating and he has noticed that he loses his temper more frequently. He did not know his father well; he died of an unknown neurological illness at an early age. What is the most likely diagnosis?

A Idiopathic Parkinson's disease
B Multisystem atrophy
C Huntington's disease
D Wilson disease
E Benign essential tremor

Chapter 14 Limb weakness

1. Which disease can cause both upper and lower motor neurone signs in the same patient?

A Guillain–Barré syndrome
B Multiple sclerosis (MS)

C Diabetic peripheral neuropathy
D Motor neuron disease (MND)
E Stroke

2. Fasciculations of muscle may be seen in:

A Motor neuron disease
B Muscular dystrophy
C Sleep
D Parkinson's disease
E A hot bath or shower

3. Signs of an upper motor neuron lesion include:

A Resting tremor
B Hypertonia
C Flexor plantar
D Reduced reflexes
E Peripheral neuropathy

Chapter 15 Limb sensory symptoms

1. The fibres of the dorsal column pathway:

A Carry information about temperature perception.
B Decussate in the midbrain.
C Are affected in the deficiency of vitamin B_1.
D When damaged might result in a positive Gower sign.
E Are spared following occlusion of the anterior spinal artery.

Chapter 16 Disorders of gait

1. A patient presents with a wide-based small-stepped gait. The most likely diagnosis is:

A Parkinson's disease
B Muscular dystrophy
C Multiple sclerosis
D Common peroneal nerve palsy
E Vascular dementia

2. A patient reports a 6-month history of tripping over his right foot. On examination he has a high-stepping gait on his right side. The most likely diagnosis is:

A Parkinson's disease
B Muscular dystrophy
C Multiple sclerosis
D Common peroneal nerve palsy
E Vascular dementia

3. A 35-year-old man has had progressive weakness in his shoulder and pelvic girdle for 10 years. When he walks, he has a waddling gait. What is the most likely diagnosis?

A Spastic hemiparesis
B Subcortical ischaemic leucoencephalopathy

C   Functional disorder
D   Common peroneal nerve lesion
E   Myopathy

4. A 25-year-old man has had difficulties walking all his life. When he walks, his legs scissor across one another. On examination, he has very stiff legs and clonus at the ankles. His reflexes are brisk and his plantars are extensor. What is the most likely diagnosis?
A   Idiopathic Parkinson's disease
B   Huntington's disease
C   Peripheral neuropathy
D   Cerebellar syndrome
E   Spastic paraparesis

5. A 30-year-old alcoholic presents with difficulty walking. On examination, he has a broad-based gait and is severely imbalanced. What is the most likely diagnosis?
A   Idiopathic Parkinson's disease
B   Huntington's disease
C   Peripheral neuropathy
D   Cerebellar syndrome
E   Spastic paraparesis

6. A 79-year-old woman with hypertension has recently had difficulty walking. Her gait is slow and shuffling and she takes very small steps. Even when she starts walking, she cannot speed up and easily comes to rest. On examination, she has pseudobulbar palsy, brisk tendon reflexes and extensor plantars. What is the most likely diagnosis?
A   Spastic hemiparesis
B   Subcortical ischaemic leucoencephalopathy
C   Functional disorder
D   Common peroneal nerve lesion
E   Idiopathic Parkinson's disease

7. A 27-year-old man presents with episodes of a sudden inability to walk. The attacks occur up to 10 times per day and are associated with twitching of his shoulder. He has fallen many times but not hurt himself. When you ask him to walk, he collapses to the floor, even though his bedside examination was normal. When he starts to walk, his gait is slow, intermittently clumsy and he has an asymmetrical posture with hunching of his right shoulder. He describes his feet as being 'stuck to the floor'. What is the most likely diagnosis?
A   Spastic hemiparesis
B   Subcortical ischaemic leucoencephalopathy
C   Functional disorder
D   Common peroneal nerve lesion
E   Myopathy

Chapter 17 The red, painful eye

1. A 52-year-old woman presents to the emergency department with severe left eye pain over the past two hours. She denies any changes in vision, nausea or vomiting. She has a past medical history of rheumatoid arthritis and takes methotrexate. Noncontact lens wearer. On examination, her heart rate is 72 bpm, her blood pressure is 118/72 mm Hg and she is afebrile The left eye is deep red and injected throughout There is pain on ocular palpation and the injected vessels do not move The application of phenylephrine drops does not blanch vessels, and the redness does not improve The visual fields and acuity of both eyes are unaffected The left eye is normal
What is the most likely diagnosis?
A   Episcleritis
B   Scleritis
C   Anterior uveitis
D   Acute angle-closure glaucoma
E   Acute keratitis

2. A 45-year-old man with a past medical history of Crohn's disease presents to his GP with a 3-day history of sudden onset dull pain in the right orbital region, red eye, lacrimation and photophobia. On examination of the right eye, there is ciliary flushing and the pupil is irregular and constricted. The left eye is normal.
What is the most appropriate management option?
A   Chloramphenicol eye drops
B   Latanoprost eye drops and urgent referral to ophthalmology
C   Saline eye drops
D   Steroid + cycloplegic eye drops and urgent referral to ophthalmology
E   Oral aciclovir

3. A 63-year-old man presents to the emergency department with a sudden left-sided painful red eye and two episodes of vomiting. The patient noticed the pain while watching television in a dark room last night. Paracetamol and ibuprofen have not helped with the pain. On examination of the left eye, there is a redness with a semidilated nonreacting pupil and hazy cornea present. The right eye is normal. The patient also wears glasses for reading and distance correction.
What is the most likely diagnosis?
A   Anterior uveitis
B   Scleritis
C   Acute angle-closure glaucoma
D   Acute keratitis
E   Primary open-angle glaucoma

4. A 28-year-old presents to the GP with a left red painful eye. She described that the redness appeared on her left eye several days ago. The patient rated the pain 8 out of 10 when asked to scale the degree of pain. She is a contact lens wearer. What is the most appropriate next step in management?
   A Aciclovir drops
   B Advice to wear contact lenses less frequently
   C Reassurance
   D Urgent 'two-week wait' ophthalmology referral
   E Same-day ophthalmology referral

5. A 52-year-old man presents to the emergency department with an acute painful left-sided red eye for the past 2 hours with an associated blurring of vision, nausea and vomiting. He also notices halos around lights and has a past medical history of hypermetropia and rheumatoid arthritis.
   On examination, his eye appears as shown in Fig. 1.

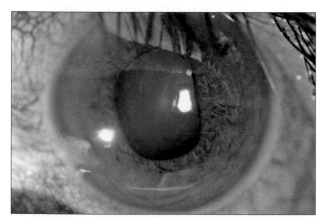

Fig. 1 (From Yanoff M, Duker JS. Ophthalmology. 6th ed. Elsevier; 2023.)

What is the most likely diagnosis?
   A Acute scleritis
   B Acute keratitis
   C Angle-closure glaucoma
   D Anterior uveitis
   E Open-angle glaucoma

Chapter 18 Gradual change in vision

1. A 78-year-old male with type 2 diabetes mellitus attends his GP surgery regarding problems with his vision. For several months he has noticed that he struggles to take notice of cars from the side of his vision. He suffers from occasional headaches but denies any vision loss, eye pain or flashes/floaters.

What is the most likely diagnosis?
   A Primary open-angle glaucoma
   B Age-related macular degeneration
   C Cataracts
   D Episcleritis
   E Acute-angle closure glaucoma

2. A 72-year-old female visits her GP with new-onset visual symptoms. She is complaining of being unable to read the newspaper properly, which is usually more difficult during the nighttime. The symptoms vary in intensity each day. Upon fundoscopy, multiple drusen are present, and the examination is otherwise normal. She is also a smoker and has no other relevant medical history.
   What is the most likely diagnosis?
   A Cataract
   B Dry age-related macular degeneration
   C Wet age-related macular degeneration
   D Presbyopia
   E Retinitis pigmentosa

3. Which of the following is not a risk factor for primary open-angle glaucoma?
   A Diabetes mellitus
   B Hypermetropia
   C Myopia
   D Family history
   E Hypertension

4. A 54-year-old female is diagnosed with primary open-angle glaucoma. How does primary open-angle glaucoma most commonly affect vision?
   A Impairs visual acuity
   B Impairs night vision
   C Impairs central vision
   D Impairs peripheral visual fields
   E Impairs colour vision, with red colour vision affected first

5. A 78-year-old male with a gradual decrease in visual acuity and difficulty while driving at night due to increased glare from headlights of oncoming cars. There are no other visual symptoms. On slit lamp examination, there is opacification of the lens in both eyes and the red reflex is obscured in both eyes. Fundoscopy revealed no abnormalities.
   Which of the following does not predispose to a cataract formation?
   A Hypocalcaemia
   B Diabetes mellitus
   C Uveitis
   D Long-term steroid use
   E Hypercalcemia

Chapter 19 Sudden change in vision

1. A 54-year-old male with chronic glaucoma goes to the emergency department with a sudden loss of vision in the right eye. He describes that while watching TV his vision suddenly became blurry in the right eye and several minutes later there was a loss of vision. There was no pain or discharge. Upon fundoscopy, there are several 'flame' haemorrhages and cotton wool spots, and examination revealed a relative pupillary defect. The left eye was normal on examination.

   What is the most likely diagnosis?
   A   Central retinal artery occlusion
   B   Central retinal vein occlusion
   C   Retinal detachment
   D   Posterior vitreous detachment
   E   Optic neuropathy

2. A 48-year-old male presented to the emergency department with a painless sudden loss of vision in the left eye. His past medical history includes atherosclerosis and is a smoker. On examination the pupils are equal and reactive to light, and normal in appearance. Upon fundoscopy, the left eye reveals a pale retina and a 'cherry-red' spot.
   What is the most likely diagnosis?
   A   Central retinal artery occlusion
   B   Central retinal vein occlusion
   C   Retinal detachment
   D   Posterior vitreous detachment
   E   Optic neuropathy

3. A 38-year-old female with a background of multiple sclerosis presents to the emergency department with an acutely painful right eye that is worse on movement. The patient had also noticed progressive vision loss over the past few days. On examination, her vision is hand movements only and there is a relative afferent pupillary defect present. The left eye is normal.
   What is the most appropriate next step in management?
   A   High-dose steroids
   B   Beta-blocker
   C   Antiplatelet
   D   Anticoagulant
   E   Antibiotics

4. A 43-year-old female presented to the emergency department with sudden painless loss of vision on the right eye. Prior to losing her vision there was dark 'floaters' seen and a 'red hue' on the right side. The patient described that the symptoms were worse when lying flat. Past medical history includes poorly controlled type 2 diabetes, proliferative diabetic retinopathy, hypertension and a previous ischaemic stroke.

   What is the most likely diagnosis?
   A   Posterior vitreous detachment
   B   Retinal detachment
   C   Central retinal artery occlusion
   D   Posterior vitreous detachment
   E   Vitreous haemorrhage

5. A 49-year-old man attends his optician for a review. He suffers from long-sightedness with no astigmatism or concurrent myopia.
   Which of the following conditions is this patient most at risk of developing in the future?
   A   Primary open-angle glaucoma
   B   Central retinal artery occlusion
   C   Cataract
   D   Optic neuritis
   E   Acute angle-closure glaucoma

Chapter 20 Eyelid problems and the bulging eye

1. A 63-year-old gentleman presents to his GP practice complaining of dry eye and epiphora (Fig. 2).

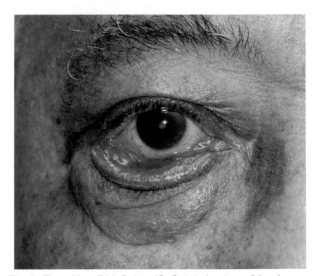

Fig. 2 (From Yanoff M, Duker JS. Ophthalmology. 6th ed. Elsevier; 2023.)

   What is the correct term to describe the eyelid pictured above?
   A   Entropion
   B   Ectropion
   C   Ptosis
   D   Anisocoria
   E   Diplopia

2. A 58-year-old lady presents to her general practitioner with an itchy scalp and greasy scaling in the nasolabial folds. The GP makes a diagnosis of seborrheic dermatitis. The lady is also complaining of bilateral itchy eyes.
What is the appropriate advice to be given to this patient for her itchy eyes?

A Lid hygiene advice and clean eyelids twice daily using a warm compress
B Urgent referral to ophthalmology
C Two-week referral to ophthalmology
D Topical low-strength steroids twice a day
E Reassure the patient and no additional advice

3. A 28-year-old male with a painful swelling of his left upper eyelid for the past 2 days. On lifting the eyelid, a yellow head pointing at the lid margin can be seen.
What is the most appropriate management for this patient?

A Analgesia and warm compress
B Topical antibiotics
C Analgesia and cold compress
D IV flucloxacillin
E Urgent referral to ophthalmology

4. A 70-year-old female presents with a 2-month history of a red swollen right upper eyelid. She remembers that initially there was a bump on the eyelid which was mildly painful and then grew bigger in size. Currently, she complains of no pain and has no associated visual symptoms.
What is the most likely diagnosis?

A Blepharitis
B Chalazion
C Hordeolum externa
D Hordeolum internum
E Entropion

5. A 69-year-old male complains of a sore right eye (Fig. 3):

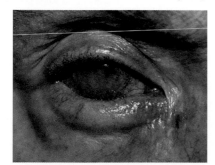

Fig. 3 (From Glynn M, Drake WM, Hutchison R. *Hutchison's Clinical Methods: An Integrated Approach to Clinical Practice.* Edinburgh, Saunders/Elsevier; 2012.)

What complication will this patient develop if left untreated?

A Corneal ulceration
B Refractive error
C Amblyopia
D Strabismus
E Wet age-related maculopathy

Chapter 21 Dementia

1. You are considering a new diagnosis of dementia. Which feature is most in keeping with dementia?
A Early hallucinations
B Progressive course
C Early disorientation
D Withdrawn behaviour
E Reversal of day night cycle

2. Which test does not need to be performed before making a diagnosis of dementia?
A Full blood count
B B_{12} and folate levels
C Head CT.
D Lumbar puncture
E Thyroid function tests

3. A 75-year-old man presents with a 6-month history of forgetfulness that is fluctuant in nature. On questioning, he reports visual hallucinations. On examination he has a slow gait.
What is the likely diagnosis?
A Lewy body dementia
B Alzheimer's disease
C Vascular dementia
D Depression
E Frontotemporal dementia

4. A 55-year-old lady is brought to the GP's surgery by her husband who reports that she has become increasingly forgetful and that her personality had changed. She is no longer as lively as she used to be and has lost her emotional response to important matters. This has been slowly getting worse over the past 12 months. During the consultation she is unable to sit still and is very fidgety. The diagnosis is most likely to be:
A Subacute sclerosing panencephalitis
B Huntington's disease
C Alzheimer's disease
D Normal pressure hydrocephalus
E Schizophrenia

5. Alzheimer's disease:
   A Commonly presents with disorientation in time and place.
   B The patient usually has insight into memory loss.
   C Typically presents with disinhibition and apathy.
   D Geographical apraxia and language deficits are often early features.
   E Patients might accuse their spouse of being an imposter (Capgras syndrome).

Chapter 22 Epilepsy

1. Of the list below, which is the safest antiepileptic drug to take during pregnancy?
   A Sodium valproate
   B Carbamazepine
   C Lamotrigine
   D Phenytoin
   E Midazolam

2. A patient is considered in status epilepticus if they have a seizure lasting longer than:
   A 1 minute
   B 5 minutes
   C 10 minutes
   D 30 minutes
   E 60 minutes

3. What is the most immediate management of a patient having a generalized seizure?
   A Resuscitation
   B Administering lorazepam
   C Blood lactate level
   D CT scan
   E Gaining a collateral history

Chapter 23 Parkinson's disease and other extrapyramidal disorders

1. A 75-year-old man was referred to the clinic querying a diagnosis of Parkinson's disease. Which features would NOT be in keeping with this condition?
   A Resting tremor
   B Arm rigidity
   C Gait ataxia
   D Small handwriting
   E Shuffling gait

2. Which of the following characteristics indicate that increased tone is due to rigidity rather than spasticity and might support a diagnosis of Parkinson's disease:
   A Tone is increased equally in flexor and extensor muscles.

B The plantar responses are extensor.
C There is a postural tremor.
D There is reduction of power in the limbs.
E There is deafness.

Chapter 24 Diseases affecting the spinal cord (myelopathy)

1. A 25-year-old woman has a 9-month history of difficulty walking. The neurological examination identified a spastic paraparesis, Five years earlier, the patient lost vision in her right eye for 4 months with some pain when her eye moved from side to side, suggestive of optic neuritis. The most likely diagnosis is:
   A Motor neuron disease
   B Myasthenia gravis
   C Multiple sclerosis
   D Peripheral neuropathy
   E Subdural haematoma

2. A 32-year-old man presented to his GP complaining of increasing weakness in his right arm and leg that had gradually developed over 7 months. He also noticed that the left-hand side of his body felt odd and different from the right. The neurological examination revealed a right-sided hemiparesis, with loss of vibration and joint position sense in the right arm and leg and loss of pinprick sensation in the left arm and leg, compatible with a Brown–Séquard syndrome. Which investigation would secure the diagnosis?
   A Nerve conduction studies
   B A lumbar puncture
   C An MRI of the cervical spinal cord
   D Syphilis serology
   E MRI of the brain

3. A 40-year-old woman from the West Indies presents with a 6-month history of progressive difficulty in walking and urinary retention. Examination reveals a spastic paraparesis. What is the most likely diagnosis?
   A Multiple sclerosis
   B Spinal tuberculoma
   C Anterior spinal artery infarct
   D Human T-cell lymphocytic virus type 1 (HTLV-1)
   E L5 radiculopathy

4. A 70-year-old man presents with weakness and numbness in both legs after walking for 100 yards, which eases on rest. The examination results are normal. What is the most likely diagnosis?
   A Spinal canal stenosis
   B Subacute combined degeneration of the cord

C Brown–Séquard syndrome
D Hereditary spastic paraparesis
E Ependymoma

5. A 23-year-old man who regularly uses cocaine presents with a sudden onset loss of power in his legs and hands. Examination reveals paraparesis with loss of pain and temperature sensation in the legs but intact fine touch sensation. What is the most likely diagnosis?
A Multiple sclerosis
B Spinal tuberculoma
C Anterior spinal artery infarct
D Human T-cell lymphocytic virus type 1 (HTLV-1)
E L5 radiculopathy

6. A 35-year-old woman with a vegan diet presents with a year's history of progressive unsteadiness on her feet. On examination, Romberg test is positive and there is paraparesis with loss of fine touch sensation up to the thighs. She has an extensor plantar response with otherwise depressed reflexes. What is the most likely diagnosis?
A Spinal canal stenosis
B Subacute combined degeneration of the cord
C Brown–Séquard syndrome
D Hereditary spastic paraparesis
E Ependymoma

7. A 28-year-old man presents after a road traffic accident with weakness in his left arm and leg. On further examination, he has loss of fine touch sensation on the left arm and leg and loss of pain sensation in the right arm and leg. What is the most likely diagnosis?
A Spinal canal stenosis
B Subacute combined degeneration of the cord
C Brown–Séquard syndrome
D Hereditary spastic paraparesis
E Ependymoma

Chapter 26 Radiculopathy and plexopathy

1. How many nerve roots are there in the cervical spine?
A 4
B 6
C 8
D 10
E 12

2. A patient presents with loss of sensation in the C8–T1 region in his right arm. There is wasting of abductor pollicis brevis and evidence of right Horner syndrome. What is the most likely diagnosis?

A Diabetic neuropathy
B Carpal tunnel syndrome
C Pancoast tumour
D Motor neuron disease
E Rheumatoid arthritis

3. A patient presents with a 2-week history of difficulty in walking and back pain. On examination, she has a loss of sensation on the dorsum of her right foot with weakness of plantar flexion. The right ankle reflex is lost. Which are the likely discs involved?
A L2/L3
B L3/L4
C L4/L5
D L5/S1
E S1/S2

4. A 43-year-old builder complains of the sudden onset of lower back pain after lifting a sack of cement. It is a sharp shooting sensation that radiates to his right leg. Compression of the right L4 nerve root:
A Causes pain over the anterior thigh and medial leg.
B Causes loss of the right ankle jerk.
C Can be confused with a common peroneal nerve lesion.
D Is usually caused by a lateral disc protrusion at L5/S1.
E Is associated with wasting of the hamstrings.

5. A 64-year-old lady visits her GP complaining of neck pain from the base of the back of her head radiating down to each shoulder. Rotation of her head to each side exacerbates symptoms and at night she finds it difficult to sleep because of neck stiffness. In cervical spondylosis:
A There may be upper motor neurone signs in the upper limbs.
B Pain is far worse during the day.
C Headaches are rare coexisting symptoms.
D Most patients have neurological signs.
E Neck traction might be helpful if the patient has upper motor neurone signs to relieve pressure from the spinal cord.

Chapter 27 Disorders of the peripheral nerves

1. A 32-year-old man presents with progressive sensory disturbance and weakness over one week that started in his feet. Prior to this, he had an episode of infective diarrhoea. What is the most likely diagnosis?
A Diabetes mellitus
B Guillain–Barré syndrome
C Excessive alcohol
D Sarcoidosis
E Myeloma

2. A 21-year-old man presents with progressive weakness in his legs since childhood. On examination, pes cavus is identified with symmetrical sensory loss up to the knee and symmetrical wasting in the distal legs. What is the most likely diagnosis?
   A   Poliomyelitis
   B   Duchenne muscular dystrophy
   C   Neurofibromatosis type 1
   D   Charcot–Marie–Tooth (CMT) disease
   E   Amyloidosis

3. A 45-year-old lady has been diagnosed with ulnar nerve compression. Which muscle should NOT be affected?
   A   Abductor digiti minimi
   B   First dorsal interosseous
   C   Abductor pollicis brevis
   D   Adductor pollicis brevis
   E   Hypothenar eminence

4. A 63-year-old woman had made an appointment to see the practice nurse in her GP's surgery. She complained of an unpleasant sensation in the toes of both feet that first started 6 months earlier and had slowly spread more proximally. She was under regular review by the practice nurse for the monitoring of diabetes, which had been diagnosed more than 10 years earlier. The characteristic sign of a sensory polyneuropathy is:
   A   Increased tone
   B   A glove and stocking sensory loss
   C   Proximal wasting
   D   Fasciculations
   E   Extensor plantars

5. A lesion to the common peroneal nerve at the fibular head causes:
   A   Weakness of plantar flexion of the foot.
   B   If long term, wasting of the quadriceps femoris.
   C   Weakness of abductor pollicis brevis.
   D   Weakness of dorsiflexion of the foot.
   E   Brisk ankle jerk.

6. A 53-year-old lady with a 13-year history of insulin-treated diabetes complained that her feet felt like blocks of ice and walking on ground felt as if she was walking on a pebble beach. Her GP diagnosed a diabetic polyneuropathy, which:
   A   Always produces symptoms.
   B   Usually causes weakness rather than sensory loss.
   C   Is unaffected by good blood glucose control.
   D   Is less common in type II diabetes.
   E   Might be associated with painless foot ulcers.

7. A cause of a demyelinating neuropathy is:
   A   Guillain–Barré syndrome
   B   Diabetes
   C   Vincristine
   D   Cryoglobulinaemia
   E   Amyloidosis

8. A 27-year-old lady who was 33 weeks pregnant would awake at night with an unpleasant and numb sensation of the right hand that would improve by shaking it repeatedly. Following an examination by her GP, she was diagnosed with carpal tunnel syndrome, which:
   A   Is associated with symptoms only in the hand.
   B   Only becomes symptomatic at night.
   C   Pinprick testing might be abnormal over the medial aspect of the middle finger.
   D   Often causes severe wasting and weakness of the whole hand.
   E   Weakness affects the first dorsal interossei more than abductor pollicis brevis.

9. The ulnar nerve:
   A   Is the main continuation of the posterior cord of the brachial plexus.
   B   Supplies the brachioradialis muscle.
   C   Runs in the spiral groove on the humerus where it is easily compressed.
   D   If damaged, usually causes numbness over the ring and little finger of the hand.
   E   Is the main motor nerve to the extensor compartments of the arm and forearm.

10. A 74-year-old male smoker has developed severe pain and weakness in his right hand. He also describes some numbness in his right arm. On examination, he has wasting and power loss in his hand involving both thenar and hypothenar eminences and sensory loss over the C8 and T1 dermatomes. Closer inspection suggests that his right eyelid is drooping and he has a small right pupil. He has also lost a stone in weight over the past month. What is the most likely diagnosis?
    A   Ulnar nerve palsy at the elbow
    B   Radial nerve palsy in the spiral groove
    C   Lower brachial plexus lesion
    D   Ulnar nerve palsy at the wrist
    E   Cervical myeloradiculopathy

11. A 25-year-old woman has noticed that, over the last 3 months, she has had increasing pain in her left arm and occasionally in her right. The pain wakes her up at night and she shakes her hands to relieve her symptoms. She

has not noticed any weakness in her hands although she has recently been prescribed thyroxine replacement for hypothyroidism. Neurological examination is normal apart from a positive Phalen test on the left side. What is the most likely diagnosis?

A   Multiple sclerosis
B   Posterior interosseous nerve palsy
C   Motor neurone disease
D   Carpal tunnel syndrome
E   Brachial neuritis (neuralgic amyotrophy)

12. A 46-year-old man had an acute onset of severe right shoulder pain that prevented him from working 6 weeks ago. Since then, he has noticed that his right shoulder has become weak. On examination, he has severe wasting and weakness of his deltoid, supraspinatus, rhomboids and biceps. The reflexes in his right arm are all diminished. He has some slight numbness over his shoulder, but it is relatively minor. What is the most likely diagnosis?

A   Multiple sclerosis
B   Posterior interosseous nerve palsy
C   Motor neurone disease
D   Carpal tunnel syndrome
E   Brachial neuritis (neuralgic amyotrophy)

13. A 59-year-old secretary has noticed that her typing was not as good as it used to be 5 months ago and took early retirement. Recently, she has noticed that she has difficulty with getting dressed because her hands feel weak. Her swallowing has also become a problem, especially when drinking tea. She suffers from cramps at night in her legs and sometimes her arms. On examination, her tongue is small and possibly has some fasciculations. She has a brisk gag reflex and jaw jerk. She has fasciculations in her hands, biceps, quadriceps and calves associated with wasting in her hands and forearms. Her reflexes are all brisk and her plantars are extensor. What is the most likely diagnosis?

A   Multiple sclerosis
B   Posterior interosseous nerve palsy
C   Motor neurone disease
D   Carpal tunnel syndrome
E   Brachial neuritis (neuralgic amyotrophy)

14. A 62-year-old woman has recently developed severe pain, especially at night, in her neck. She has also noticed that she gets shooting pains down her right arm, especially when she flexes her neck. On examination, she has weakness of her right elbow flexion and some numbness over the lateral surface of the arm. Her right biceps jerk is absent. You incidentally

notice that her walking is slow and that her triceps, knee and ankle jerks are brisk and her plantars are extensor. What is the most likely diagnosis?

A   Ulnar nerve palsy at the elbow
B   Radial nerve palsy in the spiral groove
C   Lower brachial plexus lesion
D   Ulnar nerve palsy at the wrist
E   Cervical myeloradiculopathy

Chapter 28 Disorders of the neuromuscular junction

1. A 65-year-old man with known small-cell lung cancer presents with a 6-month history of fatigable weakness in his shoulder and hip girdle. The most likely diagnosis is:

A   Myasthenia gravis
B   Vitamin D deficiency
C   Cushing disease
D   Lambert–Eaton syndrome
E   Hypothyroidism

2. A patient with the clinical suspicion of myasthenia gravis undergoes electromyography. Which finding supports the above diagnosis?

A   Fasciculations.
B   An increment in compound muscle action potentials (CMAPs) on exercise.
C   A decrement in CMAPs on exercise.
D   Decreased motor conduction velocity.
E   Prolonged H wave.

3. Which of the following drugs is not associated with myasthenia

A   Penicillamine
B   Penicillin
C   Phenytoin
D   Quinine
E   Ciprofloxacin

4. A 43-year-old lady was under review by her neurologist having presented with intermittent double vision in different directions, difficulty swallowing and weakness in her arms and legs. She had been diagnosed with myasthenia gravis which is associated with:

A   Diplopia or ptosis in over 90% of patients at some time in their illness.
B   Exercise such as repetitive shoulder abduction improves weakness.
C   Muscle cramps and myoglobinuria.
D   Type I respiratory failure.
E   Absent tendon reflexes.

Chapter 29 Disorders of skeletal muscle

1. A 6-year-old boy presents with a 4-year history of progressive difficulty in walking and jumping. His examination reveals proximal limb weakness. His creatine kinase (CK) was 18,000 U/L. What is the most likely diagnosis?
   A Myotonic dystrophy
   B Becker muscular dystrophy
   C Duchenne muscular dystrophy
   D McCardle disease
   E Mitochondrial myopathy

2. A 36-year-old electrician presents with a 3-year history of stiffness in his hands especially when using tools. More recently he has found walking on inclines difficult. Of note, he had a cataract operation 1 year ago. What is the most likely diagnosis?
   A Becker muscular dystrophy (BMD)
   B Myotonic dystrophy
   C Cushing disease
   D Mitochondrial cytopathy
   E Dermatomyositis

3. Which of the following is NOT associated with dermatomyositis?
   A A high creatine kinase (CK) level
   B Painful myopathy
   C Heliotrope rash
   D Lung cancer
   E Interstitial lung fibrosis

4. A 42-year-old woman was admitted to hospital with weakness of the arms and legs. Her muscles felt painful especially with movement and she had over the past fortnight developed considerable fatigue. A rheumatologist diagnosed polymyositis where:
   A The creatinine kinase (CK) is usually raised.
   B Swallowing is normal.
   C Patients are hyporeflexic.
   D Distal limb muscles are affected more than proximal muscles.
   E A heliotrope rash of the face and around the eyelids and extensor joint surfaces is common.

Chapter 30 Vascular diseases of the nervous system

1. A 72-year-old man presented to the A&E department with a 2-hour history of aphasia and right-sided weakness. He has had no previous strokes and had only a history of high blood pressure and diabetes, for which he takes ramipril and metformin. His admission blood pressure is 167/80 mm Hg. His computed tomography (CT) showed no evidence of an intracerebral haemorrhage. What is the most appropriate immediate management?
   A Monitoring in a hyperacute stroke unit
   B Thrombolysis
   C Thrombectomy
   D Clopidogrel
   E Warfarin

2. A 32-year-old patient presents with a stroke. On examination he had a left Horner sign and right-sided weakness. Three days previously he had sprained his neck in the gym. What is the most likely diagnosis?
   A Carotid dissection
   B Cerebral vein thrombosis
   C Subarachnoid haemorrhage
   D Lateral medullary infarct
   E Arteriovenous malformation

3. A 79-year-old woman, on warfarin for a previous deep vein thrombosis, falls and hits her head. She develops a mild headache and a fluctuating level of consciousness. What is the most likely diagnosis?
   A Subarachnoid haemorrhage
   B Acute subdural haematoma
   C Stroke
   D Sagittal sinus thrombosis
   E Extradural haematoma

4. A 67-year-old man presented to his GP complaining of a fogging of vision in the left eye, which he described as a 'curtain coming down'. It lasted a minute before returning back to normal. There were no other symptoms. The following is the most likely cause of his visual impairment:
   A Retinitis pigmentosa
   B Carotid embolism
   C Papilloedema
   D Migrainous aura
   E Glaucoma

5. A 58-year-old woman was transferred from the A&E department to the stroke ward with a diagnosis of Wallenberg (or lateral medullary) syndrome. There was a 6-year history of diabetes and an electrocardiogram in the A&E department had identified a new diagnosis of atrial fibrillation. A lesion of the lateral medulla on one side may give rise to:
   A Ipsilateral facial weakness
   B Horner syndrome
   C Contralateral weakness of the palate
   D Contralateral weakness of the tongue
   E Ipsilateral third nerve palsy

6. A 72-year-old right-handed man was admitted to the stroke unit. A computed tomography brain scan performed in the A&E department identified an infarct in the right middle cerebral artery territory. The following signs typically occur with nondominant cortical lesions:
   A Dysphasia
   B Dressing apraxia
   C Dyscalculia
   D Finger agnosia
   E Impaired discrimination between left and right

7. The following are associated with anterior circulation (carotid territory) transient ischaemic attacks (TIAs):
   A Diplopia
   B Weakness in all four limbs
   C Loss of vision in one eye (amaurosis fugax)
   D Dysphagia
   E Vertigo

8. A 58-year-old man is brought to the A&E department by ambulance having been found unconscious on the pavement outside the chemist. He was carrying his medication and prescription, which included amlodipine, metformin and simvastatin. A computed tomography (CT) of the brain identified a large intracerebral bleed. Primary intracerebral haemorrhage:
   A Can be differentiated clinically from ischaemic stroke.
   B Usually causes meningism.
   C Is often less clinically dangerous if in the posterior fossa.
   D Is usually within the internal capsule and basal ganglia in hypertensive patients.
   E Is best treated with emergency surgical evacuation.

9. A 74-year-old man with hypertension developed an acute onset of severe weakness in his right side involving his lower face, arm and leg. On examination, he has right hemiplegia with no sensory loss. What is the most likely diagnosis?
   A Lacunar infarction of the internal capsule
   B Total right middle cerebral infarction
   C Total left middle cerebral infarction
   D Basilar artery thrombosis
   E Lateral medullary syndrome

10. A 25-year-old woman was involved in a car accident and suffered a severe whiplash injury and shock but was otherwise well. The following day, she presents to the A&E department with weakness on her right side, confusion and incomprehensible speech. On examination, she has Horner syndrome on the left side, a dense right hemiplegia, dysphasia and probably a right homonymous hemianopia. Unfortunately, she becomes very drowsy and

loses consciousness over the next 24 hours and dies in the intensive treatment unit. What is the most likely diagnosis?
   A Cerebellar haemorrhage
   B Partial left middle cerebral artery infarction
   C Transient ischaemic attack
   D Posterior cerebral artery infarction
   E Internal carotid artery occlusion

11. A 66-year-old man had an acute onset of right lower facial weakness and his wife tells you that he had severe difficulties 'in stringing his words together'. It has slowly improved over the past 4 days and, when you see him, he is only complaining of slight difficulties in expressing himself fully, but he knows what he wants to say. On examination, he has a left carotid bruit and a mild expressive dysphasia. What is the most likely diagnosis?
   A Cerebellar haemorrhage
   B Partial left middle cerebral artery infarction
   C Transient ischaemic attack
   D Posterior cerebral artery infarction
   E Internal carotid artery occlusion

12. A 59-year-old man with type 2 diabetes presents to the A&E department with acute onset of vertigo and imbalance. He also has problems swallowing and the right side of his face 'feels strange'. On examination, he has Horner syndrome, loss of pain and temperature sensation on the right side, his uvula moves to the left and he has pooling of his secretions in his pharynx. He has mild left-sided weakness and right-sided dysmetria. Over the next 2 weeks, he almost makes a full recovery. What is the most likely diagnosis?
   A Lacunar infarction of the internal capsule
   B Total right middle cerebral infarction
   C Total left middle cerebral infarction
   D Basilar artery thrombosis
   E Lateral medullary syndrome

13. A 62-year-old woman with hypertension presents to the A&E department with a 4-hour history of rapidly progressive drowsiness. Her husband informs you that, prior to her becoming drowsy, she complained of a severe pain in the back of her head and she vomited twice. She tried to walk but was too unsteady. On examination, she has a Glasgow Coma Scale of 6 out of 15 and has a grossly dilated left pupil. There are no other obvious cranial nerve signs. She is too confused and drowsy to be examined properly, but she appears to be moving all her limbs. Her reflexes are brisk but symmetrical and her plantars are extensor. What is the most likely diagnosis?
   A Cerebellar haemorrhage
   B Partial left middle cerebral artery infarction

C   Transient ischaemic attack
D   Posterior cerebral artery infarction
E   Internal carotid artery occlusion

Chapter 32 Infections of the nervous system

1. A 13-year-old presents to A&E with drowsiness, with a temperature of 39°C and neck stiffness. You consider bacterial meningitis. What is the most immediate management?
   A   Lumbar puncture (LP)
   B   Intravenous cephalosporin
   C   Intravenous aciclovir
   D   Computed tomography (CT) of the head
   E   Intensive therapy unit (ITU) admission

2. A 35-year-old patient originating from India presents with new-onset seizures. A magnetic resonance imaging scan shows multiple calcified cysts. What is the most likely diagnosis?
   A   Herpes simplex virus (HSV) encephalitis
   B   Tuberculosis
   C   HIV
   D   Neurocysticercosis
   E   Syphilis

Chapter 33 Multiple sclerosis

1. A 24-year-old man is reviewed by a neurologist in the outpatient clinic and informed of a diagnosis of multiple sclerosis. He recovered from left-sided optic neuritis a year earlier and more recently had developed a progressive ataxia. Magnetic resonance imaging of the brain and spinal cord identified a number of areas of demyelination. When discussing the prognosis the patient was informed that multiple sclerosis is more likely to have a benign course if the patient:
   A   Presents with a spastic paraparesis.
   B   Presents with sensory symptoms.
   C   Is over 50 years old at the onset of symptoms.
   D   Presents with brainstem or cerebellar features.
   E   Is male.

2. The multiple sclerosis (MS) nurse specialist is counselling a 38-year-old lady who has just been given a new diagnosis of MS and discusses the different treatment options. The MS nurse informed the patient that the following medication will significantly reduce relapse rates in relapsing–remitting MS:
   A   β-Interferon
   B   Mycophenolate
   C   Steroids
   D   Methotrexate
   E   Cyclosporine

Chapter 36 Hereditary conditions affecting the nervous system

1. An 11-year-old boy presents with progressive hearing loss and bilateral vestibular schwannomas are identified on magnetic resonance imaging. What inherited condition is most likely in this case?
   A   Neurofibromatosis type 1
   B   Neurofibromatosis type 2
   C   Tuberous sclerosis
   D   Sturge–Weber syndrome
   E   Ataxic telangiectasia

2. A 17-year-old boy is admitted to the psychiatric ward of his local hospital with acute psychosis and suicidal ideation. There was an 8-year history of intractable depression. The examination is remarkable for symmetrical parkinsonism. The following supports a diagnosis of Wilson disease:
   A   The total serum copper is raised.
   B   Urinary 24-hour copper is raised.
   C   Urinary 24-hour copper is low.
   D   Penicillamine binds to copper and decreases the release of copper in the urine.
   E   Magnesium supplementation increases copper excretion in stool and reduces copper absorption in the gut.

Chapter 38 Adnexal (eyelids, lacrimal system and orbit)

1. A 53-year-old man presents to the emergency department with multiple facial lesions. The lesions appeared 48 hours ago and are tender to the touch. Several days ago, there was an episode of burning pain over the forehead. On examination, he is apyrexial. He has tenderness over the forehead. Several vesicles measuring around 4 to 5 mm are noted on the left side. Hutchinson sign is positive. What does a Hutchinson sign indicate?
   A   Ocular involvement
   B   Eruption of the vesicles
   C   Urgent IV antibiotics
   D   Ophthalmic branch involvement
   E   Use of topical steroids

2. A 5-year-old girl presents to the GP with her mother. The mother is concerned as her daughter has developed a swollen left eye over the past day. The mother noticed that the eye was swelling yesterday after she was playing in the garden. This morning the mother mentioned that her daughter was having difficulty in reading the writing in her books. There is no other past medical history.

On examination, she is pyrexial and the left eye lid is warm and erythematous, the eye seems to be protruding, and there is pain when testing eye movements The right eye appears to be normal

What is the most likely diagnosis?

A Preseptal cellulitis
B Allergic conjunctivitis
C Graves disease
D Orbital cellulitis
E Acute mastoiditis

3. A 54-year-old man presents to the emergency department with a vesicular rash around his left upper eyelid. The left eye is red and painful.
   Based on the most likely diagnosis, what should be the next step in the management of this patient?

   A Oral aciclovir
   B Oral corticosteroids + aciclovir eye drops
   C Topical corticosteroids + aciclovir eye drops
   D Oral corticosteroids
   E Aciclovir eye drops

4. A worried father brings his 5-month-old baby boy to the GP. The father describes that his son has been having recurrent eye issues. The baby has been having ongoing sticky clear discharge from both eyes. The father described that he has tried multiple drops and carried out appropriate lid hygiene advice with no good effect. On examination, the pupils are equal and reactive, no presence of any inflammatory changes on the conjunctiva, and the sclera is white. The baby has a normal gaze, and the red reflex is present. Overall, the examination was normal.
   Given the likely diagnosis, what is the best advice to give to the father?

   A Reassure the father that the condition will self-resolve by 1 year of age.
   B Urgent referral to ophthalmology.
   C Apply low-strength topical steroid eye drops twice a day.
   D The condition requires routine probing at 1 year.
   E The condition requires regular chloramphenicol eye drops.

5. A 9-year-old boy presents to the emergency department after sustaining a laceration to his left upper eyelid. On examination, he is febrile and generally unwell. The eyelid is acutely swollen, erythematous, hot and tender on palpation. There is no proptosis, visual impairment or pain when testing eye movements. The right eye is normal.

What is the most likely diagnosis?

A Bacterial conjunctivitis
B Thyroid eye disease
C Orbital cellulitis
D Preseptal cellulitis
E Blepharitis

6. A 34-year-old lady presents to her GP with a firm painless lump in her right upper eyelid for the past two months. The doctor makes a diagnosis of a chalazion (Fig. 4).

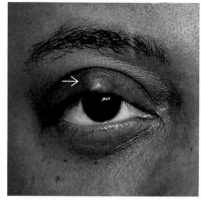

Fig. 4 (From Putnam AR, Thompson KS. *Diagnostic Pathology: Nonneoplastic Pediatrics*. 2nd ed. Elsevier; 2023.)

Which gland is affected to produce a chalazion?

A Glands of Zeis
B Glands of Moll
C Meibomian gland
D Lacrimal gland
E Thyroid gland

7. A 73-year-old male presents to the GP with a painless lesion growing over the past three months on his lower eyelid (Fig. 5).

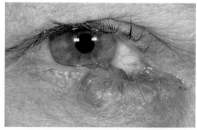

Fig. 5 (From Wojno TH. *Eyelid abnormalities*. In: Palay DA, Krachmer JH, editors. *Primary care ophthalmology*, 2nd ed. Philadelphia, Mosby; 2005.)

What is the likely diagnosis?

A   Squamous cell carcinoma
B   Melanoma
C   Basal cell carcinoma
D   Chalazion
E   Stye

8. A 35-year-old female presents to the thyroid clinic. She complains of weight loss, dizziness, sweating and increased frequency of stools. Alongside this, she complains of eye pain and diplopia. On examination, a goitre is noted (Fig. 6).

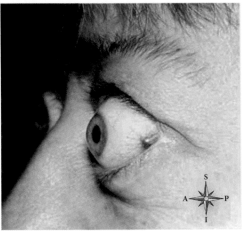

Fig. 6 (From Patton K, et al. *The Human Body in Health and Disease*. 8th ed. Elsevier; 2024.)

What is the likely diagnosis?

A   Hashimoto disease
B   Graves disease
C   Iodine deficiency
D   Toxic multinodular goitre
E   Euthyroid

Chapter 39 Anterior segment (cornea and cataract)

1. A 30-year-old male presents to emergency eye casualty with a unilateral left-sided acutely painful red eye. He describes a burning pain around the eye, photophobia and epiphora. He is not a contact lens wearer and has no other past medical history of note. Fluorescein staining is carried out (see Fig. 7).

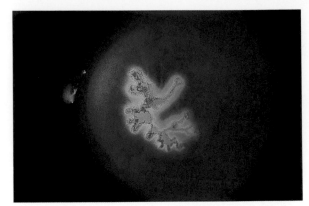

Fig. 7 (From Salmon J. *Kanski's Clinical Ophthalmology: A Systematic Approach*. 9th ed. Elsevier; 2020.)

What is the most appropriate management?

A   Topical aciclovir
B   Oral corticosteroids
C   Topical corticosteroids
D   Topical chloramphenicol
E   Artificial tears

2. A 21-year-old male presents to his GP. He has been complaining of a three-day history of soreness, redness and green discharge from his right eye. He also describes a gritty sensation in his right eye. He is a regular contact lens wearer. On examination, his right eye is red and inflamed with epiphora. The left eye is normal. Visual acuity is unaffected when wearing glasses.
What is the most appropriate management?

A   Refer for urgent same-day ophthalmology assessment.
B   Prescribe artificial tears.
C   Refer for a two-week ophthalmology assessment.
D   Prescribe chloramphenicol eye drops.
E   Prescribe corticosteroid eye drops.

3. A 78-year-old woman presented to the emergency department with an acutely painful red eye with associated loss of vision in her right eye. She described a dull ache in the morning with some redness which progressively worsened over several hours. She denies any trauma or other visual disturbances. She underwent cataract surgery on her right eye two days ago. On examination, the right eye has redness with hypopyon. She complains of severe pain when testing eye movements and visual acuity is severely reduced. The left eye is normal.
What is the most likely diagnosis?

A Herpes simplex keratitis
B Posterior vitreous detachment
C Allergic conjunctivitis
D Anterior uveitis
E Endophthalmitis

4. A 28-year-old male surfer presents to the emergency eye casualty with intense left-sided eye pain and reports the sensation of a foreign body since morning. He wears contact lenses; however he removed them since the pain started. Alongside this, he describes photophobia, epiphora and discharge. On examination, the left eye has conjunctival injection and decreased visual acuity in the left eye. Under slit lamp examination, there is a mild, regular ulceration of the left eye. The right eye is normal.
What is the most likely diagnosis?
A Conjunctivitis
B Episcleritis
C Anterior uveitis
D Acanthamoeba keratitis
E Herpes simplex keratitis

5. A 32-year-old female accountant presents to the emergency eye casualty with pain in her left eye. She describes a gritty sensation like something is stuck in her eye and increased sensitivity to light. She wears contact lenses. On slit lamp examination of her left eye, there is conjunctival injection, hypopyon and focal white infiltrates on the cornea. The right eye is normal.
What is the most likely underlying organism?
A *Chlamydia trachomatis*
B *Neisseria gonorrhoeae*
C *Pseudomonas aeruginosa*
D *Acanthamoeba*
E Herpes simplex virus

6. A 52-year-old male presents to the GP with pain in his right eye following cutting the grass in his backyard. On examination, the right eye appears red with epiphora; there appears to be a grass seed visibly lodged near his cornea. The other eye is normal.
What is the most appropriate management plan?
A Urgent same-day ophthalmology referral.
B Remove the seed at the practice and refer to ophthalmology for a review tomorrow.
C Advise eye irrigation to remove the seed and prescribe topical antibiotics.
D Advise eye irrigation and reassurance that symptoms will improve over time.
E Advise eye irrigation, prescribe topical antibiotics and analgesia.

7. A 30-year-old female mechanic visits the emergency department with a two-day history of pain and photophobia in her left eye. She also is complaining of feeling that there is something stuck in her eye. The patient admitted to not always wearing eye protection during work. There is also a vesicular rash present around the left side of the face. Slit lamp examination with fluorescein staining reveals a dendritic ulcer of the left eye. The right eye is normal.
What is the most likely diagnosis?
A Herpes simplex keratitis
B Bacterial keratitis
C Corneal foreign body
D Photokeratitis
E Corneal abrasion

8. An 80-year-old lady with type 2 diabetes presents to her GP surgery. She has been having trouble with her vision over the past few months. She described blurry vision and seeing halos around lights. No other ocular history. The doctor tells the patient that the patient has developed a cataract.
Which of the following drugs is most likely to cause a cataract?
A Metformin
B Digoxin
C Adenosine
D Corticosteroids
E Methotrexate

Chapter 40 Glaucoma

1. A 59-year-old male is seen in the ophthalmology clinic with a gradual loss of vision, mainly affecting his peripheral vision. Tonometry is carried out on both eyes which reveals an intraocular pressure of 26 mm Hg in the left eye and 25 mm Hg in the right eye. On examination through fundoscopy, there is optic disc cupping. A diagnosis of primary open-angle glaucoma is made, and a prescription for timolol eye drops is given.
What is the mechanism of action of timolol?
A Decreased uveoscleral outflow
B Increased uveoscleral outflow
C Increased production of aqueous fluid
D Decreased production of aqueous fluid
E Decreased production of aqueous fluid and increased uveoscleral outflow

2. A 68-year-old female presented to her GP surgery following a regular review at her optician. The opticians noticed raised intraocular pressure and decreased

peripheral vision. Past medical history includes asthma. The GP suspects this may be glaucoma and makes a referral to ophthalmology.

What would be an appropriate first-line treatment for this patient?

A Timolol
B Pilocarpine
C Brimonidine
D Latanoprost
E Dorzolamide

3. A 59-year-old woman presents to the emergency department with sudden unilateral right eye pain and vomiting while driving at night. The patient also complains of reduced vision in the affected eye. On examination, the right eye appeared hazy, dilated and unreactive to light. The patient usually wears glasses and is long-sighted. Tonometry reveals a raised intraocular pressure in the right eye. The left eye is normal on examination.

What investigation should be carried out next?

A Fluorescein angiography
B Optical coherence tomography
C Gonioscopy
D Fundoscopy
E Visual evoked potential

4. A 52-year-old male presents to the emergency department with an acutely painful red left eye. Alongside this, he mentioned a headache that came on around the same time the eye pain started and that his vision had worsened. On examination, the left eye has a conjunctival injection, and the cornea is hazy. Pupillary reflexes on the right eye are normal; however, the left pupil is semidilated and nonreactive.

What should the initial management of this patient be?

A Direct parasympathomimetic and β-blocker eye drops
B β-Blocker eye drops
C β-Agonist eye drops
D Direct sympathomimetic and β-blocker eye drops
E Direct sympathomimetic and β-agonist eye drops

5. A 74-year-old female presents to the emergency department with pain in her right eye. The pain started three hours ago and is associated with a severe headache around the right eye and nausea. She also described that her vision is blurred, and she is seeing rings around bright lights. On examination the right pupil is semidilated and nonreactive. There is no evidence of papilledema. Given the likely diagnosis, what is the most definitive treatment for this patient once her condition is stable?

A IV acetazolamide
B Direct sympathomimetic and β-blocker eye drops

C Laser iridotomy
D Atropine eye drops
E Direct sympathomimetic eye drops

6. An 85-year-old male presents to ophthalmology following a routine screen at his optician. The optician mentioned that he has high intraocular pressure. He has a past medical history of hypertension and type 2 diabetes mellitus. He wears prescription glasses for his short-sightedness. He is complaining of no visual symptoms at present. The ophthalmologist diagnosed him with primary open-angle glaucoma and prescribes regular latanoprost eye drops.

What is a known adverse effect of latanoprost?

A Increased eyelash length
B Hyperaemia
C Constricted pupil
D Blurred vision
E Headache

7. A 54-year-old female presents to her GP with severe pain over her left eye for the past 5 hours (Fig. 8). This is associated with a headache and nausea. She described that she had vomited several times this morning. She normally wears glasses.

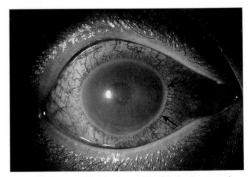

Fig. 8 (From Roberts JR, Hedges JR. *Clinical procedures in emergency medicine*. 5th ed. Philadelphia, Saunders; 2010.)

What is the most appropriate management option?

A Administer chloramphenicol eye drops.
B Reassure that the condition is self-limiting and send home.
C Same-day referral to neurology.
D Same-day referral to ophthalmology.
E Advise using eye lubricant drops twice a day.

Chapter 41 Retina

1. A 79-year-old male presented to the GP with sudden, painless loss of vision in his left eye 3 hours ago. His past

medical history includes type 2 diabetes mellitus, hypertension and dyslipidaemia. He described that there was a moment of flashes then he described what looked like 'a curtain appearing' in his peripheral vision of left eye that then moved centrally.

What is the most likely diagnosis?

A   Retinal detachment
B   Vitreous haemorrhage
C   Central retinal vein occlusion
D   Central retinal artery occlusion
E   Optic neuritis

2. A 61-year-old man presents to the emergency department with sudden, painless loss of vision in his left eye. Fundoscopy reveals the following (Fig. 9):

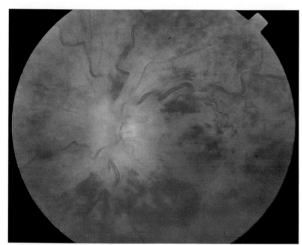

Fig. 9 (From Robertson C, Douglas G, Nicol F. *Macleod's Clinical Examination*. 12th ed. Elsevier; 2009.)

What is the most likely diagnosis?
A   Central retinal artery occlusion
B   Central retinal vein occlusion
C   Retinal detachment
D   Vitreous haemorrhage
E   Posterior vitreous detachment

3. A 42-year-old female presents to the emergency department with sudden, painless loss of vision in her right eye. Her past medical history includes hypertension, systemic lupus erythematous and is an active smoker. There is a positive relative afferent pupillary defect present. Fundoscopy reveals the following (Fig. 10):

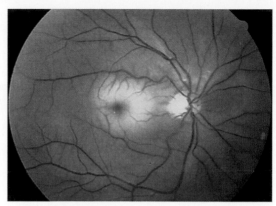

Fig. 10 (From Jankovic J, et al. *Bradley and Daroff's neurology in clinical practice*. 8th ed. Philadelphia, Elsevier; 2022.)

What is the most likely diagnosis?
A   Vitreous haemorrhage
B   Central retinal artery occlusion
C   Central retinal vein occlusion
D   Branch retinal vein occlusion
E   Retinal detachment

4. A 72-year-old male presents to his GP with a three-month history of worsening visual acuity. He describes difficulty in reading the smaller words on the newspaper and has noticed that straight lines on his wallpaper at home appear 'curvy'. He has also noticed a grey patch in his central field of vision.

What is the most likely diagnosis?
A   Diabetic retinopathy
B   Central retinal artery occlusion
C   Central retinal vein occlusion
D   Vitreous haemorrhage
E   Age-related macular degeneration

5. A 59-year-old female attends the ophthalmology department for a review as he was recently diagnosed with type 2 diabetes mellitus. A slit lamp examination was carried out which revealed cotton wool spots.

What is the likely underlying pathology causing these?
A   Retinal infarction
B   Retinal neovascularization
C   Retinal necrosis
D   Retinal detachment
E   Atrophic retinal holes

6. A 69-year-old male attends the ophthalmology department for a regular check-up. He has a past medical

history of poorly controlled hypertension. On fundoscopy, there is the presence of microaneurysms, retinal blot and flame haemorrhages, arteriovenous nipping and cotton-wool spots. Fundoscopy of the left eye is shown in Fig. 11.

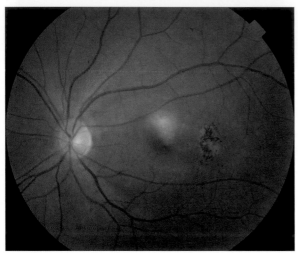

Fig. 11 (From Sadda SR, et al. *Ryan's Retina*. 7th ed. Elsevier; 2023.)

What grade of hypertensive retinopathy does this correspond to?
A   Grade I
B   Grade II
C   Grade III
D   Grade IV
E   Grade V

7. A 59-year-old female visits the ophthalmology department due to a 4-month history of gradual decline in vision. She mentioned that she has noticed a glare around objects and that her vision seems to deteriorate at night. On assessment, there is reduced central visual acuity. Amsler grid testing reveals line distortion.
Given the likely diagnosis, what changes may be present in fundoscopy for this patient?
A   Cotton wool spots
B   Pale retina
C   Papilloedema
D   Choroidal neovascularization
E   Retinal haemorrhages

8. An 81-year-old female attends an ophthalmology appointment after being referred by her general

practitioner with a new-onset gradual decline in visual acuity and metamorphopsia noted on Amsler grid testing. Past medical history includes hypertension. On fundoscopy, the ophthalmologist notices well-demarcated red patches.
Given the likely diagnosis, which of the following is the most appropriate treatment?
A   Cataract surgery
B   Low-dose steroid eye drops
C   Laser photocoagulation
D   Aspirin
E   Antivascular endothelial growth factor (anti-VEGF)

9. A 76-year-old male presents to his GP with a sudden onset of flashes and floaters in his left eye. He wears prescription glasses for short-sightedness and has a past medical history of hypertension and recurrent pulmonary embolisms. On examination, visual acuity is unchanged. Fundoscopy is unremarkable with normal optic disc and retinal vessels.
What is the most likely diagnosis?
A   Acute angle closure glaucoma
B   Posterior vitreous detachment
C   Vitreous haemorrhage
D   Central retinal artery occlusion
E   Central retinal vein occlusion

10. A 70-year-old male presents to the emergency department with sudden, painless loss of vision in his right eye. He described that the event occurred 4 hours ago and lasted approximately 2 minutes. There were no preceding symptoms present, and the patient denied any pain, nausea or any other focal neurology. Past medical history includes hypertension and type 2 diabetes. On examination, both eyes appeared normal and both pupils were equal and reactive to light.
What is the most likely diagnosis?
A   Giant cell arteritis
B   Acute angle closure glaucoma
C   Central retinal artery occlusion
D   Optic neuritis
E   Amaurosis fugax

Chapter 42 Medical ophthalmology and uveitis

1. A 29-year-old woman presents to the GP with an acutely, painful red eye. She mentioned that the pain started three days ago and has gradually worsened. There is radiation of the pain to the forehead and cheeks. Visual symptoms

include photophobia and blurred vision. She has a past medical history of systemic lupus erythematous and rheumatoid arthritis. The GP attempts to blanch the vessels in her eye using phenylephrine drops; however, no change to redness is noted.

What is the most likely diagnosis?

A Episcleritis
B Scleritis
C Bacterial conjunctivitis
D Anterior uveitis
E Viral conjunctivitis

2. An 80-year-old lady presented to the emergency department with a one-week history of a headache. The headache is predominantly around her right temple and noticed that it is worse when brushing her hair; she also noticed aching in her jaw when chewing her food. She also experienced a recent temporary loss of vision for around 2 minutes which she described as a 'dark curtain descending'.

What is the most likely finding on fundoscopy?

A Cherry red spot on the macula
B Swollen pale disc with blurred margins
C Retinal haemorrhages
D Yellow drusen
E AV nipping

3. A 78-year-old woman presented to the emergency department with a headache that started two days ago, and new onset of jaw claudication when eating his lunch. No visual symptoms are present. The doctors suspect giant cell arteritis, so start high-dose prednisolone and an appropriate biopsy is carried out. The results of the biopsy come back as normal.

What is the next step in management?

A Continue high-dose prednisolone.
B Stop the high-dose prednisolone, reassure the patient and discharge.
C CT head.
D Take additional bloods including ESR/CRP and decide whether to continue prednisolone depending on results.
E Repeat biopsy immediately.

4. A 43-year-old male presents to the emergency department with severe pain in his left eye. He also described that the pain is worse when in bright rooms. Past medical history includes Crohn's disease. On examination, the eye is shown in Fig. 12.

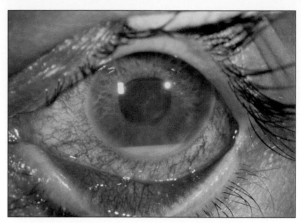

Fig. 12 (From Yanoff M, Duker J. *Ophthalmology*. 6th ed. Elsevier; 2023.)

What is the most appropriate treatment for this patient?

A Steroids and cycloplegic drops
B Chloramphenicol drops
C Lubricant eye drops
D Pilocarpine and timolol drops
E NSAID drops

5. A 54-year-old female presents to the emergency department with a left-sided headache and blurred vision in the left eye. She mentioned that when eating breakfast this morning her jaw started aching and has been feeling more tired recently. The patient also stated that she has had to change her bed sheets frequently due to night sweats.

Which of the following conditions would you expect in her past medical history?

A Fibromyalgia
B Polymyositis
C Polymyalgia rheumatica
D Osteoarthritis
E Systemic lupus erythematous

6. A 50-year-old female presents to her general practitioner with a left red eye. She describes the pain as mild and occasional irritation with some watering. She denies dryness or severe pain, with no visual symptoms. Past medical history includes rheumatoid arthritis and hypertension. On examination, her left eye was red and both pupils were equal and reactive.

What is the most likely diagnosis?

A Keratoconjunctivitis sicca
B Episcleritis

C   Scleritis
D   Anterior uveitis
E   Bacterial keratitis

7. A 78-year-old female presents to her general practitioner with a painful, erythematous blistering rash around the left side of the face. The rash is affecting the left trigeminal distribution.
What is the likely causative organism?
A   Varicella zoster virus
B   Epstein–Barr virus
C   Hepatitis C virus
D   Rabies virus
E   Coxsackie virus

8. A 49-year-old male presents to the emergency department complaining of a 2-hour history of severe pain in his right eye and photophobia. His past medical history includes ankylosing spondylitis. On examination, the pupil is small, irregular and a ring of redness spreading from the cornea of the eye. The doctor suspects acute anterior uveitis.
What does the uveal tract consist of?
A   Sclera, ciliary body and conjunctiva
B   Conjunctiva, iris and retina
C   Sclera, ciliary body and retina
D   Conjunctiva, iris and choroid
E   Iris, ciliary body and choroid

Chapter 43 Neuro-ophthalmology

1. A 29-year-old male presents to the GP with a severe headache that is worse in the mornings. The headache has been present for over a month now and over-the-counter medications do not help. Recently he has been feeling nauseous and described several episodes of vomiting. He also stated that his vision has become blurry. General examination is normal, and pupils are equal and reactive to light.
What finding is likely upon fundoscopy for this patient?
A   Cherry red spot
B   Several retinal haemorrhages
C   Retinal pigmentation
D   Blurring of the optic disc margin
E   Normal retina

2. A 48-year-old male presents to the GP complaining of a visual disturbance. Examination reveals a left homonymous hemianopia.
Where is the lesion likely to be?

A   Left optic nerve
B   Optic chiasm
C   Right optic tract
D   Left optic radiation or occipital cortex
E   Right optic nerve

3. A 36-year-old female presented to the emergency eye clinic with a 1-day history of acute vision changes, and pain in both her eyes which is exacerbated by movement. She described a 'grey cloud' in the centre of her vision. On examination, there is a relative afferent pupillary defect present and poor discrimination of colour when testing with Ishihara plates. She has a past medical history of multiple sclerosis and no other previous ophthalmological history.
What is the most likely diagnosis?
A   Retinal detachment
B   Endophthalmitis
C   Amaurosis fugax
D   Optic neuritis
E   Anterior uveitis

4. A 29-year-old female presents to the emergency department with visual disturbance. On examination, the patient has visual field abnormalities; he is unable to perceive stimuli in the inferior temporal field of his left eye and the inferior nasal field of his right eye.
What is the correct term for this visual field defect?
A   Left-sided homonymous inferior quadrantanopia
B   Right-sided homonymous inferior quadrantanopia
C   Left-sided homonymous inferior hemianopia
D   Right-sided homonymous inferior hemianopia
E   Bitemporal hemianopia

5. A 54-year-old male has been recently diagnosed with a brain tumour and is found to have a third cranial nerve palsy.
What clinical findings would be most consistent with this?
A   Downward and outward deviation of the eye, ptosis and mydriasis
B   Downward and outward deviation of the eye, ptosis and miosis
C   Abducted eye, ptosis and miosis
D   Adducted eye, ptosis and miosis
E   Miosis, ptosis, anhidrosis and exophthalmos

6. A 36-year-old female presents to the GP with a left-sided drooped eyelid. On examination, the left pupil is smaller than the right and the eyes are different colours. See Fig. 13.

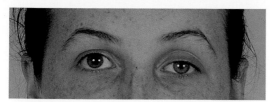

Fig. 13 (Courtesy of Shriners Hospital for Children, Philadelphia.)

Based on the presentation, what is the most likely diagnosis?

A   Third nerve palsy
B   Sixth nerve palsy
C   Fourth nerve palsy
D   Horner syndrome
E   Holmes–Adie pupil

7. A 56-year-old female is diagnosed with syphilis following several months of poor health. On examination, both pupils appear small where accommodation reflex is present but pupillary response to light is absent.
What is the most likely diagnosis?

A   Argyll–Robertson pupil
B   Horner syndrome
C   Bilateral third nerve palsy
D   Fourth nerve palsy
E   Third nerve palsy

8. A 34-year-old female presents to the emergency department with an acute loss of vision affecting her right eye, there is pain on eye movement present. She has a past medical history of multiple sclerosis and no other ophthalmological history of note.
What would be the appropriate imaging that would be recommended to confirm the suspected diagnosis?

A   MRI brain and orbits without contrast
B   CT head without contrast
C   MRI brain and orbits with contrast
D   CT head with contrast
E   MRI spine

9. A 73-year-old lady present to her general practitioner with double vision. There is an obvious squint present with the left eye pointing towards the nose. On looking to the patient's right there is no obvious squint. When the patient is asked to the left the following is seen (Fig. 14):

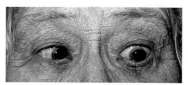

Fig. 14 (From Innes JA, Dover AR, Fairhurst K. *Macleod's Clinical Examination*. 14th ed. Elsevier; 2018.)

Which cranial nerve is affected?

A   V
B   VI
C   IV
D   III
E   II

10. A 73-year-old male presents to the emergency department complaining of visual disturbances. Examination reveals a left homonymous hemianopia. Where is the lesion likely to be?

A   Left optic nerve
B   Right optic nerve
C   Left optic tract
D   Right optic tract
E   Optic chiasm

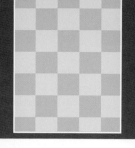

Chapter 2 The examination

1. E. Plantar extension would not be expected in a lower motor neuron lesion. Trauma, tumour and stroke can cause upper motor neuron lesions. Cogwheeling tremor is common, but not always present in Parkinson's disease. Abnormal eye movements are not seen in motor neuron disease. Patients with Parkinson's disease may not habituate to the glabellar tap.

Chapter 3 Further investigations

1. A. Individual muscle fibres. Fibrillation potentials are due to spontaneous contractions of individual muscle fibres. Fasciculation potentials represent the contractions of groups of muscle fibres supplied by a motor unit. Myasthenia gravis (a neuromuscular junction disorder) is associated with a decrement in amplitude of response on repetitive stimulation.
2. E. Polymyositis. SLE can be associated with antibodies to double-stranded DNA, complement and antinuclear factor (ANA) subtypes such as Sm, SSA, SSB and ribonucleoprotein (RNP). Sjogren syndrome can be associated with anti-Ro (SSA), anti-La (SSB) antibodies. Myasthenia gravis can be associated with anti-acetylcholine (anti-ACh) antibodies. Specific forms of Guillain–Barrè syndrome (GBS) can be associated with anti-GM1 antibodies. Polymyositis is associated with anti-Jo1 antibodies in 20% of polymyositis cases.
3. D. MRI of the spine. MRI lends itself to sensitively imaging structures close to bone such as the spinal cord and posterior fossa. CT myelography can be used to image the spinal cord; however, it is labour-intensive and now only performed in patients in whom MRI is contraindicated. Spinal arteriography images the blood vessels supplying the spinal cord, e.g., for investigation of a spinal fistula.
4. E. Tuberculous meningitis. A low CSF glucose occurs in conditions where there are cells or organisms in CSF that consume large quantities of glucose as part of their metabolism, such as bacteria, fungi, tuberculosis and neoplastic cells but not viruses or inflammation, although very high white cell counts and viral loads in the CSF can reduce the CSF glucose. Alzheimer's disease is a neurodegenerative disorder and does not cause a low CSF glucose. Ischaemic stroke can be associated with a mildly raised CSF protein but not a low glucose. During acute attacks of multiple sclerosis the lymphocyte count and protein can be raised but this is not associated with a low glucose. Guillain–Barré is typically associated with a high CSF protein in isolation due to inflammation of the proximal nerve roots.

Chapter 5 Disturbances of consciousness

1. D. 10. In this case the patient's GCS would be broken down to scoring 3 for eyes, 3 for voice and 4 for motor response, giving a total of 10.
2. C. Cardiological reflex to adrenaline.
   The following parameters are routinely tested to assess brainstem function
   - Mid-position, fully dilated, fixed and nonreactive pupils
   - Absent corneal reflexes
   - Absent oculocephalic and oculovestibular reflex
   - Absent gag reflex – no cough in response to pharyngeal or tracheal stimulation or suction
   - No grimace in response to facial pain (from firm supraorbital pressure)
   - Absent ventilatory reflexes – no spontaneous respiration even when pCO_2 rises to >6.5 kPa
   Brainstem testing is only valid in patients in whom a pathology causing irremediable brain damage is identified and the patient is not hypothermic (core body temperature above 34°C) or on depressant drugs.
3. B. Pons. Apneustic breathing, i.e., inspiration followed by prolonged pauses, is associated with pontine dysfunction. Cheyne–Stokes breathing is usually associated with basal ganglia or thalamic dysfunction.
4. A. The patient was lying in bed at the onset. Syncope is often associated with patients standing, whereas seizures can occur in any position. Jerks or convulsive movements can be seen during a syncopal episode but they are usually brief and not rhythmical. A bitten tongue (especially the side) or the inside cheek usually indicates a seizure but the tongue can be bitten (especially the tip) as a result of the fall that occurs in a true syncopal attack. Urinary incontinence is often not helpful diagnostically as it occurs

in both seizures and less often in syncope (especially if the bladder is full). Malaise is often more prolonged after a seizure but can also occur after a syncopal attack.

5. C. Typical absence seizures (previously termed 'Petit mal') are a form of generalized epilepsy that occurs in children and often resolves spontaneously with age. Children of normal intelligence can underperform at school when the absence episodes become frequent and they are missing what is being said in class. The absence attack usually lasts seconds and is not usually accompanied by any postictal confusion. The seizures tend to be relatively easily treatable. There is a distinctive 3-per-second spike and wave discharge on EEG during an attack. There is no association with an underlying structural lesion.

6. B. Lip-smacking and chewing automatisms. Temporal lobe epilepsy can be associated with epigastric rising sensations (panic-like feelings); déjà vu (simple partial seizures); various automatisms such as lip-smacking, chewing and hand wringing (focal onset impaired awareness seizures); and can secondarily generalize. Much more rarely temporal seizures may present with formed visual, olfactory and gustatory hallucinations. Adopting a 'fencing posture' is a feature of frontal lobe epilepsy. Patients who shake only the upper limbs and have repetitive conjugate eye movements often have pseudoseizures but these can reflect seizures in the frontal lobes and be difficult to diagnose.

7. E. There is a 20% chance of rebleed within the first 2 weeks. The raised pressure in subarachnoid haemorrhage (SAH) is usually communicating and it is therefore safe and sometimes necessary to perform an LP to aid diagnosis. Patients often become hypertensive and only when it becomes malignant with signs of end-organ damage or greater than 240 mm Hg systolic should hypertension be treated. Berry aneurysms are more common in the anterior circulation but are at a greater risk of rupturing in the posterior circulation. Approximately 90% of SAH can be detected on CT within the first 24 hours. The highest incidence of rebleeding is within the first 2 weeks and therefore many surgeons and radiologists advocate early treatment of aneurysms.

8. C. Absence attacks are rare in adulthood and often a patient's attacks will disappear as they get older. Poor performance at school is one possible presentation, although relatives and patients often recognize that there is a problem before this occurs.

9. E. Nonepileptic seizures are common even in patients with epilepsy. The awareness during what is apparently a generalized event and the shaking of only the upper limbs with rapid return to normality are suggestive, but

occasionally strange episodes can occur as part of frontal lobe seizures.

10. A. Vasovagal syncope often has a prodrome of impending loss of consciousness and patients can even have some myoclonic jerking of the limbs and urinary incontinence, especially if they are kept upright, which delays.

11. C. Narcolepsy often presents with excessive daytime sleepiness and hallucinations on going to sleep (hypnagogic hallucinations).

12. C. This is a typical focal seizure with loss of awareness of temporal lobe origin.

Chapter 6 Disorders of higher cerebral function

1. A. Left frontal lobe. In right-handed people the left hemisphere is dominant and this governs language. In the left frontal lobe is Broca area; if this is affected, e.g., in a stroke, speech can become nonfluent and hesitant despite comprehension of the spoken word remaining intact. In the left temporal lobe is Wernicke area, which is involved in the comprehension of speech.

2. D. Right parietal lobe. The nondominant parietal lobe is involved in the integration of somatosensory, visual and auditory information. If it is affected, patients will have visual inattention and neglect to one side of their environment. Visuospatial apraxia can also occur, where the ability to draw or build simple objects is lost. The dominant parietal lobe is involved in calculation.

3. D. Posterior cerebral arteries. The occipital lobes are principally supplied by the posterior cerebral arteries. A stroke of the occipital lobe causes a homonymous hemianopia. The occipital poles are also supplied by the middle cerebral arteries, and so central (macular) vision can sometimes be spared in an occipital stroke.

4. C. The triad of dementia, gait apraxia and urinary incontinence, especially when there is a previous history of subarachnoid haemorrhage, suggests normal pressure hydrocephalus.

5. C. New variant CJD has a slower onset than sporadic CJD and often starts nonspecifically with psychiatric features and nonspecific sensory symptoms.

6. A. A stepwise progressive deterioration in neurological function in an elderly patient with vascular risk factors suggests multiinfarct dementia, although there is considerable crossover with ischaemic leucoencephalopathy.

7. A. This is a typical presentation of Alzheimer's disease.

8. E. The patient has an excellent mini-mental state examination score and is actually able to walk to the shops and call the fire brigade but is too depressed to take an active part in life.

Chapter 7 Headache

1. E. Cluster headache. The features described are typical of cluster headache; short duration, frequent and concentrated around an eye. Glaucoma would present with a constant red eye and a loss of visual acuity. Tension headaches are usually featureless apart from pain. Migraine is associated with movement sensitivity not restlessness like cluster headaches. The patient's young age makes GCA very unlikely.

2. A. Giant cell arteritis. A new onset headache in a patient older than 50 years old should be a red flag. Giant cell arteritis typically causes systemic symptoms like fatigue, and the temporal tenderness is due to inflammation of the temporal artery. Serum erythrocyte sedimentation rate is usually raised (>50 mm/hr) in these cases and a temporal artery biopsy would confirm the diagnosis. Immediate management with steroids is imperative as permanent visual loss can occur if left untreated.

3. D. 60 minutes. A typical migrainous aura, with visual, sensory and/or motor symptoms, should last between 15 and 60 minutes.

4. B. Ptosis. A positional element to the headache and the presence of papilloedema suggest raised intracranial pressure, and urgent imaging is required to rule out secondary causes of this, e.g., tumour, cerebral vein thrombosis. Neck stiffness suggests meningism, raising the possibility of meningitis or subarachnoid haemorrhage. New onset headaches that are benign would usually start in adolescence or early adulthood. Ptosis is a nonspecific feature of a number of headache syndromes such as migraine or cluster headache.

5. B. An enlarged blind spot. Papilloedema is caused by raised intracranial pressure, which can prevent the retinal veins near the disc from pulsating. It is associated with an enlarged blind spot due to swelling of the optic disc. The optic disc may be swollen due to causes other than raised cerebrospinal fluid pressure, e.g., inflammation of the anterior part of the optic nerve or 'papillitis'. Loss of colour vision, a central scotoma and a relative afferent pupillar defect are found in optic neuritis. A small pupil is found due to a number of causes, e.g., Horner syndrome, secondary to certain drugs such as opiates.

6. A. Worsening with coughing, sneezing or bending over. Coughing, sneezing and bending over all increase intracranial pressure and worsen the headache. Fortification spectra are typical of aura associated with migraine headache. Patients with raised pressure often have a dull, progressive headache. The headache is worse on waking in the morning and on prolonged lying flat; they are better with standing in contrast to low-pressure headaches seen after lumbar puncture. Nausea and subsequent vomiting are common symptoms of increasing intracranial pressure.

7. D. Associated nausea, vertigo and photophobia. Chronic form of tension-type headache occurs most days in the month unlike migraine, which tends to occur periodically. There should be no loss of consciousness. Further investigation for a structural lesion is warranted. Standing helps headaches associated with raised intracranial pressure. A tight band-like pain around the head is the typical character of tension-type headache.

8. E. This type of headache is sudden onset and is often described as 'the worst type of pain ever felt' or as 'feeling like you have been hit over the back of the head'.

9. E. Tension headache – the lack of associated symptoms and stable nature of the headache suggest this benign type of headache.

10. C. In a patient of this demographic with these symptoms the most likely cause in meningitis. The absence of neck stiffness does not alter the working diagnosis.

11. A. The CSF confirms that the patient has bacterial meningitis, although he should have been given broad-spectrum antibiotics based on the history alone without waiting for the CSF results.

12. E. The features of raised intracranial pressure combined with a progressive course suggest a space-occupying lesion such as a neoplasm and, since he is a smoker, it is likely to be lung metastases.

13. B. The recent onset of the contraceptive pill can precipitate migraine in a susceptible individual.

14. E. The patient has had partial third nerve palsy with a sentinel bleed from a Berry aneurysm of the posterior communicating artery.

15. D. Patients who have had a stroke might complain of a headache. It is much more common with haemorrhagic strokes, but a headache should not rule out an ischaemic stroke, especially if it is a large ischaemic stroke accompanied by oedema and mass effect or if there is haemorrhagic transformation.

Chapter 9 Facial sensory loss and weakness

1. C. Is a severe, stabbing, paroxysmal pain. By definition, idiopathic trigeminal neuralgia should not be associated with neurological signs. It is not usually familial. It is usually unilateral – if bilateral then other conditions that affect the trigeminal nuclei and exit zone of the nerve need to be considered, e.g., multiple sclerosis. The pain is often paroxysmal and is triggered by touching particular parts of the face and mouth, e.g., during chewing and shaving. It is often very sensitive to the antiepileptics carbamazepine and lamotrigine. Steroids do not help in this condition.

Chapter 10 Deafness, tinnitus, dizziness and vertigo

1. D. 512 Hz. Rinne and Weber tests can be used to differentiate between conductive and sensorineural hearing loss. Both tests use a 512 Hz tuning fork. Assessment of vibration sense in the sensory examination uses a 128 Hz tuning fork.
2. B. Benign paroxysmal positional vertigo. BPPV affects the posterior semicircular canal predominantly and is experienced as sudden paroxysms of vertigo related to head movement, typically on turning over in bed. Vestibular neuronitis is usually more persistent lasting days to weeks. Tumours of the cerebellopontine angle such as acoustic neuroma are associated with sensorineural hearing loss, V and VII nerve involvement and cerebellar signs. Ménière's disease classically presents with the triad of vertigo, tinnitus and hearing loss.
3. E. Multiple sclerosis. The cochlear nerve can be affected by lesions of the cerebellopontine angle, e.g., vestibular schwannoma, arteriovenous malformation, stroke (anterior inferior cerebellar artery) and lesions of the base of the skull, e.g., infective (meningitis), inflammatory (sarcoidosis) and carcinomatous (nasopharyngeal carcinoma). Multiple sclerosis is associated with brainstem and cerebellar lesions but does not typically affect the cochlear nerve specifically.
4. B. Right-sided cerebellar features. The deafness is sensorineural and not conductive. The ipsilateral cerebellar tracts can be involved, which causes ipsilateral cerebellar signs. Lower facial weakness is an upper motor neurone deficit. Lesions at the CPA affect the facial nerve and therefore cause lower motor neurone weakness, i.e., whole of the face. Pseudobulbar dysarthria occurs in bilateral upper motor neurone deficits. A lower motor neurone bulbar dysarthria may occur due to involvement of the tenth cranial nerve. Vertigo tends to occur with acute rather than slowly progressive lesions of the vestibular system.

Chapter 11 Dysarthria, dysphonia and dysphagia

1. B. Broca area. Dysphasia is a disorder of the production or understanding of speech and not failure of articulation, or dysarthria which is seen with hypoglossal nerve, cerebellar or basal ganglia pathology.
2. B. Motor neuron disease. Pseudobulbar palsy refers to a syndrome where both sets of upper motor neurones to cranial nerve nuclei are damaged, i.e., bilateral upper motor neurone lesions. Poliomyelitis only damages the lower motor neurones. Motor neuron disease is the commonest cause of a pseudobulbar palsy due to bilateral involvement of the upper motor neurones. Huntington's disease is mostly associated with disease of the basal ganglia. Occlusion of the anterior cerebral artery causes weakness in the contralateral leg. Myasthenia gravis causes a bulbar palsy (affects the neuromuscular junction).

Chapter 13 Movement disorders

1. B. Essential tremor. Essential tremor is common, usually symmetrical and present on action and posture, e.g., holding a cup. There is usually a positive family history. The symptoms can be alleviated with alcohol. A Parkinsonian tremor is asymmetrical and present at rest, normally disappearing on movement. It is usually associated with rigidity and bradykinesia. Alcohol withdrawal is associated with a high-frequency physiological tremor. Psychogenic tremor is difficult to diagnose but is usually irregular and can be distractible or entrained.
2. D. Improved by β-blockers. Both physiological and essential tremors can respond to β-blockers. Parkinson's disease is treated with L-DOPA and deep brain stimulation. Neuroleptic medication may cause a tremor and a number of other movement disorders.
3. E. Essential tremor might be responsive to alcohol.
4. D. Any progressive abnormal movements in young patients, especially with bulbar dysfunction, suggest Wilson disease.
5. C. Most patients with idiopathic Parkinson's disease who are treated with levodopa develop peak-dose dyskinesias within 5 to 10 years of commencing treatment.
6. D. This is usually caused by a lacunar infarct in the contralateral subthalamic nucleus.
7. C. Huntington's disease typically starts with cognitive and psychiatric features and progresses to a movement disorder (usually chorea which presents with fidgety movements).

Chapter 14 Limb weakness

1. D. Motor neuron disease. Guillain–Barré is a polyneuropathy and therefore a purely lower motor neurone syndrome. MS is a disease of the central nervous system and therefore is only associated with upper motor neurone signs. MND is associated with degeneration of the anterior horn and upper motor neurone cell bodies and so causes lower and upper motor neurone signs in the same patient.

2. A. Motor neuron disease. Fasciculations are spontaneous contractions of a group of muscle fibres innervated by one axon or a 'motor unit'. Fasciculations tend to occur when the axons are damaged or the muscle becomes hyperexcitable, e.g., thyrotoxicosis. Processes that affect the central nervous system (unless it involves the anterior horn cell) or muscle do not tend to cause fasciculations. Parkinson's disease affects the basal ganglia in the central nervous system.
3. B. Hypertonia is a feature of an upper motor neuron lesion.

Chapter 15 Limb sensory symptoms

1. E. Are spared following occlusion of the anterior spinal artery. The dorsal columns carry information regarding joint position and vibration sense. The dorsal columns decussate in the lower, not the upper brainstem. B_{12} but not B_1 deficiency can cause subacute combined degeneration of the spinal cord involving the dorsal columns and the corticospinal pathways. Romberg test looks for a sensory ataxia associated with dorsal column damage. The spinal cord is mostly supplied by one anterior spinal artery that has poor anastomoses and is vulnerable to occlusion. The posterior cord, including the dorsal columns, is richly supplied by a posterior network of vessels and is therefore rarely involved following anterior spinal artery occlusion.

Chapter 16 Disorders of gait

1. E. Vascular dementia. An apraxic gait is commonly seen in severe small vessel disease. Parkinson's disease can also present with a small stepped gait, but it is usually not wide based, rather shuffling and slow. Proximal muscle weakness as in muscular dystrophy is associated with a waddling gait. Common peroneal palsy is associated with a high-stepping gait.
2. D. Common peroneal nerve palsy. Common peroneal palsy is associated with a unilateral foot drop, resulting in a high-stepping gait. Common causes include mechanical compression of the nerve and fibular fracture.
3. E. A waddling gait can occur with orthopaedic problems, but when it is symmetrical and associated with muscle weakness and wasting it is usually caused by long-standing myopathy.
4. E. This is the history of someone with a spastic paraparesis often associated with cerebral palsy.
5. D. Cerebellar disease causes a broad-based gait and it might be the only feature, especially with lesions of the cerebellar vermis.
6. B. Small, slow, shuffling steps in the context of frontal lobe disease is sometimes called *marche à petit pas*. In

contrast to Parkinson's disease, there is no festination and patients have no problem stopping once they have started to walk.
7. C. The inconsistency of his disorder and the normal bedside examination are suggestive of an underlying functional disorder.

Chapter 17 The red, painful eye

1. B. Scleritis. This is correct as a patient with a systemic connective tissue disease such as rheumatoid arthritis presenting with an acutely painful deep red eye should raise suspicion of scleritis. Acute-angle closure glaucoma although causes an acutely painful red eye commonly has features of systemic upset including nausea and vomiting, and visual acuity is reduced. Acute keratitis can also cause painful red eye; however, usually the patient will be complaining of a foreign body gritty sensation, blurry vision, discharge and photophobia; it is more likely in contact lens wearers. Anterior uveitis also presents as an acute painful red eye; however, features include a ciliary flush, hypopyon (pus in the anterior chamber) and irregular pupil. Episcleritis is least likely as classically it is not painful or less painful than scleritis; phenylephrine drops will also cause vessels to blanch and redness to improve.
2. D. Steroid + cycloplegic eye drops and urgent referral to ophthalmology. The patient is presenting with an acutely painful red eye with photophobia, and an irregular and constricted pupil. The past medical history of Crohn's disease makes anterior uveitis a likely diagnosis. The management for anterior uveitis is a steroid and cycloplegic eye drops (which dilate the pupil to relieve pain and photophobia). A diagnosis or suspicion of anterior uveitis should warrant an urgent referral to ophthalmology.
3. C. Acute angle-closure glaucoma. The patient presents with an acute painful red eye, a semidilated nonreacting pupil and a hazy cornea; there is systemic upset including vomiting. This history is suggestive of acute-angle closure glaucoma. The history describes worsening pain while watching television in a dark room which would cause mydriasis. The presence of distance glasses suggests that the patient may have hypermetropia, which is a risk factor for developing acute angle-closure glaucoma.
4. E. Same-day ophthalmology referral. Contact lens wearers with an acutely painful eye should be referred to eye casualty in the same day to rule out microbial keratitis. Assessment is usually difficult without specialist input to determine the causative organism, and reassurance at this stage would be inappropriate as keratitis is a potentially sight-threatening condition.

5. C. Angle-closure glaucoma. The image shows a red eye with a hazy cornea. There is a positive history of acute pain in the eye alongside, decreased visual acuity and systemic symptoms including nausea and vomiting. Hypermetropia is also a risk factor for the development of angle-closure glaucoma. Anterior uveitis would be considered due to rheumatoid arthritis being a risk factor for its development. However, it does not tend to be associated with systemic symptoms and visual acuity is not usually impaired from the start

Chapter 18 Gradual change in vision

1. A. Primary open-angle glaucoma. This is the correct answer. The patient describes a gradual change in vision affecting peripheral vision, as he complains of not being able to see cars from the side of his vision. He also has a risk factor for developing POAG, which is diabetes.
2. B. Dry age-related macular degeneration. The patient describes a fluctuating reduction in visual acuity, often worsening at night. These are characteristic symptoms of age-related macular degeneration. The presence of only drusen on fundoscopy confirms the diagnosis of dry age-related macular degeneration.
3. B. Hypermetropia. Primary open-angle glaucoma is associated with myopia (near-sightedness) and hypermetropia is associated with acute-angle closure glaucoma. All other options are considered risk factors for primary open-angle glaucoma.
4. **D. Impairs peripheral visual fields**

    Glaucoma causes optic neuropathy; this most commonly affects the patient's visual fields first. The peripheries are affected initially and can lead to tunnel vision if left untreated. Visual acuity can be affected but is less common.
5. E. Hypercalcemia. Hypocalcaemia predisposes one to cataract formation. All other options are risk factors that increase the likelihood of cataract formation.

Chapter 19 Sudden change in vision

1. B. Central retinal vein occlusion. The history reveals sudden painless loss of vision, retinal haemorrhages and a relative afferent pupillary defect, which suggests a central retinal vein occlusion. Similarly, a central retinal artery occlusion can be considered based on the history. However, on fundoscopy, a central retinal artery occlusion would reveal a pale retina and the presence of a cherry-red spot.
2. A. Central retinal artery occlusion. This is the correct answer as the patent describes a painless sudden loss of vision. The risk factors identified are atherosclerosis and smoking which are important to consider as they increase the likelihood of a formation of an embolus that can result in a central retinal artery occlusion. Other important findings from fundoscopy are classic signs of a central retinal artery occlusion, a pale retina and a 'cherry red' spot.
3. A. High-dose steroids. The history should raise immediate suspicion of optic neuritis. This is supported by the past medical history of multiple sclerosis. The symptoms of reduction of visual acuity, pain on movement and relative afferent pupillary defect should point towards a diagnosis of optic neuritis. Treatment of optic neuritis is the administration of high-dose steroids.
4. E. Vitreous haemorrhage. Vitreous haemorrhage is an important differential to consider with diabetic patients. Painless loss of vision with dark floaters and 'red hue' is generally a typical presentation with patients with a vitreous haemorrhage. The history describes that the symptoms are worse when lying flat, this is due to the pooling of blood within the macula thus worsening central vision. Several risk factors are identified including proliferative retinal disease, use of anticoagulants and hypertension.
5. E. Acute angle-closure glaucoma. Long-sightedness or hypermetropia is associated with an increased risk of developing acute angle-closure glaucoma. This is due to the eye being smaller and thus having shallower anterior chambers which cause their angles to be narrower.

Chapter 20 Eyelid problems and the bulging eye

1. B. Ectropion. The eyelid is drooping out, so the correct term for this malposition is ectropion.
2. A. Lid hygiene advice and clean eyelids twice daily using a warm compress. Seborrheic dermatitis can be associated with blepharitis. Therefore, lid hygiene advice and cleaning eyelids twice daily by using a warm compress with eyes closed for a 5 to 10-minute period is the correct answer.
3. A. Analgesia and warm compress. This patient has a stye. The description of a stye is outwards pointing away from the lid margin. This corresponds with an infection of the glands of the eyelid. A stye is a self-limiting condition, so management includes a hot compress to help melt away the solidified wax and allows it to drain and analgesia for symptomatic relief. Antibiotics would only be indicated if there is associated conjunctivitis.
4. B. Chalazion. The vignette describes a firm painless lump in the eyelid. This is a classic description of a chalazion or meibomian cyst. The history also suggests a previous infection of the eyelid which increases the likelihood of the development of a chalazion.

5. A. Corneal ulceration. This patient has entropion as pictured. If left untreated the patient may develop a corneal ulcer. Surgery is the definitive management. Eye lubrication and tape to pull the eyelid outward can be used while awaiting surgery.

Chapter 21 Dementia

1. B. Progressive course. A progressive clinical course is typical of evolving dementia. Although hallucinations and disorientation can occur, they are usually a late manifestation. Early hallucinations and disorientation, with a loss of circadian rhythm are more in keeping with delirium. Dementia might affect behaviour, but withdrawal is more commonly seen in pseudodementia.
2. D. Lumbar puncture. Anaemia, low B$_{12}$ or folate levels and hypothyroidism can all cause symptoms resembling dementia and are all potentially reversible. A head CT would rule out structural reasons for dementia-like symptoms, such as a subdural haemorrhage. A lumbar puncture is sometimes performed to investigate for Alzheimer's disease (although the diagnosis is normally made clinically) and to look for rarer organic causes of dementia, but this would not be routine practice.
3. A. Lewy body dementia. This patient presents with the hallmark features of Lewy body dementia including a fluctuant clinical course, prominent visual hallucinations and evidence of parkinsonism, which is usually resistant to treatment. Alzheimer's disease has a progressive course and visual hallucinations are a late feature. Vascular dementia can also have a fluctuant clinical course with a gait that resembles parkinsonism (marche à petit pas) but hallucinations are not a feature. Frontotemporal dementia can either affect behaviour (usually disinhibition) or speech content (primary progressive aphasia).
4. B. Huntington's disease. Huntington's disease often starts with subtle cognitive changes that often do not present to doctors. This is followed by chorea and dementia in middle age. Myoclonus is seen in many diseases including subacute sclerosing panencephalitis and sporadic Creutzfeldt–Jakob disease (CJD). Sporadic CJD typically presents with a rapidly progressive dementia and myoclonus, not chorea. Chorea is not a feature of Alzheimer's disease, normal pressure hydrocephalus (triad of cognitive deficit, gait apraxia and incontinence) or schizophrenia.
5. D. Geographical apraxia and language deficits are often early features. Patients who are acutely confused present with disorientation, but patients suffering from Alzheimer's disease are often initially quite well orientated. Later in the disease, patients become disorientated. Patients are often unaware of the degree of memory loss but can retain

some insight into their illness in the initial stages of the disease. Alzheimer's disease typically involves the parietal (including apraxia and aphasia) and temporal lobes initially and therefore spares the frontal lobes at presentation. Alzheimer's disease typically involves the parietal lobes causing dyspraxia and dysphasia, as well as the temporal lobes in the initial stages. The disease becomes more global as it progresses. Capgras syndrome is more in keeping with dementia with Lewy bodies.

Chapter 22 Epilepsy

1. C. Lamotrigine. Lamotrigine during pregnancy does not significantly increase birth defects and is currently favoured as a single therapy for epilepsy. Sodium valproate has been associated with a 10% risk of birth defect and reduced IQ of the child during development. Carbamazepine has been associated with increased risk of neural tube defects. Phenytoin has been associated with increased risk of cleft lip and palate and congenital heart disease. Midazolam is reserved for acute termination of seizures not seizure control.
2. B. Status epilepticus is now considered when a seizure lasts longer than 5 minutes or when seizures occur close together without recovery in between. In these cases, urgent acute management of prolonged seizures is needed.
3. A. Resuscitation. Although termination of a prolonged seizure with benzodiazepine is an important step, initial resuscitation is paramount; this includes ensuring a patent airway is maintained, breathing and circulation parameters are stable and a blood glucose level is performed. Imaging might be required if the episode is a first seizure; however, it does not form part of the immediate management. Acquiring a collateral history, if the patient's consciousness is impaired, is useful especially if the diagnosis is uncertain.

Chapter 23 Parkinson's disease and other extrapyramidal disorders

1. C. Gait ataxia. The hallmark characteristics of Parkinson's disease include an asymmetrical coarse resting tremor, asymmetrical lead-pipe rigidity of the limbs, bradykinesia (slowness of movement) and hypokinesia (small movement) seen in gait, e.g., small, shuffling steps and upper limb function, e.g., small handwriting or micrographia.
2. A. Tone is increased equally in flexor and extensor muscles. Rigidity is increased tone caused by extrapyramidal disease such as Parkinson's disease. Tone is increased throughout all movement whereas in

spasticity, tone tends to be higher in the flexors in the upper limbs and extensors in the lower limbs. Extensor plantar responses are an upper motor neurone and not extrapyramidal sign. A pill-rolling rest tremor is typical of Parkinson's disease, which is an extrapyramidal disease, not a postural tremor. Patients with Parkinson's disease are often slow but should not exhibit any limb weakness. Deafness is not a feature of Parkinson's disease.

Chapter 24 Diseases affecting the spinal cord (myelopathy)

1. C. Multiple sclerosis. This is a typical history of a relapsing-remitting illness with lesions separated in time and place, suggestive of multiple sclerosis.
2. C. An MRI of the cervical spinal cord. Brown–Séquard syndrome is associated with damage to half the spinal cord. In this case, it involves the arms and an MRI of the cervical spine would be needed. (If it had only affected the legs, the lesion could be in the cervical or thoracic spine and both would need to be scanned.) NB: If there are upper motor neurone signs, e.g., spastic paraparesis, the lesion has to be above L1 (the end of the spinal cord) and will not be in the lumbosacral spine, which is made up of nerve roots and therefore causes lower motor neurone signs only. None of the other investigations would help to make this diagnosis.
3. D. Tropical spastic paraparesis is caused by HTLV-1. HTLV-1 is endemic in equatorial Africa, South America and the Caribbean. In addition to the leg weakness, patients complain of marked urinary symptoms. Antibodies to the HTLV-1 virus can be detected in the blood.
4. A. Spinal canal stenosis can present in a number of ways: as a radiculopathy, cervical spondylotic myelopathy or, if the lumbar spine is involved, as neurogenic claudication. Patients will report calf pain, weakness and sensory disturbance that worsen with walking or prolonged standing. However, sitting or lying down improves symptoms (hence the normal examination on the couch) as the diameter of the spinal canal is enlarged by these positions.
5. C. Anterior spinal artery occlusion (ASAO) is commonly seen in the thoracic spine because it is a watershed area in terms of vascular supply. Risk factors for ASAO are identical to those of stroke, including the use of cocaine, which causes vasospasm. ASAO is sudden onset and patients complain of back pain, paralysis and loss of pain and temperature sensation below the spinal level of the infarct. Position and vibration sense are spared because the dorsal columns are not supplied by the anterior spinal artery.

6. B. Subacute combined degeneration of the cord is caused by a deficiency of vitamin B_{12}, either from diet (vegans), pernicious anaemia or absorption (gastrectomy/Crohn's disease). The deficiency causes degeneration of the dorsal and lateral white matter of the spinal cord; patients report progressive weakness, a sensory ataxia and finally paraplegia. As B_{12} deficiency also causes a peripheral neuropathy, mixed upper and lower motor neurone involvement account for upgoing plantars but depressed reflexes on examination.
7. C. Brown–Séquard syndrome is caused by a hemitransection of the spinal cord (which could be the result of or MS lesion) resulting in ipsilateral limb spasticity with upper motor neurone signs, ipsilateral loss of position and vibration sense and contralateral loss of pain and temperature sense.

Chapter 26 Radiculopathy and plexopathy

1. C. 8. Although there are only seven cervical vertebrae, there are eight cervical nerve roots because each nerve root exits above the vertebral body.
2. C. Pancoast tumour. The combination of posterior brachial plexus involvement and Horner syndrome is suspicious of an apical lung tumour. Diabetic neuropathy usually presents with progressive distal nerve involvement. Motor neuron disease should not have sensory involvement. Rheumatoid arthritis can cause radiculopathy and rarely mononeuritis but the presence of Horner syndrome is not in keeping.
3. D. L5/S1. Sensory disturbance of the dorsum of the foot suggests L5 involvement; plantar flexion weakness is due to S1 involvement. S1/S2 roots provide the reflex arc for the ankle jerk.
4. A. Causes pain over the anterior thigh and medial leg. Compression of the L4 nerve root causes pain into the thigh and medial leg rather than L5 and S1 lesions where the pain can extend into the foot. The knee jerk is supplied by L3 and L4 can therefore be reduced. The ankle jerk is innervated by S1 and should be spared. Foot drop is associated with lesions of the common peroneal nerve, which is innervated by L4 and partly L5 and therefore L4 root lesions can mimic the motor signs of a common peroneal nerve palsy, but the sensory deficit is very different. Degenerative disc disease is a common cause of lumbar radiculopathies but the level should be L4/5. The hamstrings are supplied by the sciatic nerve from L5/S1 roots. Tibialis anterior might be wasted with L4 root lesions.
5. A. There might be upper motor neurone signs in the upper limbs. Cervical spondylosis can cause compression either of the cervical spinal cord causing a cervical myelopathy

with upper motor neurone signs in the arms and legs and/or the cervical roots causing lower motor neurone signs in the arms. Pain is often worse at night. Secondary headaches are common. Most patients do not have neurological signs but have neck pain. Neck traction is contraindicated as it can lead to destabilization of the neck and subsequent cord compression.

Chapter 27 Disorders of the peripheral nerves

1. B. Guillain–Barré syndrome. The relatively acute presentation of a sensorimotor neuropathy preceded by an illness suggests Guillain–Barré syndrome. Cardiac and respiratory involvement need to be investigated if Guillain–Barré syndrome is considered. Diabetes and alcohol excess usually present over months or years. Myeloma is associated with a chronic polyneuropathy. Sarcoidosis is more associated with a (multifocal) mononeuropathy.

2. D. Charcot–Marie–Tooth disease. The long-standing history of a peripheral neuropathy since childhood strongly suggests a hereditary aetiology, with CMT the most likely. CMT1 and CMT2 have an autosomal dominant inheritance. Poliomyelitis is associated with a solely motor neuropathy. The presence of sensory symptoms makes a muscle disease such as Duchenne very unlikely. Amyloidosis has a shorter time course and more commonly associated with a painful mononeuritis.

3. C. Abductor pollicis brevis. The ulnar nerve originates from the C8–T1 roots and innervates the two medial lumbricals, adductor pollicis (which adducts the thumb), abductor digiti minimi (which abducts the little finger) and the interossei (which abduct and adduct the fingers). Abductor pollicis brevis is innervated by the median nerve.

4. B. A glove and stocking sensory loss. Sensory polyneuropathy is a disorder of the peripheral nervous system. There might be a glove and stocking sensory loss and the patient might have absent or reduced reflexes (due to reduced afferent input). In a pure sensory polyneuropathy, there should be no motor signs.

5. D. Weakness of dorsiflexion of the foot. The common peroneal nerve innervates the anterior tibialis (not quadriceps femoris) and dorsiflexes the ankle and the peronei, which evert the foot and supplies sensation to the lateral aspect of the leg and dorsum of the foot, excluding the lateral border of the foot. Plantar flexion is mediated by soleus and gastrocnemius, which are innervated by the tibial nerve. Abductor pollicis brevis is in the hand and innervated by the median nerve. The ankle reflex involves the tendon of soleus and gastrocnemius and is therefore not involved in common peroneal lesions. Tibial nerve lesions would cause a reduced, not brisk, ankle reflex.

6. E. Might be associated with painless foot ulcers. Many patients are asymptomatic and only recognize something is wrong when they are examined. The most common finding is absent ankle jerks and some distal sensory loss, especially to vibration sensation, without gross wasting or weakness. There is evidence from trials that good blood glucose control slows or even slightly improves diabetic polyneuropathy. Diabetic polyneuropathy is common in both type I and II diabetics. Small pain-carrying fibres are often affected and therefore trophic ulcers can easily occur, especially because microvascular and macrovascular arterial disease leads to ischaemia in the feet.

7. A. Guillain–Barré syndrome. It is important to recognize demyelinating neuropathies as some of them are potentially treatable. Guillain–Barré is the most common cause of an acute demyelinating neuropathy. Prolonged and/or severe demyelination might eventually cause axonal loss and therefore the patterns are often mixed. The remainder cause axonal neuropathies.

8. C. Pinprick testing might be abnormal over the medial aspect of the middle finger. Patients with carpal tunnel have paraesthesia confined to the hand but pain often extends right up the arm. There is sensory abnormality in the thumb, index and middle fingers (medial and lateral aspects) and the lateral aspect of the ring finger. Most patients have only sensory symptoms, but when wasting occurs, it predominantly affects the abductor pollicis brevis and the thenar eminence, not the whole hand. The median nerve is affected, which primarily supplies the thenar eminence including abductor pollicis brevis. The ulnar nerve supplies the first dorsal interossei.

9. D. If damaged, usually causes numbness over the ring and little finger of the hand. The radial nerve is the main branch of the posterior cord of the brachial plexus and supplies most of the muscles on the extensor surface of the arm and forearm, including brachioradialis. The radial nerve can be easily damaged, especially by pressure from misplaced crutches and by leaning an arm over a chair because it runs in the bony spiral groove of the humerus. The ulnar and median nerves supply most of the sensation to the hand.

10. C. This story is typical of a Pancoast tumour, which is usually caused by squamous cell carcinoma of the lung invading the lower brachial plexus and roots.

11. D. Young patients might have pain throughout the arm and no neurological signs, whereas older patients might have severe signs of median nerve damage with relatively few symptoms.

12. E. There is often little sensory involvement and recovery occurs over months and might not be complete.

13. C. A mixture of upper and lower motor neurone signs above and below the neck is highly suggestive of motor neurone disease.
14. E. She has signs and symptoms consistent with a right C6 radiculopathy as well as cervical myelopathy.

Chapter 28 Disorders of the neuromuscular junction

1. D. Lambert–Eaton syndrome. The presence of a new myasthenic syndrome in an older man with a history of small-cell lung cancer is suspicious of Lambert–Eaton syndrome. Lambert–Eaton syndrome preferentially affects the proximal limb girdle muscles. Myasthenia gravis would, however, be the main differential. Vitamin D deficiency, Cushing disease and hypothyroidism are all associated with a proximal myopathy, but it is usually not fatigable.
2. C. A decrement in CMAPs on exercise. A decrement of 15% in CMAP on repetitive stimulation is consistent with myasthenia gravis. Increment of CMAP is typically seen in Lambert–Eaton syndrome. Fasciculations are usually associated with peripheral motor conditions. Decreased motor conduction velocity is associated with demyelination.
3. B. Penicillin. All the other drugs are associated with drug-induced myasthenia or worsening of the symptoms in patients with known myasthenia gravis.
4. A. Diplopia or ptosis in over 90% of patients at some time in their illness. Ocular involvement in myasthenia gravis occurs in the majority of patients at some time in their disease. Symptoms are often worse towards the end of the day and after exercise and are associated with fatigable weakness of the proximal muscles of the upper limbs and cranial nerves. Muscle cramps and myoglobinuria are not associated. Patients can develop type II respiratory failure due to neuromuscular weakness surprisingly quickly and measurement of the vital capacity is an absolute requirement in any new patient presenting with bulbar myasthenia. Tendon reflexes should be present unlike Lambert–Eaton myasthenic syndrome where they are often absent at rest.

Chapter 29 Disorders of skeletal muscle

1. C. Duchenne muscular dystrophy. The presence of a significant muscle disorder from a young age strongly suggests an inherited cause. Symptoms of Duchenne muscular dystrophy usually start by age 4 years, and present as a proximal myopathy. CK levels are very high with the condition. Becker muscular dystrophy is a milder form of muscle disease that usually occurs later in life.

Myotonic dystrophy and mitochondrial myopathy are typically multisystem disorders where the eyes, heart and endocrine function are affected. McCardle disease is a metabolic myopathy where symptoms occur after exercise.

2. B. Myotonic dystrophy. This patient presents with myotonia (i.e., stiff hands) and likely proximal leg myopathy (i.e., difficulty on inclines). With the added information of cataracts at a young age, myotonic dystrophy should be considered. This is an autosomal dominant condition that demonstrates anticipation. BMD is associated with proximal muscle weakness and calf pseudohypertrophy not myotonia. Dermatomyositis presents as a painful proximal myopathy with/without typical skin changes. One would expect other multisystem symptoms with Cushing disease (e.g., fat deposition, striae) and mitochondrial cytopathy (e.g., ophthalmoplegia).
3. E. Interstitial lung fibrosis. Dermatomyositis is an inflammatory muscle disorder and as such is associated with a painful proximal myopathy and high serum CK level. Skin features such as a heliotrope rash on the face and Gottron papules on the hands may be present. In 10% of patients it is associated with lung cancer, whereas lung fibrosis is associated with polymyositis.
4. A. The CK is usually raised. The CK is usually elevated in inflammatory muscle disease and swallowing is usually affected to some degree. Patients are often hyperreflexic and not hyporeflexic, possibly due to the inflammatory changes in the muscle leading to hyperexcitability. Proximal muscles are more severely impaired in the upper and lower limbs. The heliotrope rash is associated with dermatomyositis.

Chapter 30 Vascular diseases of the nervous system

1. B. Thrombolysis. This patient has presented within 4.5 hours with a left middle cerebral artery syndrome with no contraindications to thrombolysis (e.g., recent stroke within 3 months, major surgery, international normalized ratio > 1.7). In addition, his CT shows no obvious bleed. Thus he should be considered for thrombolysis as the evidence indicates that with it he has a one in eight chance of significant improvement in morbidity. Thrombectomy may also be considered if there is radiological evidence of clot in the middle cerebral artery on CT angiogram.
2. A. Carotid dissection. This young patient has presented with a stroke following neck trauma. In addition, he has a Horner syndrome on the same side as the stroke. This makes carotid dissection a likely cause. This should be investigated with a computed tomography angiogram and if confirmed, managed with antiplatelet therapy. Cerebral

vein thrombosis can present as a stroke but usually with additional features such as severe headache or seizure. Subarachnoid haemorrhage again would present as an acute severe headache. A lateral medullary infarct caused by posterior inferior cerebellar artery occlusion can present with Horner sign but also with a specific set of other symptoms including dissociated sensory loss, vertigo and ataxia.

3. B. Acute subdural haematoma. The question outlines typical features of an acute subdural haematoma secondary to head trauma.

4. B. Carotid embolism. Amaurosis fugax is transient visual loss caused by a blockage, from whatever cause, of the ophthalmic artery or its branches to the retina. This includes carotid embolism. Retinitis pigmentosa causes progressive visual loss which usually starts in the peripheral visual field and spreads to involve central vision. Papilloedema due to raised intracranial pressure can also cause progressive visual loss starting at the periphery but can also cause transient visual loss called 'visual obscurations', which is a warning of rising intracranial pressure. Migrainous aura is associated with both positive and negative visual phenomena, which usually travels across the vision for up to 1 hour prior to the onset of the headache. Closed-angle glaucoma can be associated with transient visual loss preceding chronic visual failure.

5. B. Horner syndrome. Ipsilateral facial spinothalamic sensory loss is not weakness. The facial nucleus and nerve are in the pons. Involvement of the sympathetic tract can give rise to a Horner syndrome. The nucleus ambiguus, which is often involved in disorders of the lateral medulla, innervates the soft palate via the vagus nerve but affects the ipsilateral palate. The hypoglossal nucleus is a paramedian structure in the medulla and is therefore not affected in a lateral lesion. The third nerve nucleus is mostly in the midbrain and is therefore not affected.

6. B. Dressing apraxia. The dominant cerebral cortex is on the left in the majority of right-handed people and is specifically involved in reading, maths (dyscalculia), writing and language. Apraxia involving visuospatial tasks (e.g., dressing and drawing shapes) is a symptom of dysfunction in the nondominant right hemisphere. More subtle functions of the dominant parietal lobe include naming fingers (if abnormal, this is called a 'finger agnosia') and left–right discrimination.

7. C. Loss of vision in one eye (amaurosis fugax). Diplopia can be caused by TIAs involving the pons and midbrain supplied by the posterior circulation. Weakness of all four limbs or 'tetraparesis' is usually caused by TIAs involving the basilar artery, which supplies both corticospinal tracts in the brainstem. Amaurosis fugax is due to blockage in the ophthalmic artery or its branches. It is especially

common in the elderly and may be associated with temporal arteritis. Dysphasia (rather than dysphagia) results from lesions to the dominant frontal, parietal or temporal lobes which are supplied by the middle cerebral artery. Vertigo can be caused by lesions to the pons or cerebellum supplied by the posterior circulation.

8. D. Is usually within the internal capsule and basal ganglia in hypertensive patients. There may be distinguishing features such as headache and altered level of consciousness in a large intracerebral haemorrhage. However, usually the presentation of a haemorrhagic and ischaemic stroke is identical and can only be distinguished on imaging. Meningism only occurs if the haemorrhage extends into the subarachnoid space. A cerebellar haemorrhage in the posterior fossa is a neurological emergency and if suspected clinically, a CT scan of the head should be performed as the patient can rapidly deteriorate because of the proximity of the brainstem. Patients who are hypertensive tend to have subcortical haemorrhages in the basal ganglia, internal capsule or thalamus. Surgical evacuation is only really indicated if the haemorrhage is in the posterior fossa or is on the convexity of the brain and is having a pressure effect.

9. A. Pure motor loss is usually due to a lacunar infarct.

10. E. Complete carotid occlusion can be fatal due to postinfarction oedema. In this example, it is probably due to left carotid artery dissection following a deceleration car accident and the sympathetic fibres are involved.

11. B. His symptoms have not fully resolved after 24 hours, therefore he has not had a transient ischaemic attack. His stroke did not involve all the territory supplied by the middle cerebral artery.

12. E. The posterior inferior cerebellar artery is usually involved but patients often make a good recovery.

13. A. This woman is starting to develop transtentorial herniation with false localizing early third nerve palsy and tonsillar herniation causing drowsiness. She needs an urgent head CT and referral to neurosurgery.

Chapter 32 Infections of the nervous system

1. B. Intravenous cephalosporin. The most urgent management is intravenous treatment with a third-generation cephalosporin. An LP prior to starting antibiotic would be preferential but not if there is concern with the patient's conscious state. In any case an LP should not delay treatment. A CT of the head is only indicated if a suspected meningitis patient presents with a reduced Glasgow Coma Scale score or has evidence of focal neurology. This is mainly to rule out any contraindication for proceeding safely with an LP (e.g., evidence of brainstem coning). Aciclovir is normally used when viral encephalitis is

suspected. ITU admission may be required for monitoring or maintenance of airway due to low conscious state but should not be the first management step.

2. D. Neurocysticercosis. Seizures can be a result of HSV encephalitis, cerebral tuberculosis and neurocysticercosis. However, one would suspect additional features in HSV encephalitis such as fever, headache and confusion. If any changes are seen, it is usually in the temporal lobe. Cerebral tuberculomas can cause seizures, but they usually appear as inflammatory masses on imaging (with calcification much later on). Neurocysticercosis is the most common cause of epilepsy worldwide and calcified cysts on imaging are very suggestive of the condition. Syphilis does not usually cause seizures.

Chapter 33 Multiple sclerosis

1. B. Presents with sensory symptoms. Several studies have indicated that a poor prognosis in MS is related to male gender; a late age at onset; motor, cerebellar and sphincter involvement at onset; a progressive course at onset; a short inter-attack interval; a high number of early attacks and a relevant early residual disability.

2. A. β-Interferon. β-Interferon reduces relapses by approximately 30%. Steroids may speed up the recovery of a single episode but do not change the overall prognosis. There is no convincing evidence that methotrexate, cyclosporine or mycophenolate help in MS.

Chapter 36 Hereditary conditions affecting the nervous system

1. B. Neurofibromatosis type 2. This is an autosomal dominant condition caused by mutations in the NF2 gene and typically associated with bilateral vestibular schwannomas among other central nervous system tumours (e.g., meningioma). Neurofibromatosis type 1 is associated with neurofibromas along peripheral nerves. Tuberous sclerosis is associated with hamartomatous 'tubers' that can be a substrate for epilepsy. Sturge–Weber syndrome is associated with leptomeningeal angiomas affecting the trigeminal nerve.

2. B. Urinary 24-hour copper is raised. Total serum copper is reduced in Wilson disease because of a deficiency in the serum copper-binding protein caeruloplasmin. The reduction in caeruloplasmin leads to an increase in free, unbound copper, which is filtered at the glomerulus and therefore urinary copper levels are raised. Penicillamine treatment relies on its binding to accumulated copper and eliminating it through urine. Zinc, not magnesium, competes for copper absorption in the gut and therefore raises stool levels to help reduce dietary copper intake.

Chapter 38 Adnexal (eyelids, lacrimal system and orbit)

1. A. Ocular involvement. This patient has herpes zoster ophthalmicus, which is caused by the reactivation of the herpes zoster virus in the ophthalmic branch of the trigeminal nerve. Hutchinson sign is when there are lesions present on the tip of the nose; this is a strong indicator of ophthalmic involvement and warrants an urgent ophthalmic review.

2. D. Orbital cellulitis. This presentation is a classic description of orbital cellulitis. There is a painful, swollen eye with reduced visual acuity, proptosis and pain in the movement of the eye. The vignette suggests an infection due to pyrexia, in keeping with a diagnosis of orbital cellulitis. Preseptal cellulitis is an important differential here for a swollen eye; however, it does not cause proptosis and pain on eye movement.

3. A. Oral aciclovir. This patient has herpes zoster ophthalmicus (HZO). This is characterized by a unilateral painful rash in one or more dermatomal distributions of the trigeminal nerve. This patient should have an urgent ophthalmology review and 7 to 10 days of oral antiviral treatment, which ideally should be started within 72 hours.

4. A. Reassure the father that the condition will self-resolve by 1 year of age. The baby is likely to have congenital lacrimal duct obstruction which can cause recurrent watery/sticky discharge. This condition is usually self-resolving by 1 year of age, so reassuring and encouraging the father to massage the lacrimal duct and clean around the eye with a warm damp towel should be encouraged.

5. D. Preseptal cellulitis. The patient is likely to have an infection of the soft tissues anterior to the orbital septum secondary to the laceration. The presentation suggests preseptal cellulitis rather than orbital cellulitis, due to the absence of painful eye movement, proptosis and no impairment visual impairment.

6. C. Meibomian gland. A chalazion is also known as a meibomian cyst. It usually presents as a firm painless lump in the eyelid. Most cases resolve spontaneously but some may require surgical intervention.

7. C. Basal cell carcinoma. The picture shows a pink-coloured nodular basal cell carcinoma of the eyelid with a raised border, central ulceration and superficial telangiectatic vessels. This is the most common malignant eyelid tumour and accounts for 90% of all eyelid malignancies.

8. B. Graves disease. The symptoms described by the patient including weight loss, dizziness, sweating and increased frequency of stools suggest hyperthyroidism. The eye symptoms, diplopia and eye pain, are suggestive of thyroid eye disease, which is specific to Graves disease in this context rather than generic hyperthyroidism.

Chapter 39 Anterior segment (cornea and cataract)

1. A. Topical aciclovir. The presentation is typical of herpes simplex keratitis, which includes a painful red eye with photophobia and epiphora. The fluorescein staining reveals a dendrite with epithelial ulceration, raised edges and terminal bulbs. The treatment of herpes simplex keratitis is topical aciclovir.

2. A. Refer for urgent same-day ophthalmology assessment. This patient is a contact lens wearer who has presented with an acutely painful red eye. As a contact lens wearer, he is at risk of microbial keratitis. This must be excluded through a thorough examination via the use of a slit lamp. Microbial keratitis can lead to visual loss, hence the urgent same-day referral to ophthalmology is appropriate.

3. E. Endophthalmitis. This patient presented with an acute painful red eye and visual loss shortly after eye surgery. This makes post-operative endophthalmitis the most likely diagnosis from the options listed. This is an infection of the vitreous and aqueous humour of the eye and is a rare but important complication to think of following any form of eye surgery.

4. D. Acanthamoeba keratitis. This is a presentation of an acutely painful red eye who is also a contact lens wearer. Suspicion of an acanthamoeba infection should be raised. This infection is prominent in contact lens use in water such as swimming pools and the sea. His job as a surfer exposes him to natural bodies such as the sea and increases the likelihood that this is an acanthamoeba infection. The symptoms usually describe eye pain out of proportion to clinical findings, reduced visual acuity, redness, photophobia and discharge.

5. C. *Pseudomonas aeruginosa.* The symptoms described correspond with a diagnosis of bacterial keratitis. The key symptoms include foreign body sensation, conjunctival injection and the presence of hypopyon. The key information as to which organism is the use of contact lenses. Acanthamoeba infection would be a good differential; however, there is no mention of exposure to water, especially natural bodies such as lakes, seas or rivers.

6. A. Urgent same-day ophthalmology referral. This patient has an organic foreign body in their eye, which means they will have to be seen by an ophthalmologist on the same day to remove the foreign body due to the increased infection risk.

7. A. Herpes simplex keratitis. The presentation of foreign body sensation, pain and photophobia makes all options viable. However, the diagnostic finding of the fluorescein eye staining revealing a dendric ulcer points towards herpes simplex keratitis. Although you may think mechanics are at an increased risk of photokeratitis, it would not typically present with a foreign body sensation.

8. D. Corticosteroids. The patient has developed a cataract which is a common eye condition where there is gradual opacification of the lens. Long-term corticosteroids are known to increase the risk of developing a cataract. Other risk factors identified within the vignette are age and diabetes mellitus.

Chapter 40 Glaucoma

1. D. Decreased production of aqueous fluid. Timolol is a β-blocker that works by reducing aqueous fluid production. As primary open-angle glaucoma is a progressive optic neuropathy secondary to an increase in intraocular pressure, timolol can be used to decrease intraocular pressure.

2. D. Latanoprost. This presentation is likely to be primary open-angle glaucoma due to the increased intraocular pressure being picked up by the optometrist and the decrease in peripheral vision. The first line of management would be either timolol or latanoprost; however, timolol is a β-blocker and should be avoided in asthmatics.

3. C. Gonioscopy. This patient is suspected to have acute angle-closure glaucoma. The crucial investigation that must be performed includes gonioscopy and tonometry. A gonioscope is a specific lens that is used during a slit lamp examination to look at the iridocorneal angle, where aqueous humour is drained. In acute angle-closure glaucoma, this angle is severely reduced or closed, therefore leading to an increase in intraocular pressure.

4. A. Direct parasympathomimetic and β-blocker eye drops. The most likely diagnosis is acute angle-closure glaucoma. The symptoms described an acute, painful, nonreactive and red left eye with hazy cornea. This condition is caused by the narrowing of the iridocorneal angle, thus leading to inadequate drainage of aqueous humour and an increase in intraocular pressure. Combination eye drops should be offered. Direct parasympathomimetic eyedrops (e.g., pilocarpine) cause pupillary constriction that widens the iridocorneal angle, and β-blocker eyedrops (e.g., timolol) decrease aqueous humour production. These two drugs work together to decrease the intraocular pressure.

5. C. Laser iridotomy. The patient is likely to have acute angle-closure glaucoma. The initial treatment would be to provide intraocular pressure lower drugs. However, the definitive treatment once the condition has stabilized would be laser surgery to the iris to create a hole to allow adequate aqueous humour drainage.

6. A. Increased eyelash length. This is a known adverse effect of latanoprost. Another adverse effect of topical prostaglandin analogues to be aware is brown pigmentation of the iris.

7. D. Same-day referral to ophthalmology. This patient has suspected acute angle-closure glaucoma. The image shows conjunctival injection and a hazy cornea. The history suggests an acute painful red eye with systemic upset. The patient requires a same-day referral to ophthalmology.

Chapter 41 Retina

1. A. Retinal detachment. This patient describes a sudden painless loss of vision with a description of a 'curtain' affecting the peripheries of one eye and progressing centrally. This is characteristic of a retinal detachment. As the retina peels away from its underlying layer of support tissues, it can cause flashes as described in the vignette.

2. B. Central retinal vein occlusion. The history is of a sudden, painless loss of vision in the eye. Note the fundoscopy image shows widespread retinal haemorrhages and a swollen optic disc. The appearance of severe retinal haemorrhages can be described as a 'stormy sunset'.

3. B. Central retinal artery occlusion. This patient is complaining of sudden, painless loss of vision with an associated relative afferent pupillary defect. The fundoscopy reveals a pale retina with a cherry-red spot in the centre of the macula. This is a classic presentation of a central retinal artery occlusion (CRAO). Usually, CRAO is associated with atherosclerosis; therefore as the patient suffers from hypertension and is a current smoker, it increases the likelihood of a CRAO.

4. E. Age-related macular degeneration. The combination of age, gradual loss of vision, decrease in visual acuity and straight lines appearing 'curvy' should raise the possibility of age-related macular degeneration.

5. A. Retinal infarction. Cotton wool spots represent areas of retinal infarction that are often seen in preproliferative diabetic retinopathy. This should be emphasized to the patient and attendance at regular check-ups and compliance with antiglycaemic medications is important to prevent further microvascular damage.

6. C. Grade III. Based on the Keith–Wagner classification of hypertensive retinopathy, there is moderate hypertensive retinopathy present due to the presence of microaneurysms, retinal blot and flame-shaped haemorrhages, arteriovenous nicking and multiple cotton–wool spots. If there was the presence of papilloedema then it would be classed as grade IV and is associated with high morbidity and mortality.

7. D. Choroidal neovascularization. The history includes a 4-month history of progressive central visual loss, glares around objects and metamorphopsia on Amsler grid testing. This is likely to be related to age-related macular degeneration. From the option listed choroidal neovascularization is related to wet age-related macular degeneration.

8. E. Antivascular endothelial growth factor (anti-VEGF). This patient is likely to have wet age-related macular degeneration. The patient has characteristic signs and symptoms including a reduction in visual acuity, metamorphopsia and red patches which are likely to indicate intra/subretinal fluid leakage or haemorrhages. Anti-VEGF treatment should be initiated to prevent further leakage.

9. B. Posterior vitreous detachment. This patient has suffered from a sudden onset of flashes and floaters which are commonly caused by a posterior vitreous detachment (PVD). PVD is where the vitreous shrinks and pulls away from the retina. A risk factor for this patient is age and myopia. An important potential complication to be aware of is the possibility of the development of a retinal tear. Therefore, patients must be referred to ophthalmology urgently to assess this.

10. E. Amaurosis fugax. This patient describes a painless transient monocular blindness for a short period of time. This is likely to be amaurosis fugax. This may represent a form of a transient ischaemic attack and therefore should be treated in a similar fashion with aspirin being given.

Chapter 42 Medical ophthalmology and uveitis

1. B. Scleritis. Scleritis is a cause of red eye that is classically painful and is associated with reduced visual acuity, blurred vision and photophobia. When phenylephrine drops are applied to a red eye in scleritis the vessels do not blanch in contrast to episcleritis where there is blanching of the vessels. However, pain in episcleritis is usually mild or painless. Several risk factors are present for this patient developing scleritis which include rheumatoid arthritis and systemic lupus erythematous.

2. B. Swollen pale disc with blurred margins. This patient has temporal arteritis that has been characteristically described by the patient with a rapid onset headache with jaw claudication. There is also a description of amaurosis fugax, due to the transient visual loss. This increases the suspicion of a diagnosis of temporal arteritis. The main ocular complication with this condition is anterior ischaemic optic neuropathy which would be shown as a swollen pale disc and blurred margins on fundoscopy. This is a sight-threatening condition and so you must treat promptly with high-dose glucocorticoid steroids if suspected prior to confirmation of the diagnosis.

3. A. Continue high-dose prednisolone. This lady has symptoms suggesting giant cell arteritis/temporal arteritis. However, it's important to note that skip lesions can occur in giant cell arteritis and may show a normal biopsy. Steroids should not be discontinued as this condition may lead to irreversible blindness. There should be a rapid response to the high-dose prednisolone, if not the diagnosis should be reconsidered.

4. A. Steroids and cycloplegic drops. The diagnosis for this patient points towards acute anterior uveitis. The signs and symptoms include acute red, painful eye with associated photophobia and lacrimation. On examination, there is ciliary flush, hypopyon and an irregular pupil. This patient also suffers from an HLA-B27-associated condition, Crohn's disease, which is a risk factor for developing acute anterior uveitis. The management would be steroid eye drops to reduce inflammation, and cycloplegic eye drops to prevent the formation of adhesions between the lens and iris.

5. C. Polymyalgia rheumatica. This patient has characteristic features of temporal arteritis. Unilateral headache, jaw claudication and visual symptoms. It's important to note that temporal arteritis commonly occurs in patients with polymyalgia rheumatica.

6. C. Episcleritis. The patient describes an irritated red eye with little/no pain. Alongside this, the patient has a past medical history of rheumatoid arthritis. This points towards a diagnosis of episcleritis, which is known to be one of the ocular manifestations of rheumatoid arthritis.

7. A. Varicella-zoster virus. This patient has herpes zoster ophthalmicus, which describes the reactivation of the varicella-zoster virus in the ophthalmic division of the trigeminal nerve. This requires an urgent ophthalmic review if ocular involvement is suspected/confirmed.

8. E. Iris, ciliary body and choroid. The uveal tract consists of the iris, ciliary body and choroid. Therefore, anterior uveitis refers to inflammation of the iris, also known as iritis.

Chapter 43 Neuro-ophthalmology

1. D. Blurring of the optic disc margin. This patient has raised intracranial hypertension, with the cause unknown at this stage. This is a characteristic history of raised intracranial hypertension, a headache worse in the morning, alongside blurred vision and vomiting. The blurring of the optic disc margin is indicative of papilloedema, which is a sign of raised intracranial hypertension.

2. C. Right optic tract. The question tests your visual pathway anatomy. A left homonymous hemianopia means a visual field defect to the left, which corresponds to a lesion in the right optic tract.

3. D. Optic neuritis. The history consists of a rapidly worsening vision with colour desaturation and pain on eye movements, and the 'grey cloud' described corresponds with a central scotoma. Alongside this, the past medical history of multiple sclerosis highly suggests a diagnosis of optic neuritis.

4. A. Left-sided homonymous inferior quadrantanopia. This corresponds with the visual field defect described. As the defect described is occurring on the left eye temporally and the right eye nasally, it means the defect is left-sided. It is classed as a quadrantanopia rather than hemianopia as the defects are only occurring inferiorly.

5. A. Downward and outward deviation of the eye, ptosis and mydriasis. This patient is likely to have raised intracranial pressure secondary to the brain tumour; this can cause a third nerve palsy due to herniation. A third nerve palsy innervates the sphincter pupillae and globe muscles, except the lateral rectus and superior oblique. This results in a dilated eye and a classical 'down and out' deviation of the eye.

6. D. Horner syndrome. There is a left-sided Horner syndrome with ptosis and miosis visible. There is also the presence of heterochromia which suggests that this is congenital Horner.

7. A. Argyll–Robertson pupil. This patient is likely to have neurosyphilis which can cause a pupillary syndrome known as Argyll–Robertson pupil. This leads to a present accommodation reflex but an absent pupillary reflex.

8. C. MRI brain and orbits with contrast. This lady has suspected optic neuritis; therefore MRI brain and orbits with gadolinium contrast would be the investigation of choice. Contrast is used to highlight areas of tissues to detect leakage from blood vessels, in this case, areas of inflammation.

9. B. VI. There is weakness of the lateral rectus muscle when the patient is attempting to look left with associated diplopia. The lateral rectus muscle is supplied by the sixth cranial nerve.

10. D. Right optic tract. A left homonymous hemianopia describes a visual field defect to the right, which corresponds to the right optic tract.

OSCEs and Short Clinical Cases

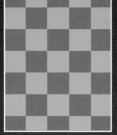

OSCEs

STATION 1

Student instructions

This patient has described facial weakness. Please perform a cranial nerve examination.

Equipment list:

- Pen torch
- Cotton wool
- Neurotip
- Tuning fork

Examiner instructions

The student has 8 minutes from the bell to examine the patient. At 8 minutes you should stop the student and use the next 3 minutes for the student to present their findings and to ask the questions below. Please use the following mark scheme to assess the student.

Introduction/consent Must include ALL below for **1 mark**: 1. Introduction with name and appropriate role 2. Confirmation of patient name and date of birth 3. Brief explanation of the examination 4. Correct position of the patient	0	1	
Ensures the patient is not in pain	0	1	
Inspects patient	0	1	
Assess visual acuity in each eye	0	1	
Assess visual fields in each eye	0	1	
Assess pupil responses Both direct and consensual = **2 marks** Direct or consensual = **1 mark** No assessment of pupil response = **0 mark**	0	1	2
Assess pupil responses – both direct and consensual (1 mark for both)	0	1	
States will perform fundoscopy (student not required to conduct)	0	1	

Assess eye movements The student asks the patient whether there is any double vision or pain present **(1 mark)** The student correctly tests all extraocular muscles by moving their finger in an 'H' pattern. **(1 mark)**	0	1	2
Assess facial sensation Light touch and pinprick The student must assess the sensory component of ALL three of the following areas and compare both sides of the face for **2 marks**: – Forehead – Cheek – Lower jaw If one area omitted or both sides not compared = **1 mark** If one area omitted and both sides not compared = **0 mark**	0	1	2
Assess muscles of mastication Masseters and pterygoids The student assesses both masseters and pterygoids for **2 marks**. Either masseters or pterygoids = **1 mark** Neither asessed = **0 mark**	0	1	2
Assess facial weakness The student asesses the following muscles: – Frontalis – Orbicularis oculi – Orbicularis oris – Buccinator All FOUR must be assessed for **2 marks** One missing = **1 mark** More than one missing = **0 mark**	0	1	2
Assess hearing on both sides	0	1	
Assess palatal movement	0	1	
Assess sternocleidomastoid and trapezius power The student assesses both sternocleidomastoid and trapezius power = **1 mark** One missing = **0 mark**	0	1	
Inspect tongue and tongue movements	0	1	
Examines professionally	0	1	

Communication – builds rapport, cooperation and explanation	0	1	2
The examiner may use judgement to score the student's communication from the following: Poor – **0 mark** Good – **1 mark** Excellent – **2 marks**			
Summarizes key findings	0	1	
Provides the correct diagnosis	0	1	

Examiner's questions: 1, 2, 3, 4, 5

Questions

1. How do you differentiate between a unilateral upper and lower motor neuron facial nerve lesion? **(2 marks)**

   An upper motor neuron facial nerve lesion will spare weakness of the upper facial muscles, as these are innervated bilaterally **(1 mark)**. By asking the patient to raise their eyebrows, this will determine if the upper motor neuron is involved (forehead spared) or the lower motor neuron (forehead involved) **(1 mark)**.

2. Which cranial nerve supplies sensation to the face? **(1 mark)**
   The trigeminal or fifth cranial nerve.

3. What does the chorda tympani branch of the facial nerve do? **(2 marks)**

   It carries taste sensation from the anterior two-thirds of the tongue **(1 mark)** and also parasympathetic innervation to the submandibular and sublingual salivary glands **(1 mark)**.

4. Name three causes of a unilateral lower motor neuron facial palsy **(3 marks)**
   The student may name any of the following: **(1 mark each)**.

   Bell palsy, Ramsay Hunt syndrome (herpes zoster infection), Lyme disease, sarcoidosis, trauma, postsurgical, acute otitis media, malignancy/tumour.

   The most common cause is Bell palsy. Ramsay Hunt syndrome is caused by herpes zoster infection, and it is important to visualize the ears and oral mucosa to assess for a vesicular rash. Patients with this syndrome can also have vestibular symptoms.

5. What treatment is given for Bell palsy? **(2 marks)**

   The main treatment given is oral steroids (prednisolone) **(1 mark)**. These should be given early from symptom onset. Furthermore, the patient should use lubricating eye drops during the day and ointment at night, and the eye should be taped shut at night to help prevent corneal abrasions **(1 mark)**.

   Total /41

STATION 2

Student instructions

This patient has described numbness in the arms. Please perform an upper limb examination.

Equipment list:

- Tendon hammer
- Neurotip
- Cotton wool
- Tuning fork (128Hz)

Examiner instructions

The student has 8 minutes from the bell to examine the patient. At 8 minutes you should stop the student and use the next 3 minutes for the student to present their findings and to ask the questions below. Please use the following mark scheme to assess the student.

Introduction/consent Must include ALL below for **1 mark**: 1. Introduction with name and appropriate role 2. Confirmation of patient name and date of birth 3. Brief explanation of the examination 4. Correct position of the patient	0	1	
Ensures the patient is not in pain	0	1	
Inspects patient	0	1	
Assess tone Assessment of ALL of the following for **1 mark** • Shoulder • Elbow • Wrist	0	1	
Assess pronator drift	0	1	
Assess power throughout the upper limbs **2 marks** – Assessment of power on both sides with communication of clear instructions. **1 mark** – Assessment of power one side at a time with poor communication. **0 marks** – if none of the above.	0	1	2
Assess upper limb reflexes Assessment of ALL three for **2 marks**: – Biceps reflex – Supinator reflex – Triceps reflex **1 mark** MAX if ALL three of the above reflexes are not assessed.	0	1	2

Assess light touch sensation	0	1	
Assess proprioception	0	1	
Assess vibration	0	1	
Assess pinprick sensation	0	1	
Assess temperature sensation	0	1	
Test for finger-nose coordination	0	1	
Test for dysdiadochokinesis	0	1	
Examines professionally	0	1	
Communication – builds rapport, cooperation and explanation	0	1	2

The examiner may use judgement to score the student's communication from the following:
Poor – **0 mark**
Good – **1 mark**
Excellent – **2 marks**

Summarizes key findings	0	1
Provides the correct diagnosis	0	1

Examiner's questions: 1, 2, 3

Questions

1. How do you differentiate between upper and lower motor neuron weakness in the limbs? **(3 marks)**
   Names three in each category = **3 marks**

   Names two in each category = **2 marks**

   Names one in each category = **1 mark**

   Upper motor neuron lesions lead to increased tone, pathologically brisk reflexes, upgoing plantars, a pyramidal pattern of weakness, clonus and pronator drift in the upper limbs.

   Lower motor neuron lesions can lead to fasciculations, muscle wasting, reduced tone, reduced or absent reflexes and mute plantars.

2. Which nerve is affected in carpal tunnel syndrome and what sensory loss does this cause in the hand? **(2 marks)**

   Carpal tunnel syndrome is caused by compression of the median nerve **(1 mark)**, which runs in the carpal tunnel at the wrist. The median nerve supplies sensation to the palm and lateral three and a half digits **(1 mark)**.

   Carpal tunnel syndrome is usually idiopathic but certain risk factors can increase the chance of developing it, including obesity, pregnancy, rheumatoid arthritis, hypothyroidism and diabetes mellitus.

3. What are the names of the pathways carrying different modalities of sensation, and what do they carry?
   (4 marks)

There are two main pathways for the appreciation of different modalities of sensation: the dorsal column pathway **(1 mark)** which carries light touch, two-point discrimination, vibration and proprioception **(1 mark)** and the spinothalamic pathway **(1 mark)** which carries pain and temperature **(1 mark)**.

Total /33

STATION 3

Student instructions

This patient has described unsteadiness on their feet. Please perform a lower limb examination.

Equipment list:

- Tendon hammer
- Neurotip
- Cotton wool
- Tuning fork (128Hz)

Examiner instructions

The student has 8 minutes from the bell to examine the patient. At 8 minutes you should stop the student and use the next 3 minutes for the student to present their findings and to ask the questions below. Please use the following mark scheme to assess the student.

Introduction/consent Must include ALL below for **1 mark**: 1. Introduction with name and appropriate role 2. Confirmation of patient name and date of birth 3. Brief explanation of the examination 4. Correct position of the patient	0	1	
Ensures the patient is not in pain	0	1	
Assess gait	0	1	
Perform Romberg test	0	1	
Inspect the lower limbs	0	1	
Assess tone	0	1	
Assess for clonus	0	1	
Assess power throughout the lower limb **2 marks** – Assessment of power on both sides with communication of clear instructions. **1 mark** – Assessment of power one side at a time with poor communication. **0 marks** – if none of the above.	0	1	2

Assess lower limb reflexes Assessment of ALL three for **2 marks**: – Knee reflex – Ankle reflex – Plantar reflex **1 mark** MAX if ALL three of the above relfexes are not assessed.	0	1	2
Assess light touch sensation	0	1	
Assess proprioception	0	1	
Assess vibration	0	1	
Assess pinprick sensation	0	1	
Assess temperature sensation	0	1	
Perform heel-shin test	0	1	
Examines professionally	0	1	
Communication – builds rapport, cooperation and explanation The examiner may use judgement to score the student's communication from the following: Poor – **0 mark** Good – **1 mark** Excellent – **2 marks**	0	1	2
Summarizes key findings	0	1	
Provides the correct diagnosis	0	1	

Examiner's questions: 1, 2, 3

Questions

1. Name four signs of cerebellar dysfunction. **(4 marks)**

   There are several signs which can demonstrate cerebellar dysfunction and they include dysarthria, nystagmus, jerky pursuits, ataxia, an intention tremor, pass-pointing/finger-nose ataxia/dysmetria, dysdiadokokinesis, heel-shin ataxia, a broad-based gait, pendular reflexes, hypotonia and the rebound phenomenon. **(1 mark each)**

2. Name four signs of Parkinson's disease. **(4 marks)**

   There are several signs of Parkinson's disease, which include hypomimia, a rest tremor, rigidity, cogwheeling rigidity, brady-kinesia/akinesia, reduced postural reflexes, a shuffling/festinant gait, reduced arm swing, a stooped posture, freezing, reduced gait initiation, hypophonia and a positive glabellar tap test. The signs are often asymmetrical. **(1 mark each)**

3. What does the Romberg test assess for? **(1 mark)**

   This assesses for impaired proprioception (a sensory ataxia).

   Total: /34

STATION 4

Student instructions

The patient has described unilateral sudden loss of vision. Please perform a fundoscopic examination, using a direct ophthalmoscope.

Equipment list:

- Ophthalmoscope
- Mydriatic eye drops

Examiner instructions

The student has 8 minutes from the bell to examine the patient. At 8 minutes you should stop the student and use the next 3 minutes for the student to present their findings and to ask the questions below. Please use the following mark scheme to assess the student.

Introduction/consent Must include ALL below for **1 mark**: 1. Introduction with name and appropriate role 2. Confirmation of patient name and date of birth 3. Brief explanation of the examination 4. Correct position of the patient	0	1	
Ensures the patient is not in pain	0	1	
Inspects patient-external eye Must include ALL below for **1 mark**: 1. Periorbital region 2. Eyelids 3. Eyes including pupils	0	1	
Preparation for fundoscopy **1 mark** for each of the following: • Instils eye drops (mentions that will add eye drops prior to ophthalmoscope examination – does not have to conduct) • Sets up ophthalmoscope correctly	0	1	2
Assessment of fundal/red reflex	0	1	
Assess pupil responses – both direct and consensual **2 marks** – Correctly identify the relative afferent pupillary defect **1 mark** – Carries out direct and consensual pupillary response	0	1	2
Assess the optic disc Student makes a comment on the following (**2 marks** for **ALL** three, **1 mark** for two comments): 1. Contour 2. Colour 3. Cup	0	1	2

Assess the retina The student methodically assesses the retina by looking at each of the four quadrants and commenting on the retinal vessels and the colour of the background. **1 mark** for assessment of ALL four quadrants. 1. Superior temporal 2. Superior nasal 3. Inferior nasal 4. Inferior temporal **1 mark** for comment on the retinal vessels and background of a **PALE RETINA**.	0	1	2
Assess the macula **1 mark** – Student states finding of 'Cherry-red spot' **0 mark** – Normal appearance of the macula	0	1	2
Repeat fundoscopy of the other eye Note the student should have started with an examination of the NORMAL eye to receive **2 marks**.	0	1	2
Examines professionally	0	1	
Communication – builds rapport, cooperation and explanation The examiner may use judgement to score the student's communication from the following: Poor – **0 mark** Good – **1 mark** Excellent – **2 marks**	0	1	2
Summarizes key findings **1 mark** for ALL three of the following: • Relative afferent pupillary defect • Pale retina • Cherry red spot	0	1	
Provides the correct diagnosis **2 marks** – Correct diagnosis: Central retinal artery occlusion **1 mark** – Branch retinal artery occlusion **0 marks** – Central retinal vein occlusion, branch retinal vein occlusion, any other incorrect diagnosis	0	1	2

Examiner's questions: 1, 2, 3, 4, 5

Questions

1. Name **THREE** risk factors for developing this diagnosis? (**3 marks – 1 mark for each**)

   Student names any **THREE** of the following:
   • Old age
   • Gender – male
   • Smoking
   • Hypertension
   • Obesity
   • Diabetes mellitus
   • Hyperlipidaemia
   • Cardiovascular disease
   • Coagulopathy

2. If this patient also presented with jaw claudication, headache and a tender, palpable temporal artery, what is the likely condition this patient is suffering from? (**1 mark**)
   Correct answer: Temporal arteritis/giant cell arteritis.

3. What investigations would you carry out for this patient? (**5 marks**)

   If giant cell arteritis is suspected the following can be a guide:

   If the patient is over 50 recommendations for initial blood tests include an erythrocyte sedimentation rate (ESR), C-reactive protein (CRP) and full blood count (FBC) alongside platelets. (**1 mark for each correct test above**)

   Temporal artery biopsy (**1 mark**)

   Other appropriate investigations could be related to atherosclerosis and emboli and can include (**all THREE for 1 mark**):
   • Cardiac echocardiogram
   • ECG
   • Carotid ultrasound

4. What is the immediate management if you suspect giant cell arteritis? (**4 marks**)
   • High-dose glucocorticoids/IV methylprednisolone/oral high-dose prednisolone (**1 mark**)
   • Temporal artery biopsy (**1 mark**)
   • Urgent ophthalmology review (**1 mark**)

   Urgent high-dose glucocorticoids should be given if suspected and the student makes it clear that it is to be given prior to confirmation of diagnosis with a temporal artery biopsy. (**1 mark**)

5. How would the signs/symptoms differ if this patient was suffering from central retinal vein occlusion? (**5 marks**)

   The student states that the symptoms would be the same, i.e., painless unilateral loss of vision. (**1 mark**)

   Differences in signs may include: (**1 mark for each**)
   • Widespread hyperaemia
   • Severe retinal haemorrhages – flame haemorrhages
   • Cotton wool spots
   • Disc/macular oedema

Total /39

STATION 5

Student instructions

The patient presents with a left red eye. Please perform a full ophthalmic examination (excluding fundoscopy).

Equipment list:

- Snellen chart
- Fine print reading chart
- Hatpin
- Pen torch

Examiner instructions

The student has 8 minutes from the bell to examine the patient. At 8 minutes you should stop the student and use the next 3 minutes for the student to present their findings and to ask the questions below. Please use the following mark scheme to assess the student.

Introduction/consent Must include ALL below for **1 mark**: Introduction with name and appropriate role Confirmation of patient name and date of birth Brief explanation of the examination	0	1	
Ensures the patient is not in pain Examiner note: The patient is not in any pain but there is some discomfort.	0	1	
Inspects patient-external eye Must include ALL below for **1 mark**: Periorbital region Eyelids Eyes including pupils Examiner note: There is redness of the left eye with mucopurulent discharge and chemosis.	0	1	
Assess visual acuity in each eye The student uses the Snellen chart appropriately – **1 mark** The student uses the near vision chart appropriately – **1 mark**	0	1	2
Assess visual fields in each eye The student uses a hatpin to appropriately assess each of the patient's visual field quadrants – **1 mark**	0	1	
Assess pupil responses – both direct and consensual (1 mark for each) Examiner note: Both pupils are equal and reactive to light – no abnormalities	0	1	2
Assess pupillary responses – accommodation	0	1	

States will perform fundoscopy (not needed)	0	1	
States would test colour vision using Ishihara plates	0	1	
Assess eye movements The student asks the patient whether there is any double vision or pain present. **(1 mark)** The student correctly tests all intraocular muscles by moving their finger in an 'H' pattern. **(1 mark)**	0	1	2
Examines professionally	0	1	
Communication – builds rapport, cooperation and explanation The examiner may use judgement to score the student's communication from the following: Poor – **0 mark** Good – **1 mark** Excellent – **2 marks**	0	1	2
Summarizes key findings **1 mark** for ALL three of the following Unilateral red eye No pain/mild discomfort Mucopurulent discharge	0	1	
Provides the correct diagnosis **2 marks** – Correct diagnosis: Bacterial conjunctivitis **1 mark** – Conjunctivitis (any type), episcleritis, any alternative diagnosis with a painless/mild discomforting unilateral red eye.	0	1	2

Examiner's questions: 1, 2, 3

Total /29

Questions

1. Name three causative organisms for bacterial conjunctivitis? **(3 marks)**

   Acute bacterial conjunctivitis is primarily caused by *Staphylococcus aureus*, *Haemophilus influenzae* and *Streptococcus pneumoniae*. **(1 mark for each correct answer)**

   Other potential organisms that are also accepted include: **(1 mark for each correct answer)**

   - *Pseudomonas aeruginosa*
   - *Moraxella lacunata*
   - *Streptococcus viridans*
   - *Proteus mirabilis*

2. What signs would be present on ophthalmic examination if the patient was suffering from viral conjunctivitis? **(4 marks)**

   The student mentions any of the following: **(1 mark for each correct answer)**

   - Follicular reaction

- Preauricular lymphadenopathy
- Watery discharge over purulent discharge
- Itchy eyes

Also, accept if the student attempts to differentiate symptoms from bacterial and viral conjunctivitis. (**1 mark each**)

- General symptoms of vital infection, e.g., fever, upper respiratory infection.
- Eyelids stuck together in the morning – more indicative of bacterial conjunctivitis.

3. What general advice would you give to a patient with bacterial conjunctivitis? (**3 marks**)

The student attempts to describe the following: (**1 mark for each**)

- Self-limiting condition – usually lasts 7 to 14 days
- Hygiene advice including handwashing, not sharing towels, etc.
- Cool compress
- Use of artificial tears
- School exclusion is not necessary

Short clinical cases

Case 1

John, a 21-year-old university student, has been found at his halls of residence unwell. He describes a headache and has been feeling under the weather for a few days. On assessment in A&E, he has a fever, photophobia, neck stiffness and Kernig sign is positive.

His observations are: HR 155 beats per minute, RR 35 breaths per minute, saturations 98% on air, capillary refill time 4 s, BP 95/58 mmHg, Temperature 39°C.

A. What do you think is the most likely diagnosis?
B. What are possible causative organisms?
C. What are the immediate management steps in this patient?
D. What treatment would you start?

Case 1 answers:

A. **Meningitis** is the most likely diagnosis with this constellation of symptoms and signs. The features of headache, photophobia and neck stiffness point to a bacterial meningitis.

B. ***Streptococcus pneumoniae* and *Neisseria meningitidis*.** The most likely causative organisms of a bacterial meningitis in an 18-year-old are *Streptococcus pneumoniae* and *Neisseria meningitidis*. *Listeria* is less likely without risk factors, such as pregnancy, age >50 years, immunocompromised patients and alcoholism.

C. **Meningitis is a medical emergency, the patient needs resuscitation. Ask for urgent help.**

- Assess and manage the Airway, Breathing, Circulation, Disability and Exposure.
- Apply high-flow oxygen, organize urgent investigations: ECG, CXR, blood tests including FBC, CRP and blood cultures, a venous blood gas and an IV cannula must be inserted.
- A lumbar puncture should be performed immediately (within the first 30 minutes of presentation) if there are no contraindications. However in patients with signs of sepsis or a meningococcal rash, do not wait for a lumbar puncture and administer antibiotics immediately after blood cultures. The lumbar puncture should test for CSF opening pressure, MCS, glucose (and paired serum glucose), protein, viral PCR, TB culture and cytology. A CT head should be performed prior to lumbar puncture if there are focal neurological signs, papilloedema, seizures or a reduced GCS, to exclude brain swelling which may predispose to cerebral herniation post lumbar puncture.

D. **Urgently start a third-generation cephalosporin**

- Also give IV aciclovir if there is a suspicion of viral meningitis.
- Add amoxicillin if there is a suspicion of or there are risk factors for *Listeria*.
- Adjunctive dexamethasone should be started in all adult patients with suspected or proven pneumococcal meningitis.

Case 2

A 74-year-old male smoker has developed severe pain and weakness in his right hand. He also describes some numbness in his right arm. On examination, he has wasting and weakness in his hand involving both thenar and hypothenar eminences and sensory loss over the C8 and T1 dermatomes. Closer inspection suggests that his right eyelid is drooping and he has a small right pupil. He has also lost a stone in weight over the past month.

A. What syndrome causing his right eyelid to droop?
B. What are the signs seen in this syndrome?
C. What is likely to be the underlying cause in this patient?
D. How many levels are involved in the pathway affected by this syndrome?

Case 2 answers:

A. **Horner syndrome.** The symptoms are very suggestive of a Horner syndrome, affecting the sympathetic pathway. In addition, the patient has a posterior brachial plexus lesion due to the same underlying cause.

B. **Unilateral miosis, a partial ptosis, anhidrosis and enophthalmos.** The characteristic features of a Horner syndrome are a unilateral miosis, a partial ptosis, anhidrosis of the ipsilateral side of the face (if the lesion is proximal to the carotid bifurcation) or anhidrosis of the medial side of the forehead only (if the lesion is distal to the bifurcation) and enophthalmos. Levator palpebrae superioris and Muller muscle both contribute to eyelid elevation, but levator palpebrae superioris is the main elevator. Levator palpebrae superioris is innervated by the oculomotor nerve, whereas Muller muscle is innervated by the sympathetic neurons. The ptosis therefore tends to be partial in Horner syndrome.

C. **Pancoast tumour.** The patient has the classical combination of a posterior brachial plexus lesion with the Horner syndrome and he is a smoker, therefore, together this points towards a Pancoast tumour (pulmonary apical lesion) being the cause of his symptoms. Pancoast tumours are usually non–small-cell lung cancers.

D. **The sympathetic pathway involves the central (first order), preganglionic (second order) and post-ganglionic (third order) nerves.** The central neuron starts in the hypothalamus and descends to the cervical spinal cord. Therefore lesions of the brainstem can lead to a Horner syndrome. The preganglionic neuron exits the spinal cord and travels in the cervical sympathetic chain synapsing in the superior cervical ganglion. Lesions of the brachial plexus or pulmonary apical lesions can affect the preganglionic neuron. The post-ganglionic neuron supplying the orbit enters the cranium with the internal carotid artery. Lesions of the carotid artery can therefore also cause a Horner syndrome, such as a carotid artery dissection.

Case 3

A 30-year-old woman presents with worsening intermittent double vision over the past 2 weeks. She has noticed that it usually comes on when she is tired at the end of the day. On examination, she has limitation of movements in most directions except on looking down with the right eye and abducting the left eye. Her pupils are normal but she has bilateral ptosis, which gets worse on sustained upgaze. She is otherwise well and has had well-controlled type 1 diabetes for 16 years.

A. What is the most likely diagnosis?
B. What antibodies can cause this syndrome?
C. What medication can be used for symptom improvement?
D. If this patient presented to A&E with deteriorating symptoms of this condition, what test must be performed urgently and why?

Case 3 answers:

A. **Myasthenia gravis.** This patient is the typical age group and sex for developing myasthenia gravis. She has an ocular presentation with double vision. The double vision tends to be worse towards the end of the day, reflecting the

fatigability seen in the disease. Ptosis also gets worse with sustained upgaze, also due to fatigue of the levator muscles.

B. **Acetylcholine receptor antibodies (AChR) and/or muscle-specific kinase antibodies (MUSK)** are the most frequently seen. AChR antibodies are present in up to 85% of patients with generalized myasthenia gravis, and 50% of ocular myasthenia gravis. Fifty percent of patients who are seronegative for AChR antibodies test positive for MUSK antibodies.

C. **Oral anticholinesterases** are used for symptom control. Of these, pyridostigmine is the most commonly used medication. The side effects include abdominal cramps and diarrhoea. The medication has a 3- to 5-hour duration of action, so it is usually given 3 to 5 times per day, depending on the patient's symptoms.

D. **Spirometry** is a critical bedside test to perform in this situation. This will give a value for the forced vital capacity, which must be measured to assess the risk of respiratory involvement and compromise. If the vital capacity is reduced, the patient must be urgently assessed by ITU, due to the possible need for intubation and artificial ventilation.

Case 4

An 85-year-old Afro-Caribbean male presented to his general practitioner with gradual onset visual loss over the past several months. He states that he was almost hit by a car last week as he did not notice the car coming towards him from his peripheral vision. He denies any pain or any other visual symptoms. Past medical history includes rheumatoid arthritis, hypertension and asthma. He takes regular amlodipine and prednisolone and has a salbutamol inhaler that he takes as required. He also wears corrective glasses for his short-sightedness. No other relevant family history.

On examination, the general appearance of both eyes and eyelids is normal, and pupils are equal and reactive to light. There is a visual field defect in peripheral vision. Appearance on fundoscopy shows a normal optic disc; however, the optic disc to cup ratio is difficult to visualize, there are visible retinal vessels, and the background is normal in colour.

A. What is the most likely diagnosis?
B. What risk factors are present for developing this condition?
C. What investigations should be carried out to diagnose this condition? What results would you expect?
D. What pharmaceutical options are available for this condition and what is the mechanism of action? What is contraindicated for this patient?

Case 4 answers:

A. **Primary open angle glaucoma** The patient has progressive loss of vision that is affecting his peripheral vision as described by the patient. He denies any flashes, floaters, pain, redness or double vision. This makes primary open angle glaucoma a very likely diagnosis.

B. **Age, Afro-Caribbean ethnicity, steroid use and myopia**

There are several risk factors but increasing age is an important one to consider, as the drainage of the aqueous humour is less efficient, leading to chronic high intraocular pressure and the symptoms described. Patients of African-Caribbean descent have been shown to have higher prevalence rates when compared to those of Caucasian descent; studies have also shown that there is earlier onset, faster rates of disease progression and more refractory to treatment. Steroids and myopia are also known risk factors for developing primary open-angle glaucoma (POAG). Other risk factors for POAG include diabetes mellitus, high intraocular pressure, central corneal thickness and a first-degree relative with POAG.

C. **Slit lamp examination, applanation tonometry, automated perimetry, gonioscopy**

The definition of primary open angle glaucoma is a diagnosis based on signs of glaucomatous optic neuropathy; this definition does not include elevated intraocular pressure (IOP).

A slit lamp examination is essential to assess the optic nerve and fundus for a baseline. Fundoscopic signs of primary open angle glaucoma include:

1. Optic disc cupping – cup-to-disc ratio >0.7 (normal is between 0.4 and 0.7), optic disc usually widens and deepens.
2. Optic disc pallor – secondary to optic disc atrophy.
3. Bayonetting of vessels.
4. Other features – cup notching and disc haemorrhages.

Goldmann applanation tonometry is the gold standard for measuring IOP. This can be elevated above normal ranges which is above or equal to 21 mmHg.

Automated perimetry which would reveal a peripheral visual field defect.

Gonioscopy can be used to look at the anterior chamber angle, by definition it should be open-normal appearing. This helps us differentiate POAG from other secondary open angle glaucomas.

A. **Prostaglandin analogues, beta-blockers, sympathomimetics, carbonic anhydrase inhibitors and miotics. Beta-blockers are contraindicated for this patient.**

The first line of eye drops suggested by NICE includes a prostaglandin analogue (such as latanoprost) or a beta-blocker (such as timolol). However, beta-blockers are contraindicated in this patient due to his past medical history of asthma. Second-line options include sympathomimetics (e.g., brimonidine), carbonic anhydrase inhibitors (e.g., dorzolamide) and miotics (e.g., pilocarpine).

The mechanism of action is as followed:

- Prostaglandin analogues – increased uveoscleral outflow
- Beta-blockers – reduced aqueous humour production
- Sympathomimetics – reduced aqueous humour production and increased uveoscleral outflow
- Carbonic anhydrase inhibitor – reduced aqueous humour production
- Miotics – increased uveoscleral outflow

Case 5 Keratitis

A 32-year-old female beach lifeguard presented to her emergency department with a painful red eye. She mentioned that her right eye has been red and painful for the past day. This is associated with watery discharge and a gritty sensation. She has no other relevant past medical history and takes no regular medication. She wears daily contact lenses and has no other ocular history.

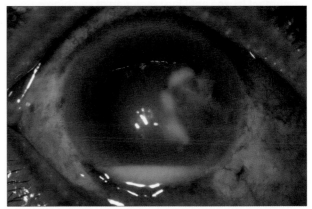

Fig. Case 5 (From Ophthalmology, 6th ed. Elsevier; 2023.)

On inspection, the right eye is pictured above (Fig. Case 5):

Further examination reveals that pupils are equal and reactive to light, but the patient is in discomfort when light is shone in the right eye. Eye movements are normal.

A. What is the likely diagnosis? Describe the image. What signs can be seen to support this diagnosis?
B. What are the possible causative organisms? What is the most likely?
C. What is the immediate management for this patient?
D. What complications may arise secondary to this condition?

Case 5 answers:

A. **Bacterial keratitis**

This patient has presented with a unilateral painful red eye associated with epiphora and photophobia. This patient is a lifeguard and a daily contact lens wearer which suggests that there is natural body exposure; these are significant risk factors for the underlying pathology. The image reveals conjunctival injection with a hypopyon present within the anterior chamber and infiltration of the central cornea (corneal ulceration). The signs and symptoms are highly suggestive of a diagnosis of bacterial keratitis.

B. ***Pseudomonas aeruginosa, Streptococcus pneumoniae, Staphylococcus aureus* – Most likely: *Pseudomonas aeruginosa***

The causative organisms for bacterial keratitis include *Staphylococci, Streptococci and Pseudomonas*. The most causative organism of bacterial keratitis is *Staphylococcus aureus*. However, the vignette suggests natural body exposure and daily contact lens use which is highly suggestive of a *Pseudomonas aeruginosa* infection.

C. **Immediate referral to ophthalmology, topical antibiotics, cycloplegics and advice to stop wearing contact lenses until the resolution of symptoms.**

Any contact lens wearer with an acutely red painful eye should be referred to eye casualty for a thorough assessment of microbial keratitis. Topical antibiotics should be started if there is a confirmation of bacterial keratitis, typically quinolones are used first line. Cycloplegics (e.g., cyclopentolate) can be considered to help with pain management. Advice to stop contact lens use until the resolution of symptoms is very important.

D. **Residual corneal scarring, corneal perforation, endophthalmitis, visual loss**

These are the potential complications of bacterial keratitis. Endophthalmitis is a purulent inflammation of the intraocular fluid, which includes the aqueous and vitreous humour. This is an ophthalmic emergency that would cause the patient to present with an acute red eye, alongside blurred vision, swollen lid, epiphora and photophobia.

Glossary

Acalculia Difficulty in performing simple mental arithmetic.

Ageusia Loss of taste sensation.

Agnosia Deficit of higher sensory processing caused by impaired recognition.

Agraphaesthesia Loss of the ability to recognize numbers or letters traced on the skin.

Akathisia Feeling of inner restlessness associated with repetitive movements of a purposeless nature.

Akinesia Inability to initiate a voluntary movement.

Amyotrophy Wasting of muscle.

Anarthria Inability to articulate.

Anisocoria Unequal pupil size.

Anosognosia Patient's unawareness of their illness.

Apraxia Inability to perform a motor sequence with preserved motor, sensory and coordination functions.

Astereognosis Inability to recognize an object placed in the hand with eyes closed and intact peripheral sensation.

Athetosis Involuntary movements characterized by slow writhing purposeless movements.

Aura A neurological phenomenon occurring seconds to minutes before a migraine headache or epileptic seizure.

Ballismus Wild flailing movements of the limbs.

Broca aphasia Nonfluent, slow, laboured effortful speech, but patient can recognize errors in own speech. Comprehension often preserved for simple material. Repetition, reading, writing and naming impaired, but naming may be helped by contextual cues.

Cataplexy Sudden loss of lower limb tone leading to falls without loss of consciousness.

Chemosis Conjunctival oedema.

Chorea Involuntary hyperkinetic movement disorder associated with jerky, restlessness, purposeless movements, which move from one part of the body to another in an unpredictable way.

Coma A state of unresponsiveness to verbal or mechanical stimuli.

Conjugate gaze palsy A disorder affecting the ability to move both eyes in the same direction. These palsies can affect gaze in a horizontal, upward or downward direction.

Cotton wool spot A white fluffy lesion due to a superficial retinal infarction.

Crowding phenomenon Individual letters can be read better than a whole line; most commonly seen in ambylopic patients.

Déjà vu An inappropriate feeling of overfamiliarization with the environment.

Delirium A neurobehavioural syndrome associated with problems with attention.

Dementia Loss of intellectual functions leading to impaired function or behaviour.

Diplopia Double vision.

Dissociated sensory loss Impairment of some, but not all, sensory modalities.

Dysdiadochokinesia Difficulty in performing rapid alternating movements.

Dysgeusia A distortion of the sense of taste.

Dyskinesia Excessive involuntary movements (e.g., chorea, athetosis).

Dysmetria Abnormal control of range of movement.

Dysphagia Difficulty swallowing.

Dysphonia Disorder of volume, pitch or quality of voice due to dysfunction of the larynx.

Dystonia Sustained involuntary muscle contraction.

Ectopic lentis Dislocated lens.

Encephalopathy General term for diffuse disturbance of brain function.

Fasciculation Rapid, flickering movements within a muscle associated with spontaneous activity of a motor unit. Sometimes described as 'worms under the skin'.

Fibrillation Spontaneous contraction of single muscle fibres. These cannot be seen by the eye and are detected electrophysiologically.

Flare Increased protein in the anterior chamber fluid, permitting visualization of the slit-lamp beam.

Floaters Visual perception of dots or spots which may seem to 'swim' or shift location when the position of gaze is shifted.

Fovea An area of the retina corresponding to central vision, located temporal and slightly inferior to the centre of the optic disc.

Glossary

Frontal release signs A group of reflexes that are usually absent in healthy adults but may be found following a wide range of disorders of the central nervous system. Their anatomical localization is vague, even though they are still referred to as the 'frontal release signs'; 'primitive reflexes' may be a more appropriate term as it suggests that these are reflexes that are inhibited as the brain develops.

Gait apraxia The inability/impairment to walk despite preserved motor sensory and coordination functions. It usually occurs with lesions of the frontal lobes and its white matter connections.

Glabellar tap reflex Tap on the forehead produces blinking, which habituates in most people. If this fails to habituate, then it used to be felt that it was a useful diagnostic sign of idiopathic Parkinson disease. Unfortunately, it is often positive in normal aged individuals and in other extrapyramidal disorders and is, therefore, usually not clinically useful.

'Glove and sock' sensory/motor loss The loss of sensation and power in a polyneuropathy is typically worse distally than proximally. This is often referred to as 'glove and stocking' but the loss rarely extends up to the midthigh and usually stops midcalf.

Gower sign A typical movement made by a patient with proximal lower limb weakness where the arms are used to 'climb up' the legs to stand from lying on the floor.

Hard exudates Deep retinal lipid, often glistening yellow in appearance.

Hemianopia A defect of one-half of the visual field.

Horner syndrome Partial ptosis, meiosis and anhydrosis associated with dysfunction in the sympathetic supply to the eye.

Hypemetropia (long sighted) The eye is too short or the refractive power too weak to bring objects at distance or near into clear focus (without the use of accommodation).

Hyphaema Blood in the anterior chamber.

Hypomimia Reduction of voluntary facial expression.

Hypopyon Layer of white blood cells inferiorly in the anterior chamber.

Hyposmia A decreased sense of smell.

Internuclear ophthalmoplegia Failure or slowing of adduction during horizontal conjugate gaze with or without gaze-evoked nystagmus in the abducting eye secondary to a lesion in the medial longitudinal fasciculus.

Jacksonian march Sequential spread of a simple partial usually motor seizure (e.g., hand, elbow then shoulder), which may terminate spontaneously or with a secondary generalized seizure.

Kayser–Fleischer rings Green/brown deposits of copper in Descemet membrane, which can usually only be seen with slit-lamp examination and is highly suggestive of Wilson disease.

Keratic precipitates Lymphocytic cellular aggregates that form on the corneal endothelium, often inferiorly, in a base-down triangular pattern.

Kernig sign Pain in the lower back and neck and resistance to passive extension of the knee when the thigh is flexed secondary to meningitis.

Leukocoria A grossly visible white pupil.

Lhermitte sign Electric shock-like sensation down the arms and legs following flexion of the neck due to a lesion within the cervical cord.

Locked-in syndrome Severe damage to the ventral pons causing loss of the ascending and descending tracts to the spinal cord, pons and medulla so that the patient can only move the eyes, often vertically, and blink. It is usually caused by basilar artery thrombosis.

Macula An area four disc diameters in size centred at the posterior part of the retina.

Marche à petits pas Small-stepped, often wide-based, shuffling gait without a flexed posture or festination of idiopathic Parkinson disease caused by bilateral frontal cortical or white matter damage usually secondary to small vessel disease.

Marcus Gunn pupil Delay or failure of constriction of a pupil to direct light due to a lesion in the optic nerve.

Micrographia Small handwriting. This is often seen in idiopathic Parkinson disease and starts normally, but fatigues and becomes small.

Miosis Constriction of the pupil.

Mydriasis Dilatation of the pupil.

Myelopathy A disorder of the spinal cord which is usually associated with a sensory level near the level of the lesion, upper motor neuron weakness below the lesion, sometimes lower motor neuron signs at the level of the lesion and sphincter disturbance.

Myoclonus Involuntary 'shock-like' contraction resulting in a jerking movement, usually of the limbs, trunk or neck.

Myopia (short sighted) The eye is too long or the refractive power too great to bring objects at a distance clearly into focus.

Myotonia Inability to relax a muscle following contraction.

Neglect Inability to respond to or attend to a sensory stimulus.

Nystagmus Rhythmic oscillations or tremors of the eyes that occur independently of normal movements.

Oculocephalic response (doll's eye movements) The eyes remain fixated on an object when the head is passively moved, which is a sign of an intact pontine brainstem reflex.

Oculocephalic response (doll's eye movements) The eyes remain fixated on an object when the head is passively moved, which is a sign of an intact pontine brainstem reflex.

Optic neuritis Inflammation of the optic nerve.

Optokinetic nystagmus A physiological involuntary conjugate pursuit eye movement in response to a moving object with a return saccade when the object disappears out of vision (e.g., looking out of a moving train).

Papilloedema Optic disc swelling produced by increased intracranial pressure.

Paraplegia Severe/total weakness of both legs.

Parkinsonism A constellation of signs associated with some or all of the features of bradykinesia, rigidity, tremor and postural instability.

Peripapillary Surrounding the optic disc.

Peripheral iridectomy Removal of a portion of the peripheral iris.

Pes cavus High arched feet due to imbalance in the muscular contractions acting on the feet usually associated with genetic neuropathies (e.g., Charcot–Marie–Tooth), or due to an early neurological insult (e.g., cerebral palsy).

Phalen sign Tingling in the distribution of the median nerve when the wrist is forced flexed at 90 degrees; it is associated with carpal tunnel syndrome.

Phonophobia Dislike or fear of loud noises.

Photophobia Ocular pain on exposure to light.

Posterior synechiae Adhesions between the iris and the anterior lens capsule.

Proptosis Protrusion of the globe from the bony orbit.

Pseudobulbar palsy Impairment of bilateral corticobulbar fibres associated with dysphagia, dysarthria, brisk jaw jerk, slow and spastic tongue and exaggerated gag reflex.

Pseudodementia Global impairment of cognitive functions due to affective disorders (anxiety/depression), which mimics dementia caused by organic pathology (e.g., Alzheimer disease).

Ptosis Drooping of the upper Eyelid.

Punctum The opening of the tear drainage system in the eyelid margin.

Pyramidal Synonymous with corticospinal and upper motor neuron.

Quadrantanopia Loss of a quarter of the visual field.

Quadriplegia Total or severe loss of power in all four limbs.

Radiculopathy Disorder of the nerve roots causing sensory loss in the corresponding dermatome, motor loss in the corresponding myotome, reflex loss and pain in a radicular distribution.

Retinitis Retinal inflammation.

Rhegmatogenous retinal detachment Detachment of the retina as a result of a retinal tear or hole.

Rigidity Increased resistance to passive movement that is equal throughout the range of movement and is associated with extrapyramidal disease.

Romberg sign Increase in unsteadiness when a standing patient closes their eyes; it is associated with proprioceptive loss to the feet.

Saccades Rapid movements of the eyes, which move the focus from one point to another.

Scleritis Inflammation of the sclera (white coat of the eye).

Scotoma An area in the visual field with a loss of sensitivity.

Spasticity Increased resistance to passive movement at a joint that varies with amplitude and velocity and is associated with a lesion in the upper motor neuron.

Strabismus Ocular misalignment.

Supranuclear gaze palsy Impairment of the supranuclear connections to the nuclei of the nerves supplying the extraocular muscles leading to preservation of reflex, but loss of voluntary, eye movements.

Syncope Loss of consciousness.

Tandem gait The ability to walk in a straight line with one foot in front of the other. This is impaired in midline cerebellar disorders.

Tinel sign Paraesthesia following tapping of a trapped or regenerating peripheral nerve.

Todd paresis Transient localized weakness following a seizure usually lasting seconds or minutes.

Trabeculectomy Surgery to improve aqueous outflow and reduce intraocular pressure in glaucoma patients.

Uhthoff phenomenon Worsening of visual acuity with exercise or other causes of increased body temperature in optic neuritis related to temperature sensitivity of demyelinated axons.

Upper motor neuron The cell in the primary motor cortex that projects its axon down through the internal capsule and spinal cord to synapse with the lower motor neuron.

Vegetative state Clinical syndrome associated with extensive loss of cognitive function but preserved vegetative function (e.g., respiration and autonomic). It has a very poor prognosis.

Wernicke aphasia Fluent aphasia with phonemic and semantic paraphasias; impaired comprehension; impaired repetition and severely impaired naming, reading and writing.

Index